Interpretation of Endoscopic Biopsy - Gastritis, Gastropathies and Beyond

Kim Vaiphei

Interpretation of Endoscopic Biopsy - Gastritis, Gastropathies and Beyond

Springer

Kim Vaiphei
Department of Histopathology
Post Graduate Institute of Medical Education and Research
Chandigarh, India

ISBN 978-981-16-6025-2 ISBN 978-981-16-6026-9 (eBook)
https://doi.org/10.1007/978-981-16-6026-9

This Springer imprint is published by the registered company Springer Nature Singapore Pte Ltd.
The registered company address is: 152 Beach Road, #21-01/04 Gateway East, Singapore 189721, Singapore

I dedicate all to my late parents who taught me the values of Integrity, Hard work and Faith in Almighty

Preface

This book is a small attempt to make my contribution to the vast ocean of gastrointestinal pathology. It has been my intention for quite a few years to formulate in black and white the little knowledge I acquire in my day-to-day academic activities. This wish of mine got materialized in disguise. During the lockdown period of the first wave followed by the second wave of pandemic, I manage to dedicate my working hours in fulfilling my desire of writing. In my personal experience, interpretation of gastric biopsy has a very casual attitude. This is one such area where most pathologists consider it to be simple and fit for the inexperienced junior most residents. This attitude leads to overlooking many of simple as well as specialized morphological changes that may be present in a given biopsy, resulting in underdiagnosis of many interesting and rare conditions. I have tried to highlight many such conditions with a simple approach, possibly in repeated manner under different chapters. Stomach is one such organ where anything we ingest gets accumulated for processing, thereby the gastric mucosa gets exposed to all the good, the bad and the ugly ones. As a highly vascularized organ, it tends to react strongly resulting in all the clinical symptoms that are associated with any upper GI problems. The kind of response depends on the type of the irritant, and the resulting pathology in gastric mucosa, hence, may not be similar for all irritants. Interpretating any tissue biopsy, it is advisable to pay attention to clinical parameters, including age and sex of the patients. For a comprehensive interpretation, it is almost mandatory to have knowledge of the endoscopic features and other radiological parameters. It is equally important to have good communication with the treating physician. Medical science, like any other, is a very rapidly growing subject with new technology and changing spectra in disease profiles. Upkeeping with recent and latest knowledge must accompany any routine practice.

Intention of bringing out this book is for the benefit of post graduate students, fellows and practicing pathologists. I have tried to make the writings and presentations in the most possible simplified approach with many representative photographs, clinical material and endoscopic features.

Chandigarh, India Kim Vaiphei

Acknowledgements

First of all, my acknowledgement goes to my students who have been the pillar behind my constant and relentless efforts to improve myself. I am also indebted to all known and unknown patients whose biopsy materials have been utilized in order to make this small book materialized. I am also grateful to may departmental technical and other supporting staffs, who are all the time ready to help me out. I also like to thank Dr Jimil Shah, Assistant Professor, Department of Gastroenterology, for providing me with the endoscopic pictures. The last but not the least, I like to highlight the constant support of my family in completing this very small and primitive endeavour of mine.

Contents

List of Abbreviations

AB-PAS	Alcian Blue Periodic Acid Schiff
AdenoCa	Adeno carcinoma
AFP	Alpha feto protein
AG	Atrophic gastritis
AIG	Autoimmune gastritis
AJCC	American Joint Committee on Cancer
APC	Adenomatous polyposis coli
BL	Burkitt's lymphoma
Cag A	Cytotoxin associated antigen A
CCKB	Cholecystokinin B
CD	Crohn's disease
CG	Collagenous gastritis
CEA	Carcino embryonic antigen
CKD	Chronic kidney disease
CLO	Campylobacter-like organism
DT	Differentiated type
DGC	Diffuse gastric cancer
DLBCL	Diffuse large B cell lymphoma
Dup A	Duodenal ulcer promoting gene A protein
ECL	Enterochromaffin like
EGC	Early gastric cancer
ELISA	Enzyme-linked immunosorbent assay
EMR	Endoscopic mucosal resection
EG	Erosive gastritis
ERCP	Endoscopic retrograde cholangiopancreatography
ESD	Endoscopic submucosal dissection
EUS	Endoscopic ultrasonography
FEG	Focally enhanced gastritis
FGP	Fundic gland polyps
FISH	Fluorescent in situ hybridization
FliD	Hook-associated protein 2 homologue
FPM	Filter paper mount
GA-FG	Gastric adeno Ca with fundic gland type
GA-CCD	Gastric adenocarcinoma with chief cell differentiation
GAED	Gastric adenocarcinoma with enteroblastic differentiation
GAVE	Gastric Antral Vascular Ectasia
GC	Gastric cancer

GCLS	Gastric (adeno)carcinoma with lymphoid stroma
GCP	Gastritis cystica profunda
GFTD	Dysplasia of gastric foveola
GIM	Gastric intestinal metaplasia
GERD	Gastro-oesophageal reflux disease
GEJ	Gastro-oesophageal junction
G cell	Gastrin releasing cell
GI	Gastrointestinal
GG	Granulomatous gastritis
GVHD	Graft versus host disease
H	Helicobacter
HAS	Hepatoid adenocarcinoma of stomach
HCG	Human chorionic gonadotropin
HDGC	Hereditary gastric cancer
HE	Haematoxylin eosin
HG	Hyperplastic gastropathies
HGD	High-grade dysplasia
HH	*Helicobacter heilmannii*
HP	*Helicobacter pylori*
H. pylori	*Helicobacter pylori*
HpNGC	*H. pylori* negative gastric cancer
HSCT	Homologous stem cell transplant
HSP	Heat shock protein
IBD	Inflammatory bowel disease
IgA	Immunoglobulin A
ICD	International Classification of Diseases
IHC	Immunohistochemistry
IM	Intestinal metaplasia
JGCA	Japanese Gastric Cancer Association
LGD	Low-grade dysplasia
MALT	Mucosa associated lymphoid tissue
MANEC	Mixed adeno neuro endocrine carcinoma
MD	Ménétrier's disease
MGC	Mucinous gastric cancer
MIE	Metaplastic intestinal epithelium
MiNEN	Mixed neuroendocrine non-neuroendocrine neoplasm
miRNA	Micro RNA
MMR	Mismatch repair
MRI	Magnetic resonance imaging
MT	Mixed-type
MUC	Mucin
MZL	Marginal zone lymphoma
Nap A	Neutrophil activating protein
NEC	Neuroendocrine carcinoma
NET	Neuroendocrine tumour
NMGC	Non-mucinous gastric carcinoma
NSAID	Non-steroidal anti-inflammatory drugs
OGP	Oxyntic gland polyp/adenoma

OipA	Outer inflammatory protein A
OLGA	Operative link for gastritis assessment
OLGIM	Operative link on gastric intestinal metaplasia
PAP	Peroxidase anti-peroxidase
PCC	Poorly cohesive carcinoma
PG	Phlegmonous gastritis
PGA	Pyloric gland adenoma
PGL	Primary gastric lymphoma
PHG	Portal hypertensive gastropathy
PUD	Peptic ulcer disease
RUT	Rapid urease test
ROS	Reactive oxygen species
SAT	Stool antigen test
SRC	Signet ring cell
TNM	Tumour node metastasis
UBT	Urea breath test
UC	Ulcerative colitis
UDT	Undifferentiated type
UICC	International Union Against Cancer
Vag A	Vacuolating cytotoxin
WHO	World Health Organization
ZE	Zollinger–Ellison

General Principles of Endoscopic Gastric Biopsy and Specimen Handling

1

1.1 Introduction

Diseases involving the proximal segment of the digestive tract is a common problem and frequently observed disorder by the practising gastroenterologists as it hampers normal lifestyle of the affected individual [1–3]. These problems reduce the effective output in any society and also add significantly to high public health expenditure [4, 5]. The clinical symptoms related to these conditions are not specific, may not be truly projecting the underlying condition. Routine workup to determine the underlying pathology may include routine investigations, ultrasonography, radiology, and endoscopic examination. Endoscopy is indicated only when a patient presents with an alarming symptom or in elderly individuals [6].

Various types of diseases may involve gastric mucosa, which includes both malignant and non-malignant diseases. Frequently observed diseases include gastric mucosal inflammation related to infectious and injurious agents, and diseases that may primarily affect blood vessels. Gastric mucosa may also be affected by both neoplastic and non-neoplastic polypoidal mucosal outgrowths. These mucosal outgrowths may be composed of neoplastic mucosal epithelium showing variable grades of dysplasia and frank carcinomatous changes. The non-neoplastic mucosal growth may be composed of various types of tissue which are inherently of gastric mucosal in origin like hyperplastic mucosa of variable grades and types, that may be associated with metaplastic and dysplastic epithelium. Or these may be composed of inflamed mucosa which may dominantly be of inflammatory granulation tissue and granulomas intermixed with a variable amount of native gastric epithelium [7]. Endoscopy is a technique that is essential for a complete work-up of any individual with major complaints associated with upper segment of the digestive tract. By this technique, the gastroenterologists are enabled to get mucosal biopsy from different chosen sites of gastric mucosa for histopathological examination. These mucosal samples contribute to making a definitive diagnosis and are of much help in monitoring treatment response [8]. Histological examination of the mucosal fragments obtained from the normal looking area of the gastric mucosa may reveal presence of microscopic disorder [6, 9]. Such interventions can be expensive approach though there are minimal complications associated with the procedure [10]. In advanced countries, expenses incurred for gastroduodenoscopy procedures may add up to quite a few billion dollars [9]. A substantial number of gastric and other sites are subjected to biopsy though the mucosa may appear normal and the additional cost for such type of biopsy has not been well analyzed.

K. Vaiphei, *Interpretation of Endoscopic Biopsy - Gastritis, Gastropathies and Beyond*,
https://doi.org/10.1007/978-981-16-6026-9_1

1.2 Biopsy Sampling Techniques

Numerous methods and devices have been developed for tissue sampling during gastrointestinal endoscopy, including pinch biopsy, brush cytology, endoscopic ultrasound-guided fine needle aspiration, true cut needle biopsy, snare excision, suction biopsy, endoscopic mucosal resection and combinations of techniques [11]. Endoscopy has progressed over the last 150 years and it was Kussmaul who had used the first gastroscopy in 1868 [12]. Since then, there have been many modifications and advancements. The primitive instrument initially was a stiff metallic pipe using candles as the light source. Currently available highly sophisticated endoscopes utilizing fibre optics speak volumes of the capability of human beings [13].

1.3 Endoscopes

Currently available endoscopes are flexible instruments combine with fibre optics and charge-coupled devices to facilitate illumination and visualization of inaccessible sites of hollow organs. It consists of a tip, an insertion tube and a control section. This model comes with many advanced features of impeccable images and high magnification inbuilt camera to study the mucosa better enhancing vascular pattern. Gastroscopes used to examine the upper gastrointestinal tract, have a wider bore in order to accommodate additional accessories for the purpose of administering treatments [14]. In any endoscopy laboratory, maintenance of cleanliness and hygiene by proper sterilization, disinfection and storage practices. These steps are essential in order to prevent contamination and spread of infection from one patient to another and also amongst the health workers.

References

1. Tack J, Talley NJ, Camilleri M, et al. Functional gastroduodenal disorders. Gastroenterol. 2006;130:1466–79.
2. Kurata JH, Nogawa AN, Everhart JE. A prospective study of dyspepsia in primary care. Dig Dis Sci. 2002;47:797–803.
3. Dent J, El-Serag HB, Wallander MA, et al. Epidemiology of gastro-oesophageal reflux disease: a systematic review. Gut. 2005;54:710–7.
4. van Zanten SV, Wahlqvist P, Talley NJ, et al. Randomised clinical trial: the burden of illness of uninvestigated dyspepsia before and after treatment with esomeprazole—results from the STARS II study. Alim Pharm Ther. 2011;34:714–23.
5. Lacy BE, Weiser KT, Kennedy AT, et al. Functional dyspepsia: the economic impact to patients. Alim Pharm Ther. 2013;38:170–7.
6. Talley NJ, Vakil N. Guidelines for the management of dyspepsia. Am J Gastroenterol. 2005;100:2324–37.
7. Memon F, Baloch K, Memon AA. Upper gastrointestinal endoscopic biopsy; morphological spectrum of lesions. Professional Med J. 2015;22:1574–9.
8. Krishnappa R, Horakerappa MS, Karar MA, et al. A study on histopathologic spectrum of upper gastrointestinal tract endoscopic biopsies. Int J Med Res Health Sci. 2013;2:418–24.
9. Peery AF, Dellon ES, Lund J, et al. Burden of gastrointestinal disease in the United States: 2012 update. Gastroenterol. 2012;143:1179–87.
10. Harewood GC. Economic comparison of current endoscopic practices: Barrett's surveillance vs. ulcerative colitis surveillance vs. biopsy for sprue vs. biopsy for microscopic colitis. Dig Dis Sci. 2004;49:1808–14.
11. Barkun A, Liu J, Carpenter S, et al. Update on endoscopic tissue sampling devices. Gastrointest Endosc. 2006;63:741–5.
12. Kluge F, Seidler E. Zur Erstanwendung der Ösophago- und Gastroskopie: Briefe von Adolf Kussmaul und seinen Mitarbeitern. Medizinhist J. 1986;21:288–307.
13. Achord JL. The history of gastrointestinal endoscopy. In: Ginsberg GG, Kochman ML, Norton ID, Gostout CJ, editors. Clinical gastrointestinal endoscopy. 2nd ed. St. Louis, Missouri: Elsevier Saunders; 2012. p. 5–11.
14. Kohli DR, Baillie J. How endoscopes work. In: Chandrasekhara V, Elmunzer BJ, Khashab MA, et al., editors. Clinical gastrointestinal endoscopy. 3rd ed. Elsevier; 2019. p. 24–31.

2 Endoscopic Features of Normal and Abnormal Gastric Mucosa

Almost all gastric biopsies are sampled under endoscopic guidance, it is appropriate that a pathologist should also have knowledge of the endoscopic pictures of gastric mucosa under different circumstances. Describing the endoscopic features of inflammatory mucosal changes may be a tricky situation. There are innumerable published materials with different views dealing with this subject with no well-defined terminology and many different ways of interpretations of the observations [1]. Some Gastroenterologists question legitimacy in utilizing the term Gastritis as an endoscopic descriptive feature in gastric mucosal inflammatory changes, or whether this term should only be used for the histological description of demonstrable inflammatory changes.

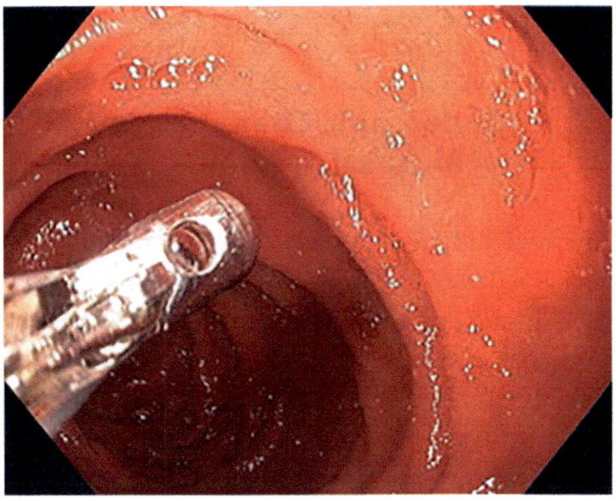

Fig. 2.1 The picture shows an endoscopic view of normal gastric mucosa

2.1 Normal Gastric Mucosa—Description of Endoscopy

Description of appearance of a normal gastric mucosa may be a matter of controversy, as endoscopists see variable grades of alterations, especially in healthy middle-aged and elderly individuals. Hence describing an endoscopically normal gastric mucosa may be of a wide range of pink shades, smoothness, and lustre (Fig. 2.1). Antrum mucosal folds are irregular and relatively less prominent compared to body mucosa and do not disappear completely even with excessive air insufflation (Fig. 2.2) [1]. Occasionally, there can be a few mucosal folds along the roof of the pyloric channel forming incomplete arches. Remaining proximal component of the stomach forming the major component has prominent well-formed mucosal folds or rugae. These are arranged uniformly and individual mucosal folds measure not more than 5 mm across. Normal gastric mucosal folds yield easily on insufflation and may totally disappear. Normal stomach mucosa otherwise is not covered by any form of exudate [1–4].

K. Vaiphei, *Interpretation of Endoscopic Biopsy - Gastritis, Gastropathies and Beyond*,
https://doi.org/10.1007/978-981-16-6026-9_2

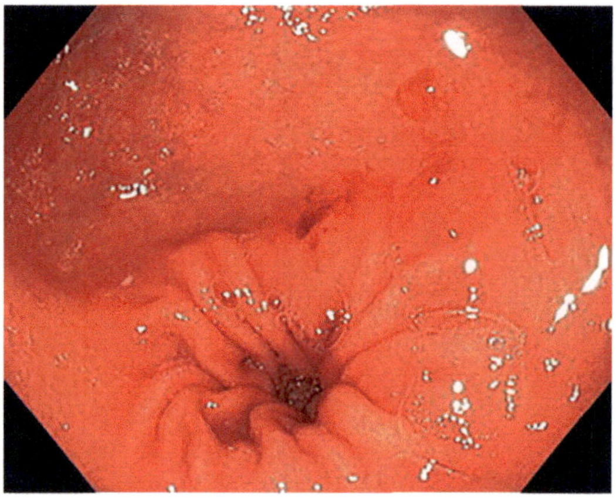

Fig. 2.2 Endoscopic view of gastric pyloric antrum showing a patch of haemorrhagic area in the mucosa

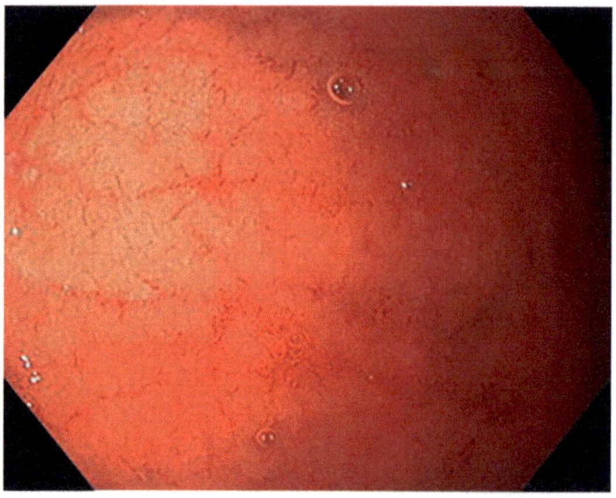

Fig. 2.3 Endoscopic picture of gastric mucosa showing mosaic pattern due to prominence of the vascular marking along with small patches of pinpoint congested mucosa to indicate gastritis

2.2 Endoscopic Characterization of Mucosal Inflammation

Mucosal inflammation on endoscopic examination is indicated by the presence of visible alterations in the appearance of gastric mucosa as the result of changes in vascular component and inflammatory cell infiltration. And the diagnosis of an inflamed mucosa is entertained when the mucosa shows variable degrees of oedema, punctate or confluent erythema, friability, punctate or confluent exudate, erosions in small focus, or maybe in multiple areas in confluents (Figs. 2.3 and 2.4). These changes may be observed as flat or raised lesions along with prominent or flattened rugae folds. All these may be associated with variable grades prominent vascular marking that may be seen forming mosaic patterns (Fig. 2.3). The intramural bleeding spots may be in the form of punctate or petechiae, or confluent ecchymosis that may result in raised mucosal nodularity which may be fine or coarse [5, 6]. Mild-to-moderately oedematous mucosa may be difficult to perceive in endoscopic examination, only when oedema is extensive, it may be identifiable with confidence and the mucosa appears somewhat paler or whiter accompanied by accentuation of the normal mucosal hexagonal pattern [1]. Mild erythema is diagnosed when there are patchy areas of mucosa discernible as redder than adjacent mucosa (Figs. 2.3, 2.4) [7]. When the

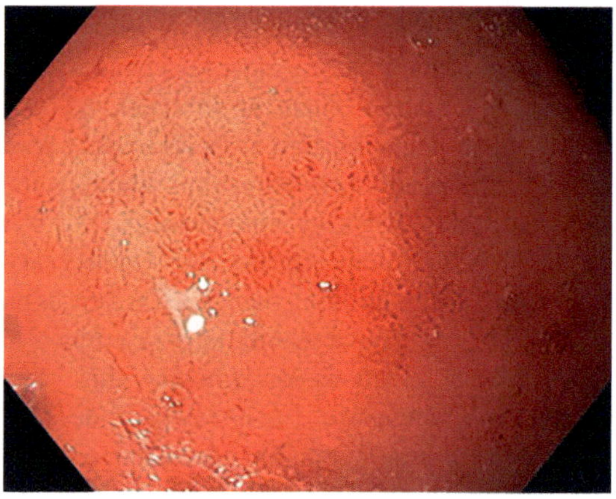

Fig. 2.4 Another endoscopic picture of gastritis where many more conglomerates of small multiple mucosal congested areas

mucosa is obviously discoloured that may be in patches may be graded as moderate erythema, severe degree of mucosal changes may be observed when the mucosa appears grossly blood red [1]. These erythematous areas on magnification are observed to be composed of many haemorrhagic spots of 1–3 mm in sizes laced with fine pinkish speckles, which may be seen involving the antrum or body mucosa or may be more diffuse. In the antral mucosa, sometimes the erosions may be seen as streaks of red spots. Friable mucosa causes punctate haemorrhages and frank oozes to minimal touch [5, 6]. A severely friable mucosa tends to be markedly swollen, congested and readily bleeds, and may be covered by grey yellowish, deep red or almost blackish friable necrotic exudate. It may be difficult to differentiate these exudates from gastric content. The exudates tend to present in clusters of fibres or may adhere to the mucosa resulting in a mound-like appearance. Presence just a few reddish areas are graded as mild, when seen as small groups or clusters are graded as moderate and larger areas covered with exudates are graded as severe [3, 8]. *Helicobacter pylori* infection may result in whitish small discoloured areas of exudates in antral mucosa and the duodenal bulb mucosa. Similar changes may also be artefactually produced by reflection of the white light which tends to be brighter and not well outlined [9]. A superficial mucosal break represents erosion, which may be superficial or flat, may represent a superficial necrotic mucosa and tends to be surrounded by a thin rim of congestion, the deeper muscularis mucosae at histological examination. Erosion covered by inflammatory exudate or larger haemorrhagic spots measuring up-to 10 mm size will not be difficult to identify. These lesions may be seen in isolation or in numerous. Erosions may be deeper and larger making it difficult to differentiate from more superficially located ulcers and if the depth of the mucosal injury is more than 1 mm then qualifies for ulcer. An elevated lesion having a centrally placed mucosal defect is known as varioliform erosion, usually seen in corpus, may also involve antrum, may be superimposed with mucosal folds. It may be solitary or few or numerous in numbers [9, 10].

During the process of endoscopic examination, variation in the thickness of the gastric mucosal fold may be seen, which may be of variable thickness. Abnormally thicken folds are resistant to insufflation and do not show a significant change in their size. Mucosal fold thickness may range from 5 mm to more than 10 mm. The thicken folds may be superimposed by nodular irregularities. In contrast to these mucosal changes, there may be gross atrophy or thinning of the mucosal folds, sometimes there may be totally flattened gastric rugae. This abnormal loss of mucosal fold most frequently involves the gastric body mucosa with a few remnants of small mucosal elevations. Along with the mucosal thinning, the branching vascular markings become prominent and easily visible, which may be associated with slightly protuberant vessels [1, 11, 12].

2.3 Biopsy Forceps

There are various types of biopsy forceps available for routine utilization. There are biopsy forceps which allow only one bite and others that allow two bites in one go. Cold biopsy forceps usually allow only one bite at a time. Another variant of biopsy forceps is the one that has a needle fitted in between the two cups that are opposed to each other and can take two bites in one go. Because of these advantages this particular forceps is equipped with, this is the most frequently utilized one and offers the advantage of targeted sampling of the preferred site by stabilizing the forceps cups with the help of the needle the first specimen while collecting the second specimen in one go [12, 13]. These forceps are equipped with variably designed cups that may have jigsaw margins with or without fenestration, and that may be round, oval, or elongated. The larger biopsy forceps can sample bigger tissue piece having deeper areas of the mucosa, double or more than double the size compared to that of a standard-sized forceps [14, 15]. There are specially designed forceps with accessory channel allowing to take multiple bites of four or more tissue pieces. Some of the forceps are specially designed with a swing jaw, rotatable channels, and angulated ones [15]. There are many types of biopsy forceps, some of which may be heated up to desirable temperature and may be used simultaneously for biopsy and tissue coagulation. This type is not being favoured for routinely used as it produces coagulative defects in the biopsy sample [16]. GI mucosal polyps are removed with snares and these snares may have different types of shapes. There are a wide range of choices in the snare types, some are re-usable. They may be variable sizes and they may also be made with different types of materials [16–18].

Similarly, the instruments usable for brush cytology may be flexible having single or multiple channels with a wide range of brush sizes. These instruments may be of variable stiffness with or without a guide wire. The size of the outer sheaths recommended for ERCP ranges from 6 to 8 F [19–21]. Aspiration cytology has not gained wide acceptance. It may be carried out using a hollow bore needle and the size of the retractable needle may range from 7.5 to 22 gauge for ERCP that may be fitted to a catheter having a ball tip. The direction of the needle may be directly viewed under fluoroscopic guidance [22, 23].

2.4 Endoscopic Biopsy Techniques

Most of the endoscopic biopsies are carried out with pinch biopsy forceps that can fit into a 2.8-mm channel and can sample 4–8 mm size mucosal fragment. A smaller-size forceps used for young children can be fitted into 2.2 mm channel [24]. A pinch biopsy usually contains the gastric mucosa along with the muscularis mucosa. The yield depends upon the size of the forceps used, the angle and extends firmness of the force applied on the forceps while taking the biopsy placed against the mucosa and the optimal angle of the forceps. However, in gastric biopsy specially for gastric body biopsy with thicker mucosal folds or in situation associated increase mucosal fold thickness, it may be difficult to take a bite into the full mucosa using pinch forceps [25]. The whole thickness of the gastric mucosa may be successfully sampled using larger cup forceps having a channel size of 3.6–3.7 mm, which are usually used for therapeutic purposes. The size of the mucosal biopsy obtained with this forceps maybe 6 or more mm in size and may not necessarily include the deeper tissue and are equally safe for the patients. But larger the size of the mucosal fragments, the pathologists are at advantage as it provides more mucosa to examine under the microscope and is useful for surveillance tissue sampling and also easier for orientation for the histotechnologists in the pathology laboratory [26]. The third technique of biopsy is the utilization of electrically heated hot biopsy forceps and these forceps are insulated. This type of biopsy forceps usually produces extensive cautery artefacts, which often makes histologic interpretation difficult. Besides, this technique carries may be associated with hollow organ leakage as the result of cauterized tissue and residual tissue on follow-up biopsy tends to give a false positive interpretation for dysplasia [27–29].

In the snare procedure, a wire loop is placed around the targeted mucosal polyp allowing the lesion to be cut in one piece. This technique has been primarily designed for removing any polyps anywhere in the gastrointestinal tract especially polyps present in colon. Depending upon the size of the polyp in target, different size snares may be used. This technique may be utilized along with electrocautery [30, 31]. Excised polyps may be placed on the snare loop or can be transported across the suction channel separately or along with the endoscope. This method is usable for any size polyp [30]. Polyp with a well-defined pedicle is cut along the base usually using the hot snare technique where a quantified current is passed through a metal wire. In contrast to the hot snare technique, cold snare polypectomy is carried out without the electrical current, thereby avoiding all the complications that may arise in the hot snare technique. However, cold snaring is associated with higher chances of bleeding [32].

2.5 Endoscopic Mucosal Resection

Neoplastic or pre-neoplastic growth confined either to the mucosa or to submucosa is dissected out using Endoscopic Mucosal Resection (EMR), which in short may be described as the lift and the cut technique [31]. The technique involves expansion of the submucosal space by injecting liquid thereby also reducing chances of injury to the muscular layer by cautery. The depth of the invasion by the growth is the main factor for patient selection for EMR and is assessed with the help of endoscopic ultrasonography (EUS) [33]. The most commonly used liquids for injecting into submucosa are saline, diluted epinephrine with saline, saline (3.5%), dextrose (50%), or sodium hyaluronate [31]. Failure to lift mucosal lesions by this technique may be an indicator for the involvement of deeper gastric wall of the stomach [34]. The protruding lesion in the lifted-up portion of the mucosa is removed with the help of a snare [35]. Orientation of the resected specimen using markings is an important step for proper sampling and reporting for optimal tumour staging by assessing depth of invasion and resection margins. EMR allows the endoscopist one piece resection of the early malignant lesion, which usually is between 15 and 20 mm in size [36]. In situations where the deep margins show infiltration by the tumour, the patient will be subjected to gastrectomy [37].

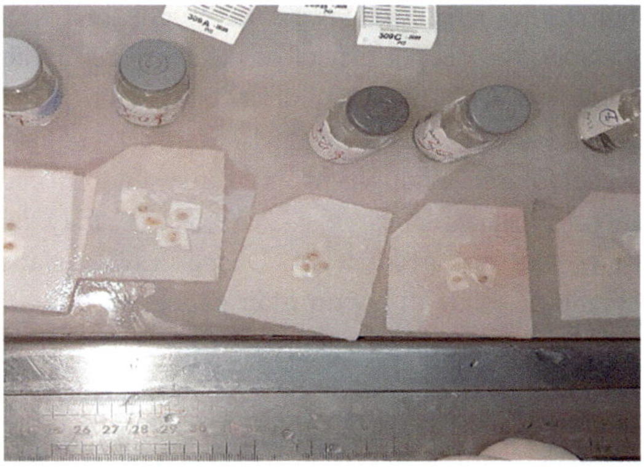

Fig. 2.5 Photograph showing filter paper mount endoscopic mucosal pieces on larger size filter papers displayed on grossing table along with the labelled vials in which the biopsies were submitted to Histopathology Laboratory; each sample has different numbers of filter paper mounted specimens, some having more than one tissue piece and some with no tissue on filter paper. The tissue piece may be inked or may also be processed as such

2.6 Handling of Endoscopic Biopsy

Most of the time endoscopic biopsies from stomach tends to be sampled from multiple sites and different areas of the stomach. Normal gastric mucosa in endoscopic examination is pinkish and velvety with regularly dispersed fine vascular networks. The gastric mucosa is thrown into regularly placed straight mucosal folds with smooth surface, the folds are about 5 mm thick. Mucosa is also covered by mucus layer usually present mainly along the great curvature of gastric body. Normally blood vessels are also visible. These collecting venules exhibit a regular pattern, i.e., starfish-like red spots arranged regularly in fundic mucosa and also along the lesser curvature. Diameter of these venules is just a few mm and are mostly regular size. All biopsy sampled from different areas should be ideally put into differently labelled vials containing adequate amount of 10% buffered formalin (Fig. 2.5). Each vial should be handled separately during the whole course of processing in the pathology laboratory till the step of staining and while making histopathology reporting as well.

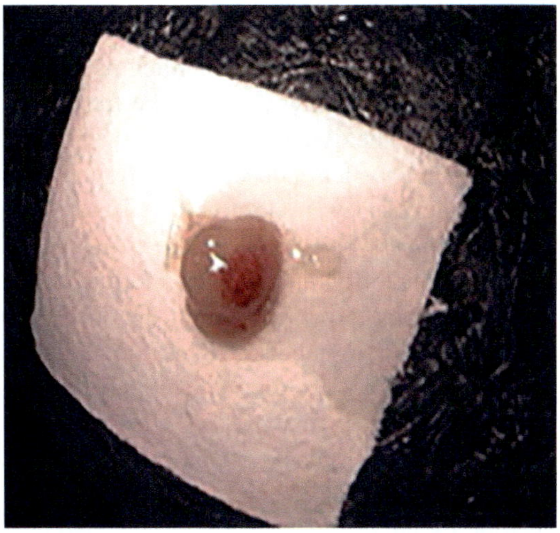

Fig. 2.6 Close-up photograph of one such filter mounted specimen to show the character that is mainly composed of necrotic material

All endoscopic biopsies should preferably be oriented and to be mounted on filter paper immediately as a bedside activity in the endoscopic room (Fig. 2.6). Mounting on filter paper is a process that needs to be expertized and to be carried out in the endoscopy room immediately after the fresh tissue is released either from the forceps on a clean smooth surface tabletop. The mucosal fragment should be optimally stretched using needles or pins and to be placed flat on filter papers with the mucosal surface facing upwards.

Sometimes when there is gastric mucosal erosion of ulcer, the deeper aspect of the biopsy may be identified with the help of a hand lens. Filter paper should be cut into ~10 mm size square pieces, large enough to hold the endoscopic biopsy tissue pieces (Fig. 2.6). Tissue may be inked but not necessarily. Deeper raw surface should be made to lay on filter paper, which will adhere firmly with tissue plasma protein present on the cute surface. Once the specimen is mounted, it is to be put into the vial containing adequate volume (at least 10 times the approximate volume of the tissue pieces) of 10% buffered formalin and appropriately labelling of the vial to be carried out. Tissue penetration of the buffered formalin takes place at the rate of 1 mm per hour [31, 38]. Formalin fixation produces optimally maintained tissue morphology, suitable for microscopic examination using various types of stains including immunohistochemistry. These tissues may also be utilized for molecular study and fluorescent stains [31, 39, 40]. The biopsy piece that has been placed on filter paper will remain adherent to filter paper as the freshly cut raw surface of the tissue is rich in plasma protein, which is an excellent adhesive. While grossing, the mounted tissues are not to be dislodged from the filter papers and to be grossed as such. It should be made routine to count the number of filter paper pieces present within the submitted vial and also the number of tissue fragments on the filter papers; sometimes there may be discrepancies between the two, as all filter paper mounted specimens may not be mucosal tissue fragments as it can be faecal matter, mucous or necrotic tissue, or one filter paper may also bear more than one tissue piece (Fig. 2.7). This step of mounting on filter paper is necessary for fixing the tissue piece in a properly spread-out state, thereby making edgewise embedding of the biopsy in the paraffin block easy. Edgewise embedding of the biopsy will help to get a full thickness of the mucosa for histological examination under the microscope. Important to remember at this point is that the technical staff of the pathology laboratory or histo-technician who will be handling these filter paper-mounted specimens, should be aware of handling methodology of filter paper-mounted samples (Fig. 2.8). There are certain careful steps like tone should avoid shaking of the vial containing the fresh tissue before it gets fixed, as there may be fragmentation of the friable tissue, detachment or sloughing out the surface lining epithelium [41, 42]. Endoscopic tissue may be stored at −20 or − 80 degree centigrade, or specified fixative may be handled according to the guidelines of the specified test. Unfixed fresh tissues are required for flow cytometry and microbial culture. The first few pieces of tissue should be preferably submitted for microbial culture to reduce contamination. For electron microscopy, fresh tissue should be put into vials containing 2% glutaraldehyde, otherwise, formalin-fixed tissue may also be used for electron microscopy [31].

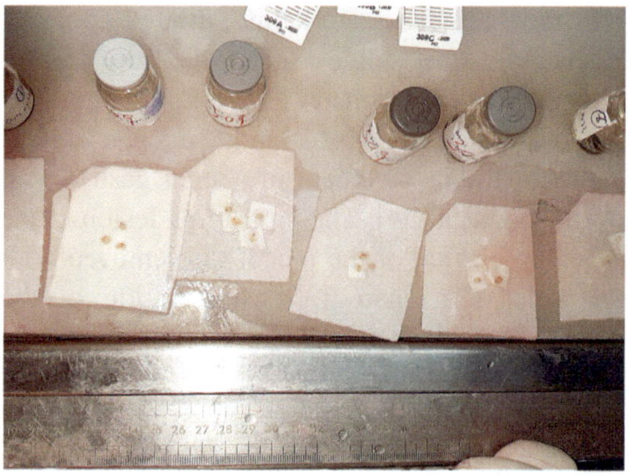

Fig. 2.7 Another photograph showing the filter-mounted endoscopic tissue pieces after being placed on larger filter papers for processing. If one closely examines each biopsy individually, it will be obviously seen that the first biopsy on the left having three tissue pieces has not been mounted on filter paper, i.e., unmounted tissue bits. And the next one with four filter papers with discoloured areas does not have any recognizable tissue bits. Similar filter papers with no tissue bits are also identifiable in the next two biopsies

Sometimes a practising endoscopist likes to know how many biopsy tissue pieces are to be taken in a certain condition. Number of endoscopic biopsy tissue to be sampled may vary depending upon the type of mucosal lesion observed in the endoscopic examination. There are few studies in gastric cancers in which percentage of the definitive diagnosis of carcinoma was significantly higher if the number of tissue

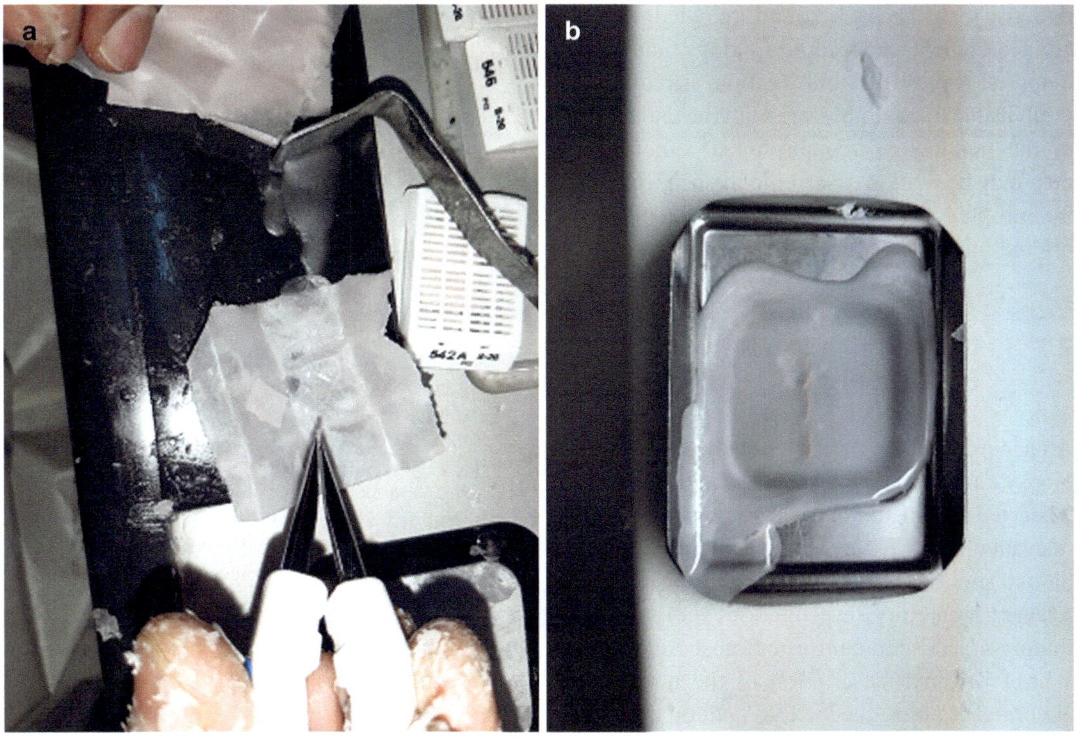

Fig. 2.8 This photograph shows the process of embedding the processed endoscopic biopsy mounted on filter paper in (**a**). In A, the trained technician is seen picking up the oriented tissue from the filter paper mount, and embedding/placing the tissue fragments edgewise within the molten paraffin wax arranged regularly by placing them close to each other with proper spacing in a metallic tissue mould in (**b**)

pieces sampled were two or more compared to single tissue piece sampling from endoscopically visible lesions. Increasing the number of tissue pieces by more than two did not show any significantly different diagnostic yield [43, 44].

In the updated Sydney classification, it has been documented that mapping studies by taking four biopsy tissues, two from antrum and body each help in assessing the correct status of *H. pylori* infection [45]. Besides these four biopsies, a biopsy from incisura angularis was added as this site is believed to be affected early in the process of development of atrophic gastritis and subsequently followed by histological evidence of goblet cell in development of gastric cancer [46]. Sydney classification has provided an easy concept in understanding the histological parameters by diagrammatic representation of the grades of mucosal changes taking place in the evolution of gastritis of the extent of chronic inflammatory cell infiltration, neutrophil infiltration, and gastric glands destruction and loss, extend of replacement fibrosis and goblet cell metaplasia and presence of HP [47]. In order to carry out gradings of the mucosal changes, biopsies are to be taken from different segments of the stomach and every biopsy from a particular segment is to be put into a separately labelled vial so that it can be read and interpreted separately [43, 44, 46]. While putting the biopsy tissue fragments, it should be made mandatory to orient and mount them on tissue paper for an optimal histological evaluation [45], which may be done with difficulty in cases of small pinch biopsies. It may be accomplished easily with larger biopsies. While examining the haematoxylin and eosin-stained sections, it is advisable to match between the description of the tissue fragments during grossing and number of tissue fragments observed in the ribbon sections. This is an important step as it helps to examine all the tissue fragments present under the microscope. Interpretation is best carried out with the background knowledge of the clinical history, endoscopic findings, and site of biopsies. Any further information, if required, it is advisable to communicate with the endoscopist or the treating gastroenterologist; otherwise, a note may be written describing the needful below the morphological description and the diagnosis offered in the histopathological report form.

2.7 Communication Between Endoscopist and Pathologist

An accurate and appropriate interpretation of the biopsy can be achieved and executed better only when the histopathologist has knowledge of the relevant clinical history, endoscopic findings, and biopsy site. Clinical history should also include relevant laboratory investigations and radiology findings. Endoscopic information should include a brief narrative description of the normal and abnormal features like the fold pattern, any nodularity or thickening or both, polyps, masses, erosions, ulcers or vascular patterns, and any abnormal-looking area specifying the sites. Also, not to be forgotten, is history of intake of drug or any chemical irritant specifying the duration of intake and type of drug.

Acknowledgement All the endoscopic pictures are courtesy of Dr. Jimil Shah, Assistant Professor, Department of Gastroenterology, Post Graduate Institute of Medical Education and Research, Chandigarh, India, Pin—160012.

References

1. Tytgat GNJ. The Sydney system: endoscopic division. Endoscopic appearances in gastritis/duodenitis. J Gastroenterol Hepatol. 1991;6:223–34.
2. Jang JY. The past, present, and future of image-enhanced endoscopy. Clin Endosc. 2015;48:466–75.
3. Yang JM, Chen L, Fan YL, et al. Endoscopic patterns of gastric mucosa and its clinicopathological significance. World J Gastroenterol. 2003;9:2552–6.
4. Anagnostopoulos GK, Yao K, Kaye P, et al. High-resolution magnification endoscopy can reliably identify normal gastric mucosa, helicobacter pylori-associated gastritis, and gastric atrophy. Endoscopy. 2007;39:202–7.
5. Qi Q, Guo C, Ji R, et al. Diagnostic performance of magnifying endoscopy for helicobacter pylori infection: a meta-analysis. PLoS One. 2016;11:e0168201.
6. Hussain I, Ang TL. Evidence based review of the impact of image enhanced endoscopy in the diagnosis of gastric disorders. World J Gastrointest Endosc. 2016;8:741–55.
7. Tytgat GNJ, Hofer S, Rauws EAJ. Endoscopic and histologic aspects of gastritis. In: Malfertheiner P, Ditschuneit H, editors. Helicobacter pylori, gastritis and peptic ulcer. Berlin and Heidelberg: Springer; 1990.
8. Tahara T, Shibata T, Nakamura M, et al. Gastric mucosal pattern by using magnifying narrow-band imaging endoscopy clearly distinguishes histological and serological severity of chronic gastritis. Gastrointest Endosc. 2009;70:246–53.
9. Lee SY. Endoscopic gastritis, serum pepsinogen assay, and helicobacter pylori infection. Korean J Intern Med. 2016;31:835–44.
10. Maratka Z. Endoscopic diagnosis and terminology of erosions and similar mucosal lesions. Gastrointest Endosc. 1996;43:633–6.
11. Mihara M, Haruma K, Kamada T, et al. The role of endoscopic findings for the diagnosis of helicobacter pylori infection: evaluation in a country with high prevalence of atrophic gastritis. Helicobacter. 1999;4:40–8.
12. Mao T, Wang Y, Yin F, et al. Association of Endoscopic Features of gastric mucosa with helicobacter pylori infection in Chinese patients. Gastroenterol Res Pract. 2016;2016:6539639.
13. Bernstein DE, Barkin JS, Reiner DK, et al. Standard biopsy forceps versus large-capacity forceps with and without needle. Gastrointest Endosc. 1995;41:573–6.
14. Faigel DO, Eisen GM, Baron TH, et al. Tissue sampling and analysis. Gastrointest Endosc. 2003;57:811–6.
15. Levine DS, Blount PL, Rudolph RE, et al. Safety of a systematic endoscopic biopsy protocol in patients with Barrett's esophagus. Am J Gastroenterol. 2000;95:1152–7.
16. Gilbert DA, DiMarino AJ, Jensen DM, et al. Status evaluation: hot biopsy forceps. Gastrointest Endosc. 1992;38:753–6.
17. Carpenter S, Petersen BT, Chuttani R, et al. ASGE technology status evaluation report: polypectomy devices. Gastrointest Endosc. 2007;65:741–9.
18. Fyock CJ, Draganov PV. Colonoscopic polypectomy and associated techniques. World J Gastroenterol. 2010;16:3630–7.
19. Shroff CP, Nanivadekar SA. Endoscopic brushing cytology and biopsy in the diagnosis of upper gastrointestinal tract lesions. A study of 350 cases. Acta Cytol. 1988;32:455–60.
20. de Bellis M, Sherman S, Fogel EL, et al. Tissue sampling at ERCP in suspected malignant biliary strictures (part 1). Gastrointest Endosc. 2002;56:552–61.

21. de Bellis M, Sherman S, Fogel EL, et al. Tissue sampling at ERCP in suspected malignant biliary strictures (part 2). Gastrointest Endosc. 2002;56:720–30.
22. Ito H, Inoue H, Ryozawa S, et al. Fine-needle aspiration biopsy and endoscopic ultrasound for pretreatment pathological diagnosis of gastric gastrointestinal stromal tumors. Gastroenterol Res Pract. 2012;2012:1–6.
23. American Society for Gastrointestinal Endoscopy guidelines. Biliary and pancreatic sampling devices during ERCP. Gastrointest Endosc. 1996;43:775–8.
24. Ladas SD, Tsamouri M, Kouvidou C, et al. Effect of forceps size and mode of orientation on endoscopic small bowel biopsy evaluation. Gastrointest Endosc. 1994;40:51–5.
25. Weinstein WM. Mucosal biopsy techniques and interaction with the pathologist. Gastrointest Endosc Clin N Am. 2000;10:555–72.
26. Bernstein DE, Barkin JS, Reiner DK, et al. Standard biopsy forceps versus large-capacity forceps with and without needle. Gastrointest Endosc. 1995;41:573–6.
27. Gilbert DA, DiMarino AJ, Jensen DM, et al. Status evaluation: hot biopsy forceps. American Society for Gastrointestinal Endoscopy. Technology assessment committee. Gastrointest Endosc. 1992;38:753–6.
28. Wadas DD, Sanowski RA. Complications of the hot biopsy forceps technique. Gastrointest Endosc. 1988;34:32–7.
29. Peluso F, Goldner F. Follow-up of hot biopsy forceps treatment of diminutive colonic polyps. Gastrointest Endosc. 1991;37:604–6.
30. McAfee JH, Katon RM. Tiny snares prove safe and effective for removal of diminutive colorectal polyps. Gastrointest Endosc. 1994;40:301–3.
31. Jacobson BC, Crawford JM, Farraye FA. Chapter 1—GI tract endoscopic and tissue processing techniques and Normal histology. In: Odze RD, Goldblum JR, editors. Surgical pathology of the GI tract, liver, biliary tract, and pancreas. 2nd ed. W.B. Saunders; 2009. p. 3–30.
32. East JE. Resection techniques for small colonic polyps: cold forceps polypectomy, hot biopsy, cold snare and hot snare. Video J Encycl GI Endosc. 2013;1:401–2.
33. Soetikno RM, Inoue H, Chang KJ. Endoscopic mucosal resection. Current concepts. Gastrointest Endosc Clin N Am. 2000;10:595–617.
34. Uno Y, Munakata A. The non-lifting sign of invasive colon cancer. Gastrointest Endosc. 1994;40:485–9.
35. Inoue H, Takeshita K, Hori H, et al. Endoscopic mucosal resection with a cap-fitted pan-endoscope for oesophagus, stomach, and colon mucosal lesions. Gastrointest Endosc. 1993;39:58–62.
36. Tanabe S, Koizumi W, Kokutou M, et al. Usefulness of endoscopic aspiration mucosectomy as compared with strip biopsy for the treatment of gastric mucosal cancer. Gastrointest Endosc. 1999;50:819–22.
37. Kojima T, Parra-Blanco A, Takahashi H, et al. Outcome of endoscopic mucosal resection for early gastric cancer: review of the Japanese literature. Gastrointest Endosc. 1998;48:550–4.
38. Fox CH, Johnson FB, Whiting J, et al. Formaldehyde fixation. J Histochem Cytochem. 1985;33:845–53.
39. van Beers EH, Joosse SA, Ligtenberg MJ, et al. A multiplex PCR predictor for aCGH success of FFPE samples. Br J Cancer. 2006;94:333–7.
40. Lips EH, Dierssen JW, van Eijk R, et al. Reliable high-throughput genotyping and loss-of-heterozygosity detection in formalin-fixed, paraffin-embedded tumors using single nucleotide polymorphism arrays. Cancer Res. 2005;65:10188–91.
41. Chatterjee S. Artefacts in histopathology. J Oral Maxillofac Pathol. 2014;18(Suppl 1):S111–6.
42. Khan S, Tijare M, Jain M, et al. Artifacts in histopathology: a potential cause of misinterpretation. Res Rev J Dent Scie. 2014;2:23–31.
43. Nishitani M, Yoshida N, Tsuji S, et al. Optimal number of endoscopic biopsies for diagnosis of early gastric cancer. Endosc Int Open. 2019;07:E1683–90.
44. Choi Y, Choi HS, Jeon WK, et al. Optimal number of endoscopic biopsies in diagnosis of advanced gastric and colorectal cancer. J Korean Med Sci. 2012;27:36–9.
45. Dixon MF, Genta R, Yardley J, et al. Classification and grading of gastritis, the updated Sydney system. Am J Surg Pathol. 1996;20:1161–81.
46. Park YH, Kim N. Review of atrophic gastritis and intestinal metaplasia as a premalignant lesion of gastric cancer. J Cancer Prev. 2015;20:25–40.
47. Sipponen P, Price AB. The Sydney system for classification of gastritis 20 years ago. J Gastroenterol Hepatol. 2011;26(Suppl 1):31–4.

Normal Gastric Mucosa

3

Assessment may be carried out by compartmentalizing the mucosa into different segments as the morphological changes are not diffuse. Normal gastric mucosa seldom has any amount of inflammatory cell, though a few scattered mononuclear cells and one or two eosinophils may be taken as within normal limits. Gastric mucosa is also affected by normal ageing process. There may be few scattered small lymphoid aggregates in the deeper portion of lamina propria in biopsies from individuals who are above 50 years of age. Biopsy from gastric cardia is seldom routinely carried out unless there is focal lesion. Length of cardia is variable may range from 1 to 15 mm [1]. Some authors, however, believe that there is no cardia mucosa as such and it develops over the years due to acid reflux and length of which gradually increases with ageing. Before addressing the controversial issues, I like to refer to the normal cardia mucosa of the stomach. It is a narrow area of the gastric mucosa separating distal oesophageal squamous mucosa from fundic mucosa [2]. In 1961, Hayward had proposed that normal human oesophagus at its lower end measuring about 2 cm long is lined by mucus type of columnar epithelium (Fig. 3.1). This short segment of columnar mucosa lies between the stratified squamous mucosa of the oesophagus and fundic mucosa of the stomach [3]. At this point, I like to refer to original studies with contradictory observations. The first one was a study by Öberg et al. [4]. They had examined 334 consecutive endoscopic biopsies obtained from two critical sites, i.e., at and below oesophagogastric junction in patients who had presented with symptoms of foregut disease. Of these, 74% had either cardiac-type (mucus type of glands with gastric type of mucosal lining epithelium) or oxyntocardiac-type mucosa (similar to cardiac type of mucosa, however, the glands have a mixture of mucus type and oxyntic type of cells) in addition to normal oesophageal mucosa and gastric body/fundic type of mucosa and, only in 26% of patients had fundic gastric mucosa in addition to the normal oesophageal mucosa. People who would likely

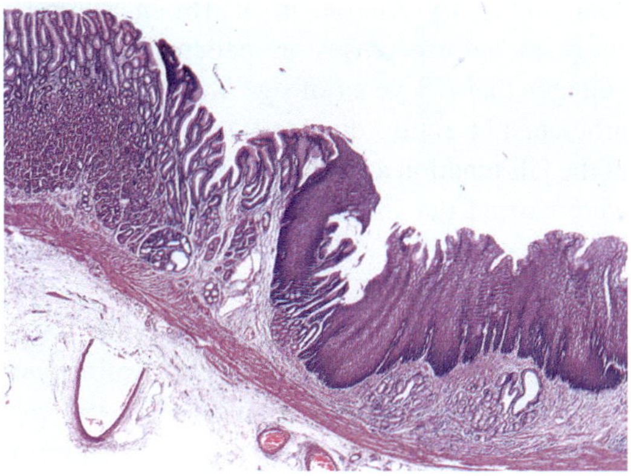

Fig. 3.1 Medium power photomicrograph of gastro-oesophageal junction to show relatively normal cardia mucosa with cardiac simple glands and normal stratified squamous lining mucosa of the oesophagus with the few clusters of submucosal glands (Haematoxylin eosin, ×250)

K. Vaiphei, *Interpretation of Endoscopic Biopsy - Gastritis, Gastropathies and Beyond*,
https://doi.org/10.1007/978-981-16-6026-9_3

develop GERD based on abnormal study of 24 h acid output test and also the ones with shorter oesophageal length had cardiac type or oxyntocardiac type mucosae in oesophageal gastric junction biopsy [5]. These authors hence believed that the columnar mucosa present in an endoscopically normal GE junction comprising of gastric cardia and body type mucosae could be a metaplastic mucosa of the distal oesophagus [5]. Oberg et al. carried out a prospective study in autopsy cases who were younger than 20 years of age and they observed a lack of cardiac type or oxyntocardiac type mucosae in the transition zone of GE junction [4]. This observation was contradicted by Kilgore et al. [6] in a similar study in autopsy cases in patients who were younger than 18 years of age with no upper GI problem like reflux disease. Detail examination of the GE junction and the mucosa on either sides were carried out in all cases. All cases showed appropriate gastric cardiac mucosa on the inferior aspect of the GE junction and the cardiac type of mucosa was present in the limited area ranging from 0.1 to 0.4 cm. This observation confirms the hypothesis of presence of gastric cardiac mucosa from birth. The surface has a bit of villous configuration and the mucosa is relatively thinner than the body mucosa and more like the antral mucosa. The gastric pits depth with mucosal thickness is about 1:1. The gastric foveolae and the cardiac glands are not very regularly arranged like in the rest of the stomach with loose stroma. The surface lining is similar to other parts of the stomach, i.e., tall columnar mucous cells where the nuclei are placed towards the basal portion. Lamina propria contains simple tubular glands and no or minimal inflammatory cells, occasionally a few biopsies may have a few fires of smooth muscle as extension from muscularis mucosae, which will be just a normal variation. Seldom there will be parietal cells amongst the cuboidal to columnar lining of the simple tubular glands in cardia mucosa. The gastric pits or foveola are shorter than that of pyloric antral mucosa.

The thickest mucosa of the stomach is that of fundus and body. Due to their inherent similarities, fundic and body mucosa are described together. Gastric fundus is the portion of the stomach that is above the level off gastro-oesophageal junction (GEJ). Body extends from the level of GEJ and fundus downward to the transverse segment of the antrum. Histologically type of gastric mucosa roughly corresponds to the gross divisions. However, there is no clear-cut identifiable division amongst the different segments of the stomach, one type of mucosa merges with the other types [7]. Grossly the gastric fundus has the most prominent mucosa folds or rugae, which is prominent in empty state as it is responsible distensibility of the stomach. Rugae become less prominent as it reaches antrum and tends to firmly adherent to the underlying muscle. In between the mucosal folds, there are finer shallow furrows called areae gastricae giving almost a mosaic pattern of areas measuring 1–5 mm in diameter, which can be seen the best with the help of a hand lens. These undulations are not affected by stretching of the gastric wall or mucosa, they are an intrinsic component of the mucosa is an intrinsic feature and is not altered by stretching or contraction of the gastric wall.

Under light microscopy, gastric mucosa has a lining of tall columnar mucous type of epithelium showing regularly placed undulating surface intervened by pits or foveolae, lined by similar tall columnar mucus-secreting epithelium. These surface lining epithelial cells are similar in all the mucosal zones. Specialized gastric glands depending upon the different segments of the stomach, open into the base of the gastric pits (Fig. 3.2). The bases of the specialized gastric glands abut upon the surface of muscularis mucosae. Between the pits/foveolae and the gastric glands is the lamina propria. Tall columnar mucus type of cells along the surface epithelium and gastric pits have basally placed round nucleus with finely stippled chromatin and the cytoplasm is filled with neutral periodic acid Schiff positive mucin. Electron microscopy shows a layer of glycocalyx with stubby microvilli along the surface. Gastric mucus is in two forms—one secreted by the surface lining mucus-type columnar epithelial cells, which is insoluble form and its main purpose is to protect the surface by forming a thick layer. The second form is the soluble form secreted by the gastric glands. The mucus neck

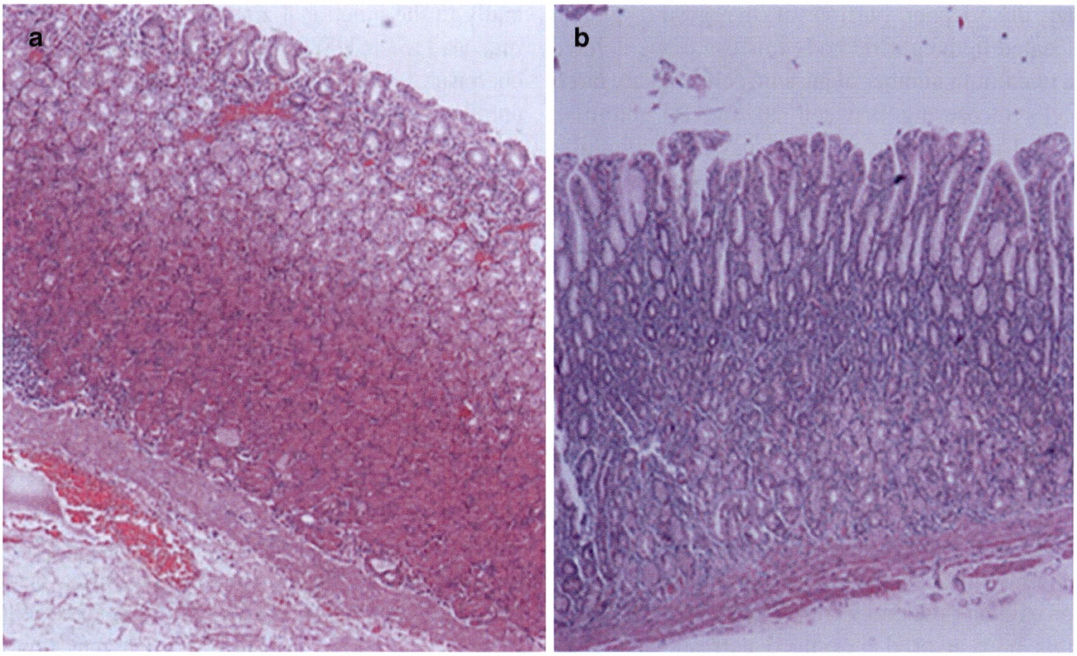

Fig. 3.2 (**a**) Medium power photomicrograph representing gastric body and fundic mucosa. Except for the upper one-fourth to one-fifth, the remaining portion of mucosa contains tightly packed specialized gastric glands. Majority of the cells visible are parietal cells seen as polygonal cells with eosinophilic cytoplasm, no visible lamina propria component. The surface lining is columnar mucous cells (Haematoxylin eosin, ×250). (**b**) Medium power photomicrograph of pyloric antrum showing the depth of foveolae limiting to less than half the thickness of the mucosa and the lower two-third of the mucosa occupied by tightly packed mucous glands. No or minimally visible lamina propria component. The surface lining is columnar mucous cells (Haematoxylin and eosin, ×250)

cells may secrete small amounts of sulfomucin and sialomucin [8]. Soluble mucins have lubricating property and the insoluble fragment act as a barrier for gastric mucosa from dispersing the gastric juice into the mucosa [9]. Another view suggests that mucus might have some protective function, but actual mucosal barrier is formed by the continuous layer of columnar surface mucus cells and the tight junctions between adjacent cells [10]. Gastric mucosa is a very active organ metabolically. The gastric surface mucus epithelial cells have very high regenerative activity and get replaced normally every few days to within a week's time [11]. The specialized cells present in gastric body mucosa have a slower turnover rate than the mucous epithelial cells and take place every 1–3 years [12]. Length of the gastric pits/foveolae in fundus and body mucosa are shorter than the rest and elsewhere and form just about a quarter of the full mucosal thickness. The specialized glands are arranged in a tubular pattern and do not have the twisting tube-like pattern of other parts of the stomach. The specialized glands are composed of bluish-looking chief cells mainly in the basal portion intermixed with pinkish or eosinophilic parietal cells. Toward the isthmic portion, the glands are mainly composed of parietal cells intermixed with the mucous lining epithelial cells. Any amount of mucus type of cells, if identified amongst the specialized fundic and body glands, that will be indicative metaplasia as a part and partial of mucosa undergoing atrophy changes. Scattered neuroendocrine cells (enterochromaffin and a few enterochromaffin-like cells) identifiable as smaller cells having pale cytoplasm can be seen along the basal zone in between the other specialized cells [13]. Mucous neck cells are lesser in number in gastric fundic and body mucosa. They are mainly located at the interphase between the gastric glands and foveolar pits. Upper portion of the gastric glands located in the gastric body mucosa tends to have a maximum number of parietal cells that are large cells measuring between 20 and 35 microns, round to pyramidal in shape having acidophilic cytoplasm with centrally placed round nucleus. These cells produce blood group-specific substances, intrinsic factors, and hydrochloric acid [14]. The lower half of the body glands dominantly contain chief cell population. These cells have basophilic refractile granules with a basal nucleus and secrete pepsinogen. Proximal portion of gastric body mucosa contains more of chief cells whereas the distal portion contains more of parietal cells [15].

The pyloric mucosa is present distal to the body mucosa and the pylorus portion becomes slightly horizontal giving a triangular zone lying proximal to the duodenum. The transverseness of this portion of the stomach corresponds to its function where mixing of the ingested food particles with the gastric juice secreted by the fundus and body mucosa takes place. Pyloric sphincter ends abruptly by telescoping into first part of the duodenum, and obviously the character of the mucosa from the gastric type to the duodenal type is distinctly different in appearance, i.e., longitudinal mucosal folds in pylorus and circumferentially placed mucosal folds in duodenum. In the pyloric antral zone, the gastric pits occupy approximately 50% of the mucosa and the deeper 50% mucosa contains the antral glands. The antral mucus glands are twisted in circular shape with occasional branching, and are rather relatively loosely packed with more amount of intervening lamina propria. The packing of the glands is looser in the cardiac mucosa with more lamina propria helping in differentiating histologically between the two sites. The cells of the mucous glands have ill-defined cell membrane with pale vacuolated cytoplasm differentiating the cells of the foveolar glands from the surface epithelial mucous cells. Antral mucosa may infrequently have scattered parietal cells singly or in a small group intermixed with the mucous cells, especially in the junctional zone of antrum and body mucosa [15, 16]. With the help of immunohistochemistry, endocrine cells are identified in the antral mucosa and body mucosa contains somatostatin-producing D cells, serotonin-secreting enterochromaffin, and enterochromaffin-like cells have been identified [17].

The surface lining mucus epithelial cells of the gastric mucosa, and epithelial cells of the pits/foveolae and glands rest on a basement membrane, which is similar to that seen elsewhere in the body. The structural integrity of the gastric mucosa is maintained by lamina propria consisting of fine reticulin framework, collagen and elastic tissue along with scattered capillaries, venules, lymphatics and naked nerve fibres [16]. There may be few scattered smooth muscle fibres extending from the muscularis mucosae. These fibres get condensed underneath the basement membrane. Lamina propria is sparse in the deeper portion of the mucosa as the main component is formed by the specialized gastric glands. In contrast to this, the superficial portion that lies in between the gastric pits appears to be more prominent as there is no glandular component. It contains a mixture of cells, i.e. scattered fibroblasts intermixed very occasional histiocytes, plasma cells and lymphocytes, very infrequently normally there may be occasional polymorphs and mast cells. Lymphoid tissue is on the whole very sparse in stomach mucosa [16]. Lamina propria also contains capillaries, arterioles, lymphatics and non-myelinated nerve fibres and a few smooth muscle fibres extension from muscularis mucosa into the lamina propria occasionally reaching the superficial portion of mucosa [7]. Isolated lymphocytes occasionally may be seen and are dominantly B cell type and plasma cells secrete IgA. Just scattered intraepithelial lymphocytes may be occasionally seen but much lesser than in small intestine. A few of the IEL and lamina propria lymphocytes may be T cell type. Lymphoid follicles occasionally may be found in the deeper portion of the lamina propria and tend to be age-related changes [16].

References

1. Sarbia M, Donner A, Gabbert HE. Histopathology of the gastroesophageal junction: a study on 36 operation specimens. Am J Surg Pathol. 2002;26:1207–12.
2. Owen DA. Stomach. In: Sternberg SS, editor. Histology for pathologists. New York: Raven Press; 1992. p. 533–45.
3. Hayward J. The lower end of the esophagus. Thorax. 1961;16:36–41.
4. Öberg S, Peters JH, DeMeester TR, et al. Inflammation and specialized intestinal metaplasia of cardiac mucosa is a manifestation of gastroesophageal reflux disease. Ann Surg. 1997;226:522–32.
5. Goldblum JR. Inflammation and intestinal metaplasia of the gastric cardia: helicobacter pylori, gastroesophageal reflux disease, or both. Dig Dis. 2000;18:14–9.
6. Kilgore SP, Ormsby AH, Gramlich TL, et al. The gastric cardia is not a metaplastic mucosa secondary to gastroesophageal reflux disease. Gastroenterol. 1999;116:A213.
7. Owen DA. Normal histology of the stomach. Am J Surg Pathol. 1986;10:48–61.
8. Filipe MI. Mucins in the gastro-intestinal epithelium: a review. Invest Cell Pathol. 1979;2:195–216.
9. Allen A, Flemström G, Garner A, et al. Gastroduodenal Mucosal Protection. Physiol Rev. 1993;73:823–57.
10. Piper DW. Mucus: chemistry and characteristics. In: Sircus W, Smith AN, editors. Scientific foundations of gastroenterology. Philadelphia: W.B. Saunders; 1980. p. 333–43.
11. Eastwood GL. Gastrointestinal epithelial renewal. Gastroenterol. 1977;72(5 Pt 1):962–75.
12. Winawer SJ, Lipkin M. Cell proliferation kinetics in the gastrointestinal tract of man. IV. Cell renewal in the Intestinalized gastric mucosa. J Natl Cancer Inst. 1969;42:9–17.
13. Voutilainen M, Juhola M, Pitkänen R, et al. Immunohistochemical study of neuroendocrine cells at the gastric cardia mucosa. J Clin Pathol. 2002;55:767–9.
14. Goldstein AMB, Brothers MR, Davis EA Jr. The architecture of the superficial layer of the gastric mucosa. J Anat. 1969;104:539–51.
15. Hogben CAM, Kent TH, Woodward PA, et al. Quantitative histology of the gastric mucosa: man, dog, cat, Guinea pig, and frog. Gastroenterology. 1974;67:1143–54.
16. Genta RM, Hamner HW, Graham DY. Gastric lymphoid follicles in helicobacter pylori infection: frequency, distribution, and response to triple therapy. Hum Pathol. 1993;24:577–83.
17. Lechago J. The endocrine cells of the digestive tract. Am J Surg Pathol. 1987;11(suppl 1):63–70.

4 Interpretation of Endoscopic Biopsy

The next important step is reading and interpretation of the biopsy. It is important to question oneself—is it fundamentally essential to follow the published criteria for interpreting gastric biopsy amended by a group like the original Sydney and the modified classification of gastritis [1, 2]. These criteria are cumbersome and lengthy for routine day-to-day diagnostic use though it gives a complete graded clinic-histological diagnosis. For all practical purposes, a histopathological report should be crisp, informative and to the point in a descriptive format and should be easily communicable with the treating physician. In order to have uniformity, the format for reporting may be according to the format described by World Health Organisation the International Statistical Classification of Diseases and Related Health Problems tenth Revision (ICD-10)-WHO Version, Chapter XI Diseases of the digestive system (K00–K93) for non-tumorous condition [3].

Able to identify correctly the appropriately identified site of a biopsy under the microscope is the first and foremost important step in the diagnostic approach, taking care to examine all the biopsy fragments and all the ribbon sections (Fig. 4.1) in a systematic way. Examination of endoscopic biopsy is time-consuming activity. Absence of any significant feature does not rule out any particular condition in small biopsy whereas positive finding in small biopsy is important. Small biopsies are carried out for a diagnostic purpose and planning of further management, not for staging or more detailed categorization of any particular condition. It is wise to defer from making any definitive diagnosis if quality of the

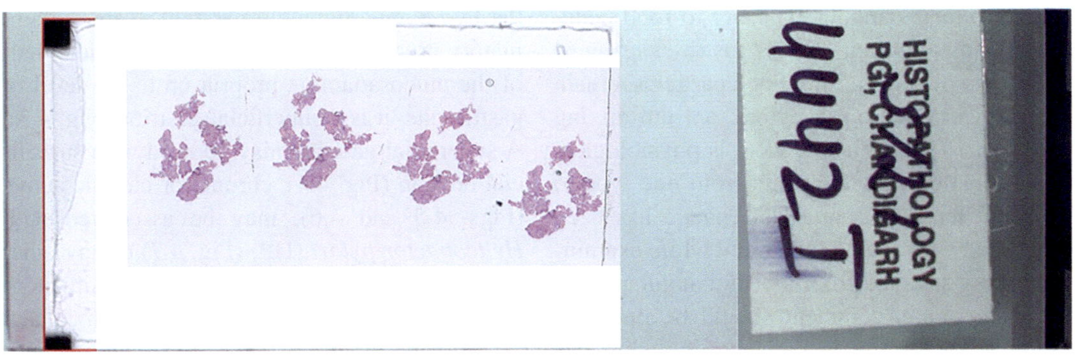

Fig. 4.1 Photograph of a glass slide bearing ribbon sections of multiple endoscopic biopsy tissue pieces, stained with haematoxylin eosin

K. Vaiphei, *Interpretation of Endoscopic Biopsy - Gastritis, Gastropathies and Beyond*,
https://doi.org/10.1007/978-981-16-6026-9_4

sample is inappropriate or inadequate. Most gastric biopsies sampled from abnormal appearing mucosa tend to show inflammation, even normal appearing mucosa on endoscopy may show a variable degree of mucosal inflammation in histology. Inflammatory changes may be of various types and grades, maybe with identifiable causative agent or organism. An adequate endoscopic biopsy should be composed of mucosa with muscularis mucosae. Submucosa will only be a part of the biopsy if the endoscopist has made extra effort to take a deep bite, or in a situation where the ongoing pathology extends beyond the mucosa involving the submucosa.

While interpreting, biopsy along the lesser curvature, the gastric glands are affected by ageing process. There is gradual extension of the antral type of mucosa along the lesser curvature beginning from incisura angularis upward gradually toward the GEJ. Hence, a biopsy taken from a normal looking mucosa from lesser curvature of the body region may be misinterpreted as showing evidence of atrophy [4]. If the histological feature of atrophy is present only in the biopsy sample from the lesser curvature and the individual is in his or her fifth decade or above, and the endoscopic examination being essentially within normal limits, it is most likely to be age-related changes, rather than true atrophic gastritis, and needs to be correlated with the biopsies taken from other areas of the body. However, replacement of the body type mucosa by antral type along the gastric canal may be related to long standing exposure to food material pasing through from gastro-esophageal spincter to pyloric antrum. Food particles remain for a longer duration in pyloric antrum mixing with gastric juice. Hence, there is physiological transformation over the years from one type to another. Hence, this mucosal change has been associated with ageing factor and while examining biopsy sampled from incisura angularis and lesser curvature, comment should be made on the presence of any metaplastic epithelium or dysplasia or malignancy. This particular segment may be more prone to neoplastic changes due to the presence of mucosal atrophy, which is believed to be the precursor lesion of neoplastic mucosa according to Correa's hypothesis of gastric cancer [5].

One may start examination of the mucosa from surface lining epithelium going along gastric pits commenting on their appearances and integrity of the foveolar epithelium. Normally mucous type of epithelium is tall columnar with basally placed nuclei, which may look slightly mucodepleted in the neck regenerative zone. There may be a certain degree of undulation or villiform appearance of the surface in biopsies taken from pyloric antrum and cardia regions which are normal for the sites (Fig. 4.2). Biopsies sampled from body and fundus can be identified with shorter length foveolae and presence of pinkish easily identifiable parietal cells (Fig. 4.2). Presence of friability may be indicated by denudation of the surface lining and dissociated or fragmented foveolae, which needs to be differentiated from artefacts. In truly friable mucosa, there will be mucosal oedema and vascular congestion, occasionally extravasated red blood cells and scattered sparse neutrophils.

The next one may be the lamina propria. Lamina propria in gastric biopsies may be divided into two compartments—(i) inflammation involving the superficial portion extending from the surface lining to the level of gastric pits/foveola with no involvement of specialized gastric glands, (ii) inflammation involving both superficial and deeper halves including the specialized gastric glands extending to the level of muscularis mucosae. It is essential to interpret the involvement of the two compartments separately. If the inflammatory process involves only the superficial half of the mucosa/lamina propria up to the level of gastric pits, it is a superficial gastritis (Fig. 4.3). A superficial gastritis may be mild with superficial erosion (Fig. 4.4), chronic or chronic active (Figs. 4.5 and 4.6), may be associated with *Helicobactor pylori* (HP) (Fig. 4.7) or any other infective or non-infective agent. In this situation, the specialized gastric glands remain intact. Occasionally, there may be age-related changes in the form of one or two lymphoid follicles in the deeper part of the lamina propria, without any other significant changes. Inflammatory cells may involve the mucosa in full thickness with

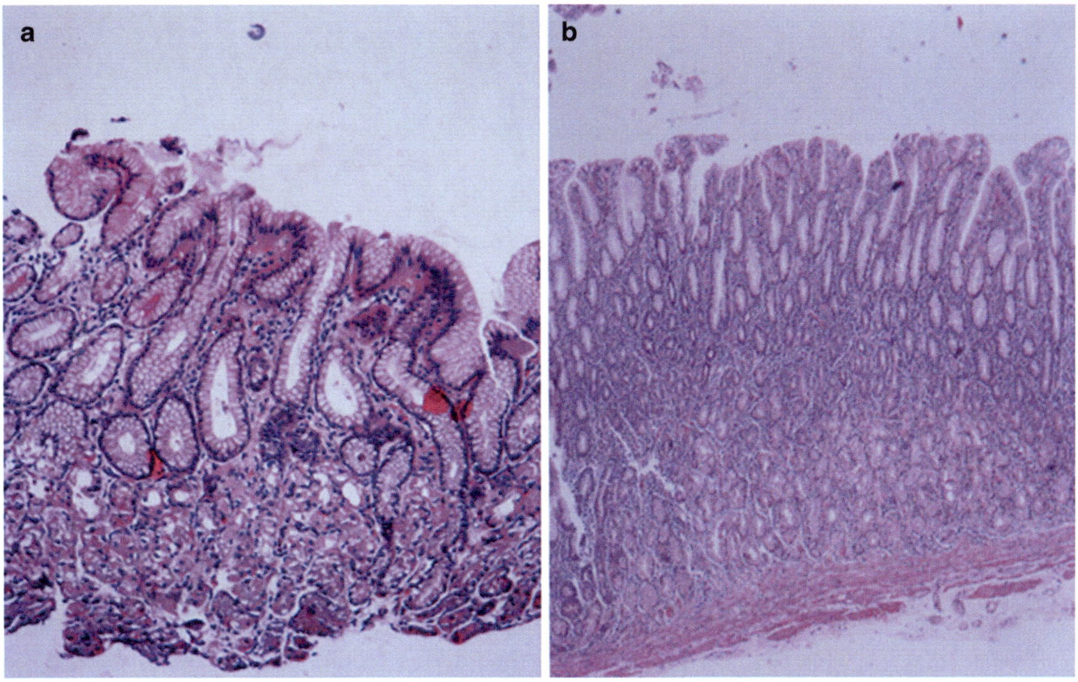

Fig. 4.2 Photomicrographs of antral biopsies showing, **a**—mild chronic inflammatory cell infiltration dominantly in the superficial half of lamina propria (HE, x200). **b**—Similar grade of chronic inflammatory cell infiltration in lamina propria, to be note is the prominent villous configuration of the surface epithelium (HE, x150)

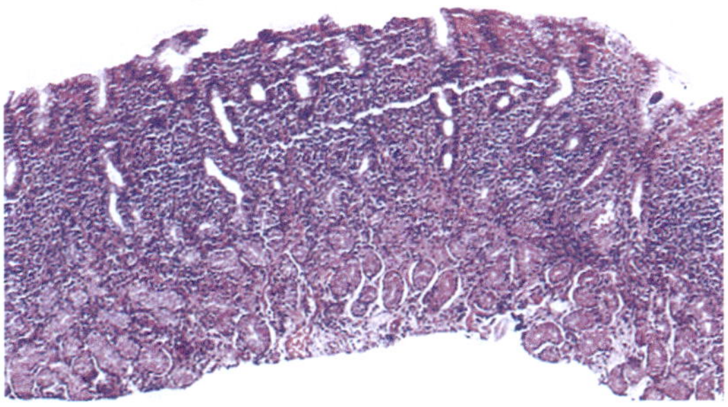

Fig. 4.3 A classic picture of a chronic superficial gastritis of antral biopsy where the moderate-to-heavy chronic inflammatory cells are limited to the superficial half of the mucosa with relatively well preserved antral mucous glands. Gastric pits or foveolae are widely spaced by the inflammatory cells (HE x200)

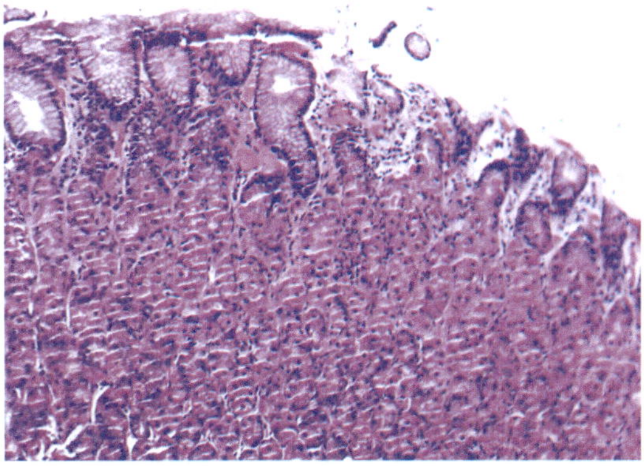

Fig. 4.4 A photomicrograph of the body mucosa showing erosion of the surface lining epithelium with oedema of the underneath lamina propria and collection of a few lymphomononuclear cells corresponding to the site of erosion along with congested and dilated capillaries. The specialized glands are well preserved (HE, x300)

disorganization of gastric glands, which may be diffuse or patchy and focal. Loss of glands indicated by infiltration by inflammatory cells with glandular destruction may be of variable extend. True destruction and loss of glands need to be differentiated from increased spacing between the glands by inflammatory cell infiltration, which frequently may be observed in acute fulminant gastritis and chronic active gastritis with lymphoid follicles. Typing the infiltrating inflammatory cells is important for the morphological diagnosis of disease activity which is indicated

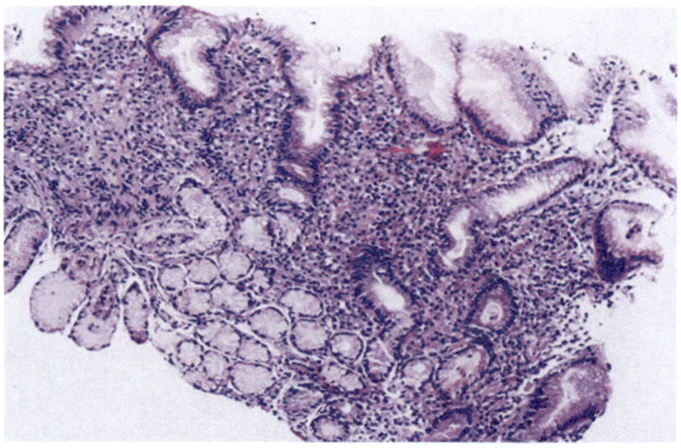

Fig. 4.5 Photomicrograph of antral biopsy showing heavy mucosal inflammation dominantly comprising of chronic inflammatory cells. Inflammatory cells are heavier towards the superficial half in between the hyperplastic and coiled foveolae. There is true reduction in the number of antral mucous glands. Important point to be noted is the true reduction as an indicator for atrophy and apparent reduction due to heavy inflammatory cell infiltration (HE, x200)

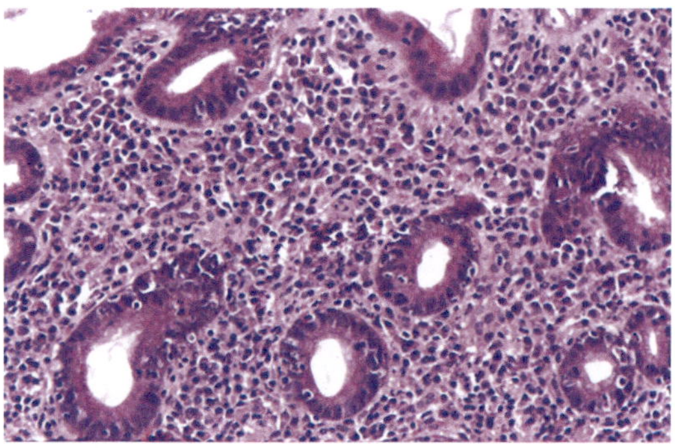

Fig. 4.6 Antral biopsy showing heavy inflammatory cell infiltration dominantly composed of plasma cells, few scattered neutrophils infiltrating the epithelial cells with destruction is also noted associated with depletion of the mucin (HE, x400)

usually by neutrophils (Figs. 4.8–4.10). Alternatively, there may be eosinophil or lymphocyte dominant infiltration of the destroyed glands, which will equally amount for disease activity. Eosinophil tends to be present quite frequently in any endoscopic biopsy (Fig. 4.11) and diagnosis of eosinophilic gastritis or eosinophilic gastroenteritis will not be wise to offer randomly. Any mucosal injury associated with gastric acid tends to have eosinophils amongst the inflammatory cells. In chronic gastritis, there may be prominence of lymphoid follicles in lamina pro-

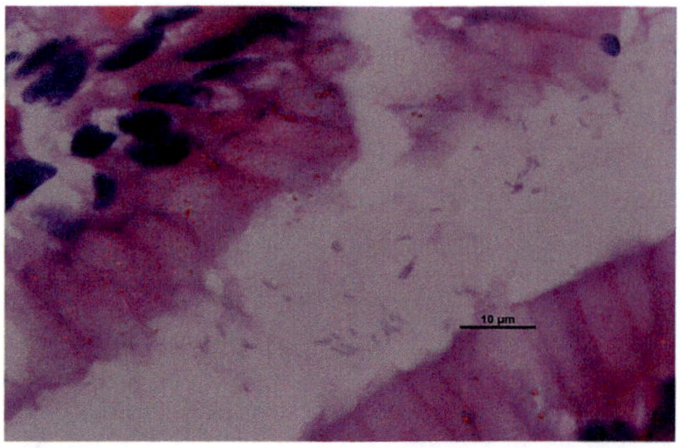

Fig. 4.7 An oil immersion image of a gastric biopsy to show collections of *H. pylori* on the luminal aspect of the gastric foveola seen as single or in small groups (HE, x1000)

pria with other inflammatory cells and is considered to be associated with chronic HP infection. Though autoimmune gastritis is a rare condition in our country, isolated cases may crop up anytime during routine practice and it needs to be considered in all patients with diffuse mucosal inflammation with destruction or loss of parietal cells. These patients may also have co-existing inflammation of the pyloric antrum by HP infection.

Interpretation of gastric body and fundic mucosal biopsies may be different from that of antral biopsy, with similarity in the patterns and types of inflammation. In fundic and body biopsy, it is essential to pay attention to the type of specialized cells lining the glands, which normally are parietal and chief cells. Atrophic gastritis refers to any situation where there is patchy or diffuse replacement fibrosis of the lamina propria, with minimal or any amounts of inflammatory cells usually chronic, with mucous metaplastic or cystic dilated glands (Fig. 4.12). Destruction of the specialized glands may be variable and sometimes, there may not significant loss of glands as only the epithelial cell component of the glands differs as they are lined by mucus cells, which is an indicative of atrophy changes. Hence, in atrophic gastritis, mucosa may not be thinner than normal, rather may be thicker due to associated inflammation, foveolar hyperplasia and metaplastic epithelium and glands with cystic dilatation (Fig. 4.13). Biopsy

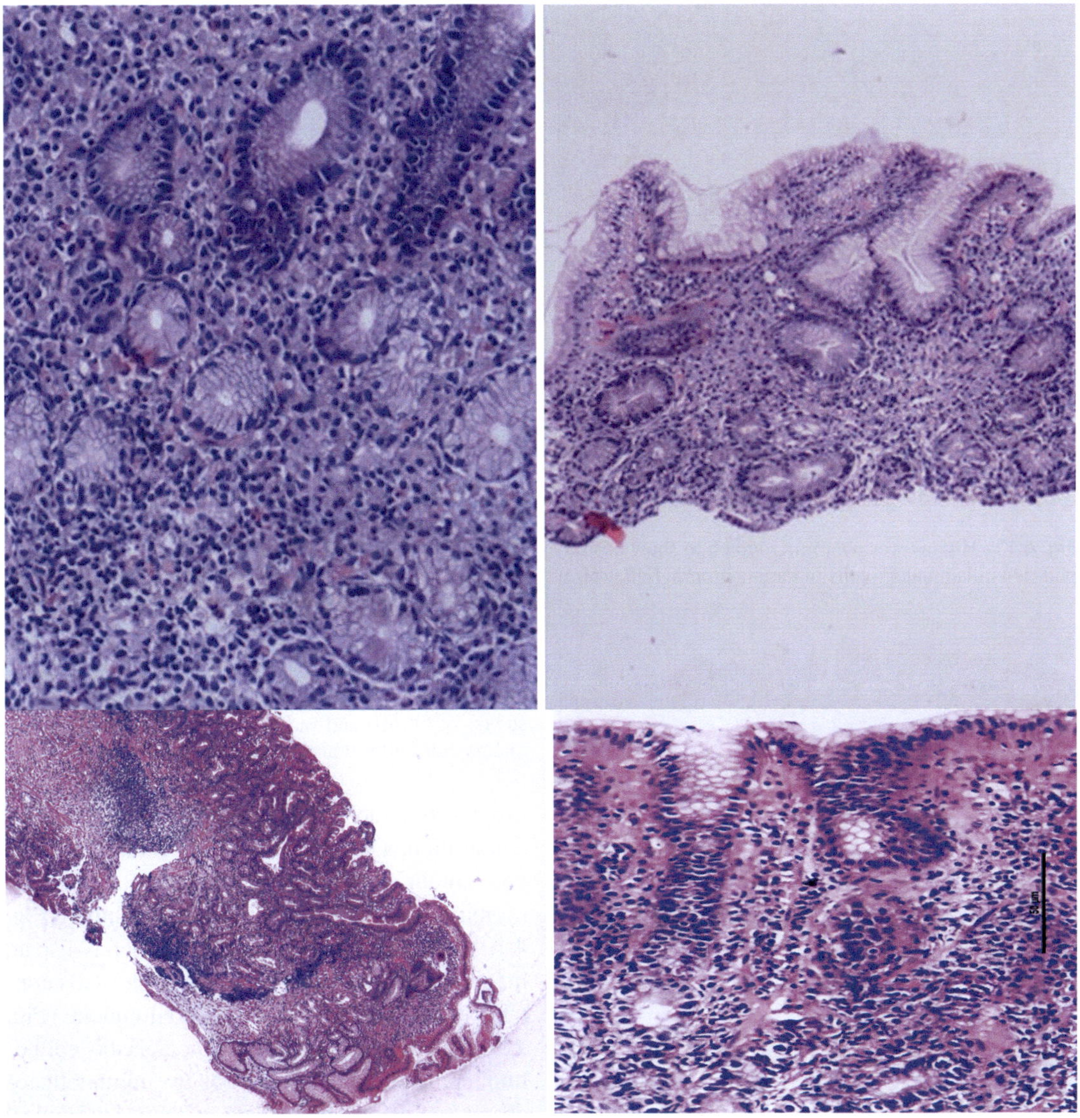

Figs. 4.8–4.10 All the microphotographs of gastric biopsies show heavy mucosal inflammatory cells dominantly of lymphoplasmacytic cells with varying grades of glandular loss, lymphoid follicle, foveolar hyperplasia and lamina propria patchy fibrosis (HE, x250)

from the gastric cardia is seldom performed except when there is a localized lesion. The simple tubular glands of the cardia may show changes similar to other segments of the gastric mucosa.

Intestinal metaplasia (IM) is not an uncommon feature in a setting of chronic gastritis or atrophic gastritis (Figs. 4.14 (A + B) and 4.15). IM is a patchy and a focal disease, due to which it may not be picked-up in a given mucosal biopsy, even if sampling has been carried out from multiple sites. Hence, missing IM may be a frequent phenomenon in routine practice. Besides, the metaplastic epithelial cells may not show the characteristic appearance of goblet cells but having more of bubbly and vacuolated cytoplasm, known as globoid cells. In such situation, it is all the time the best to carry out a double histochemistry staining like alcian blue periodic acid Schiff

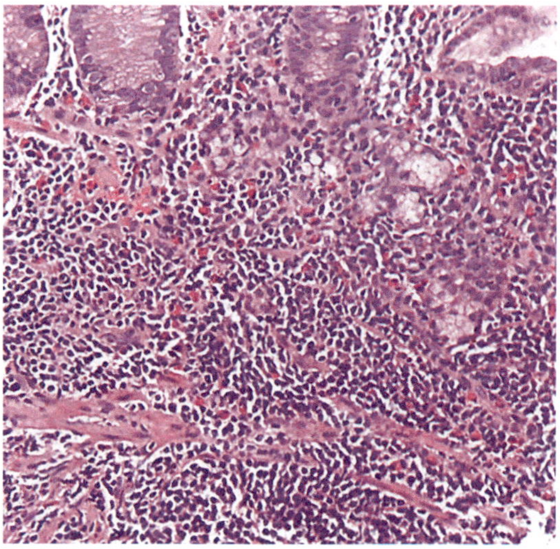

Fig. 4.11 High power photomicrograph to show eosinophil rich inflammatory cells in lamina propria (HE, x500)

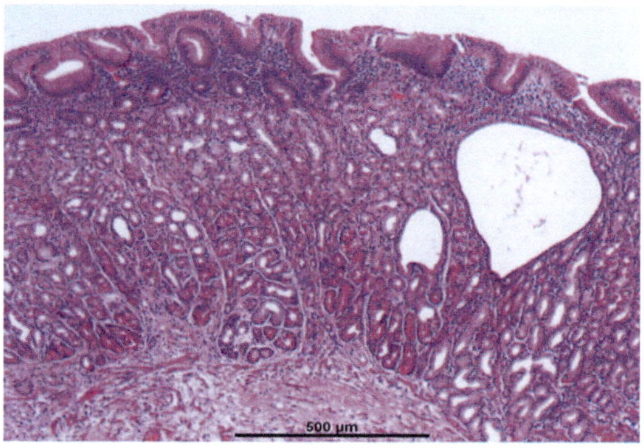

Fig. 4.12 Photomicrograph of gastric biopsy of body mucosa showing varying grades of glandular loss as indicated by fine streaks of fibrosis and cystically dilated glands and variable amount of chronic inflammatory cell infiltration in lamina propria (HE, x250)

(AB-PAS) in the same section to study the pattern of PAS and AB positivity (Figs. 4.16 and 4.17). Intestinal metaplastic epithelium may be of three types—(i) complete type where the metaplastic epithelium includes goblet cells intermixed with absorptive cells and Paneth cells (Fig. 4.18). Goblet cells are easily identifiable as they are AB positive mainly composed of sialomucin; (ii) incomplete metaplasia where absorptive cells are absent and there is mixture of cells containing neutral or gastric type of mucin intermixed with sialomucin containing cells having bubbly look-

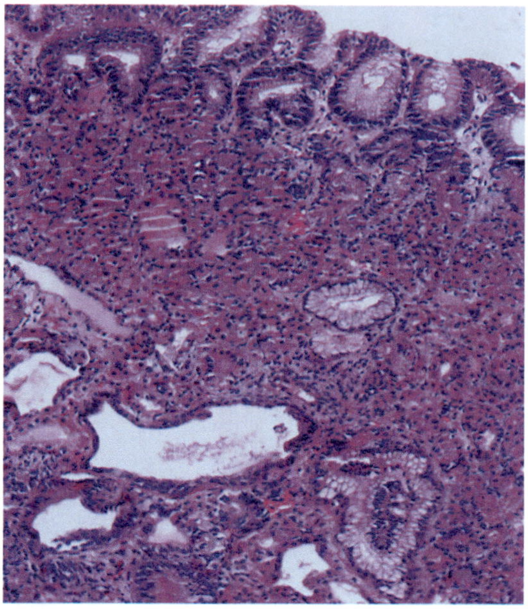

Fig. 4.13 Photomicrograph of gastric body mucosal biopsy showing varying grades of glandular loss, many cystically dilated glands, mucous gland metaplay, patchy streaks of fibrosis and variable amount of chronic inflammatory cell infiltration in lamina propria (HE, x250)

ing microvescicles taking up a purplish magenta colouration, i.e. an intermediate colour between blue colour of sialomucin and magenta colour of normal gastric mucin in AB-PAS staining [Fig. 4.19 (A + B)]; (iii) the third group which is also an incomplete metaplasia where the goblet cells contain sulphomucin in place of sialomucin (Fig. 4.20). Demonstration of the metaplastic epithelium may also be carried out by immunohistochemistry using appropriate primary antibodies. Normal gastric mucosal cells react positively with MUC1, MUC5AC and MUC6 whereas MUC2 is negative. In intestinal metaplastic epithelium, the metaplastic cells react with MUC2 and all metaplastic cells will exhibit positive staining [6, 7]. Intestinal metaplasia in the background of atrophic gastritis is taken as one of the histological evidences of an intermediate lesion in the development of gastric cancer. By the time a gastric mucosa develops IM, there may not be evidence of HP infection due to changing milieu in the gastric luminal environment, though HP could be the initiating factor. These mucosal changes may be associated with dysplasia or intramucosal carci-

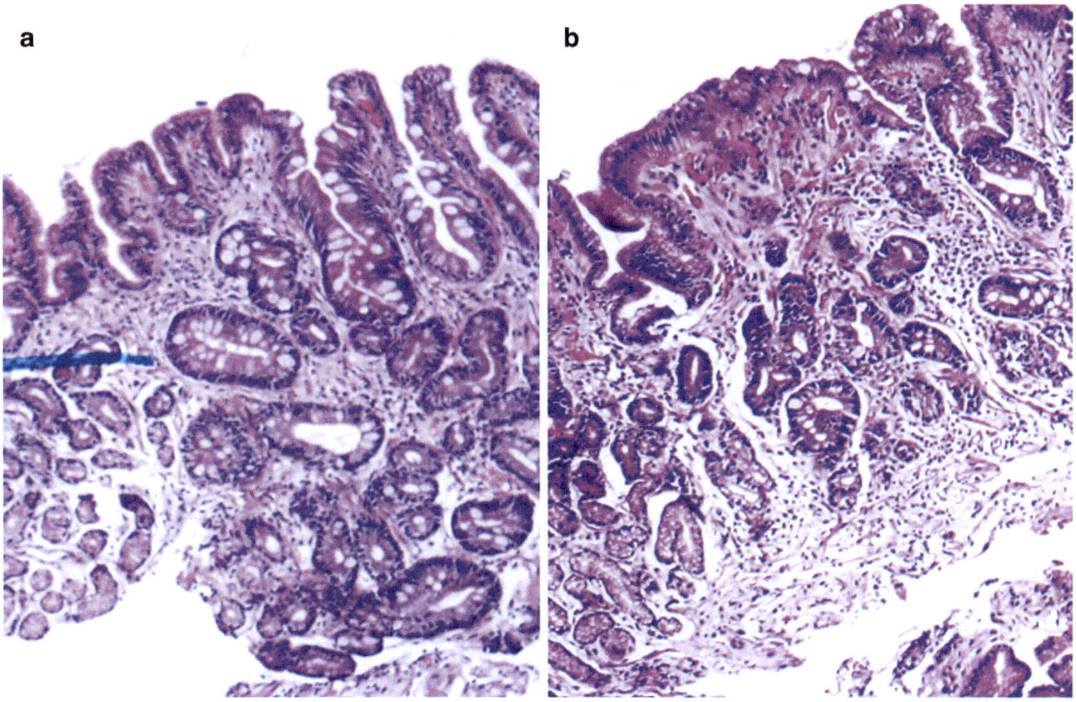

Fig. 4.14 (A + B) Photomicrographs of gastric antral biopsies showing loss of glands and replacement fibrosis of lamina propria along with variable extend of intestinal metaplasia in both the biopsies; **A**—metaplastic epithelium is seen in larger extend involving full thickness of the mucosa and in **B**—the metaplastic epithelium is more confined to smaller area compared to Fig. **A** (HE, x300)

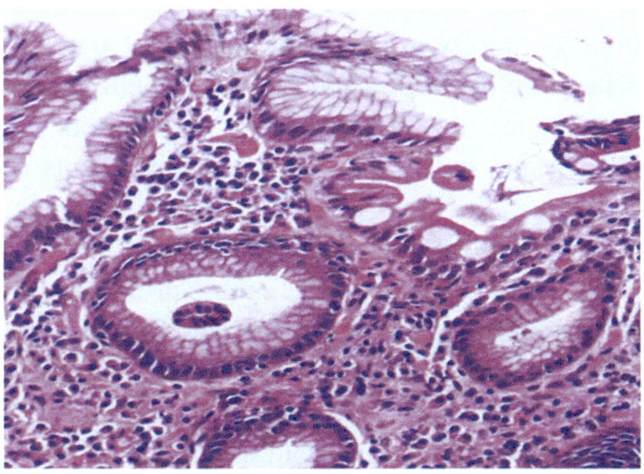

Fig. 4.15 High-power photomicrograph of gastric biopsy showing moderately heavy chronic inflammatory cell infiltration of lamina propria with disorganization of the glands and foveolar hyperplasia. The surface epithelium is showing undulation with a patch of goblet cell and absorptive cell metaplasia (HE, x500)

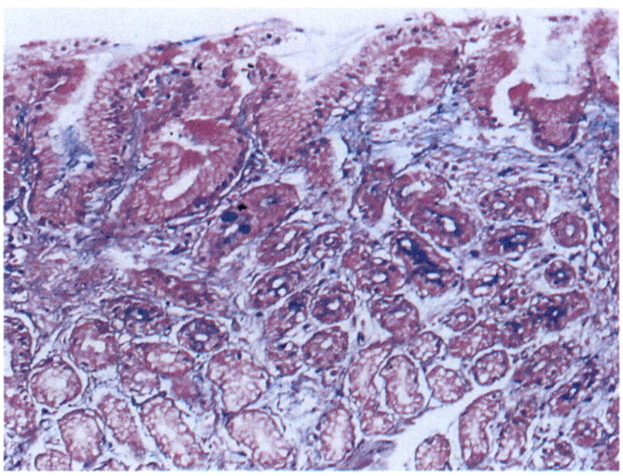

Fig. 4.16 The photomicrograph of alcian blue PAS stained section highlighting positively stained goblet cells and stroma due to presence of abundant acid mucopolysaccharide as a part and partial of the metaplastic process and lamina propria fibrosis (Alcian blue PAS, x200)

noma satisfying Correa's cascade [5, 8], or enterochromaffin like (ECL) cell proliferation and neoplasm [9].

Gastric biopsy may be grouped appropriately according to the format proposed by latest Sydney classification by grading extend of mucosal

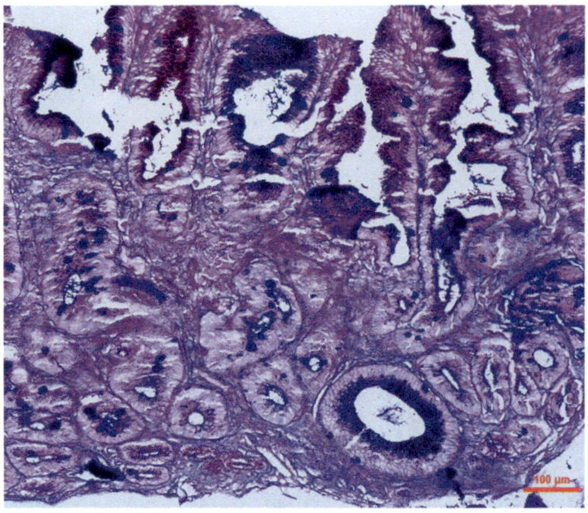

Fig. 4.17 A photomicrograph of alcian blue PAS stained section indicating significant villous transformation of the gastric surface epithelium. There are four patterns of positively stained cells in addition to alcian blue positive stroma. Goblet cells are highlighted quite well. In addition, there are PAS positive dark magenta colour gastric lining epithelium and some of the columnar epithelial cells have stained positively for alcian blue indicating the changed in the pH of the mucin contained. And the fourth character of the positively stained cells are the ones that have taken up intermediate colour between blue and dark magenta colour indicating an early alteration in the pH of the neutral mucin (alcian blue PAS, x300)

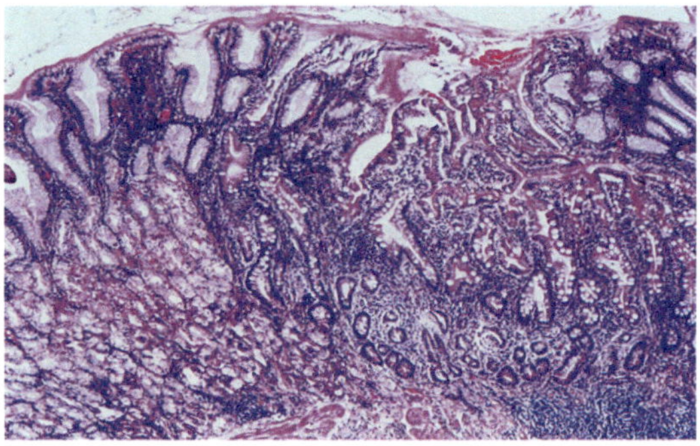

Fig. 4.18 Medium power photomicrograph of a gastric mucosa showing two distinctly different morphology. In the left 1/3rd area, it gives appearance of a conventional chronic gastritis of antral mucosa. The right 2/3rd has the appearance of a small intestinal mucosa with villous configuration with total loss of pyloric gland. The surface lining epithelium is composed of absorptive cells intermixed with goblet cells and Paneth cells. Lamina propria is relatively lack of fibrosis, however, shows many lymphoid follicles (HE, x300)

inflammatory cell infiltration, presence of HP, mucosal glandular loss and goblet and absorptive cell type metaplasia. These changes were translated into mild, moderate and heavy inflammation subjectively assessing extend of infiltration and changes observed under the microscope [10, 11]. There is poor agreement among the histopathologists regarding the recognition and utilization of the Sydney system. A few years later, there was another study supporting this method of grading for gastritis [12], which was followed by another proposal suggesting the gradings into two groups of low and high grades [13]. Rubio [14], more recently have proposed another way of scoring gastritis in a simplified manner depending upon the extend mucosal inflammatory cell infiltration, presence of HP, glandular loss and presence of goblet cells. Based on these criteria, biopsies were identified as the ones with focal lesion or grade 1, and changes occupying the whole of the biopsy specimen observed under the microscopy or grade 2 changes. He further stated that a biopsy specimen with grade 2 changes is more likely to be widespread mucosal changes. Rubio also believed that this system would permit the GI physician to be able to monitor treatment outcome in follow-up biopsies. In biopsies with metaplastic epithelium or poorly oriented or tangential cut, the histopathology report should make mention of all the features observed including the status of the surface and lateral sides of mucosa in recuts or serial sections. And if the surface lining epithelium is visible in the serial sections, specify number of sections where the lining can be seen. A score 0 is allotted for a normal biopsy [14].

When a focus of chronic gastritis is associated with intestinal metaplasia (IM) in a single biopsy warrants further biopsy from multiple sites of the stomach to map extend of the metaplasia, which may be carried out according the modified Sydney classifications [2]. Operative Link for Gastritis Assessment (OLGA) has proposed a system, i.e. OLGA staging system, for the histological changes associated with chronic gastritis and gastric atrophy by arranging morphological features with a scale ranging from OLGA stage 0

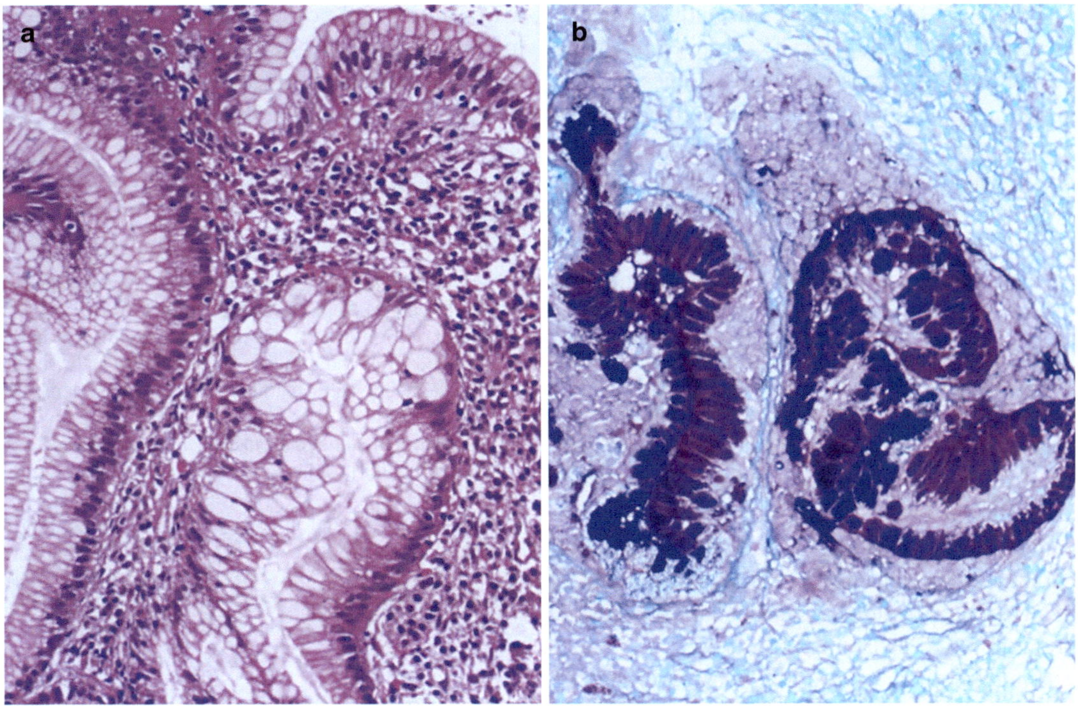

Fig. 4.19 (A + B) **A**—High-power photomicrograph of a gastric biopsy showing undulation of the surface epithelium and a grossly disorganised architecture along with chronic inflammatory cells in the lamina propria due to associated atrophy changes. The hyperplastic foveolae are lined by cells which are larger than the conventional tall columnar mucous type epithelium and cytoplasm of which appear bubbly due to cytoplasmic vacuolisation giving the appearance of goblet cell (HE, x500). **B**—high photomicrograph of alcian blue PAS stain section showing different patterns of positively stain cells with bubbly cytoplasm termed as globoid cells. To be noted is the bluish tinged of the lamina propria stroma (Alcian blue PAS, x500)

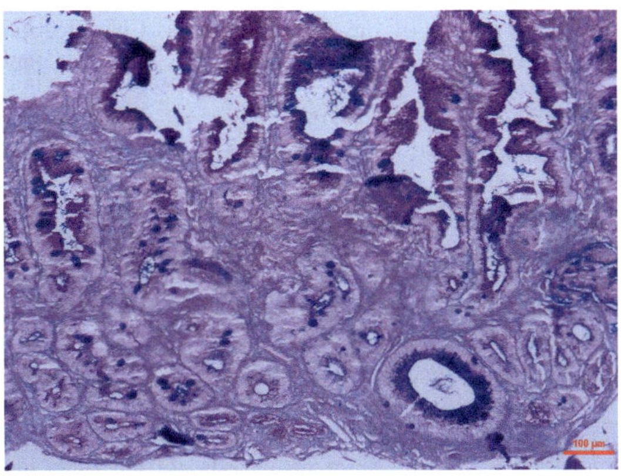

Fig. 4.20 Medium power micrograph showing positive staining for alcian blue at pH1 indicating the mucin to be sulphomucin type (Alcian blue at pH1)

to OLGA stage IV with an increasing risk for the development of gastric cancer (GC) [15]. OLGA system simply identifies the risk for cancer in biopsies showing features of atrophic gastritis. This is an attempt to make the treating clinician to be aware of the warning signs so that a tailored protocol for further investigation of the patient may be carried out. This method of assessment has been further upgraded by the same group in their followed-up study [16]. Usually the focus where there is associated IM in a single biopsy warrants further biopsy from multiple sites of the stomach to map extent of the metaplasia, which may be carried out according the modified Sydney classifications [2] and OLGA [15].

Evidences have shown a correlation between the extent of atrophy with risk of development of gastric cancer. Advancing gastritis stages express increasing extent of atrophy in histological studies in antral and corpus biopsies. Patients who had revealed stages III and IV of OLGA staging in gastric biopsies, though were less in number, are reportedly at higher risk of development of GC [17, 18]. In addition, these groups of patients, i.e. OLGA stages III and IV mucosal changes, have been observed to express consistently markers associated with high-risk biopsies [19, 20]. These group of patients have been found to have consistently high serology levels of pepsinogen. As a result of documentation of constant interrelationship between morphological biopsy evidence and serologic findings, serologic parameters for pepsinogen has been rationalized as an essential parameter in secondary prevention program of GC screening [18].

Interpretations of atrophy changes in gastric mucosal biopsies have shown low interobserver agreement even with the routine utilization of the visual analogue system provided by Updated Sydney [17, 18]. This has created a potential shortcoming in OLGA staging system and is based on the extend of the atrophic change sin gastric biopsy [11, 21–23]. Presence of metaplastic intestinal epithelium (MIE) in gastric biopsy is defined as the replacement of mucous type of columnar epithelium by cells composed of absorptive type intermixed with goblet cells that may be with or without Paneth cells [24]. Due to the presence of well-defined histological features in MIE, there is high degree of agreement amongst the various histopathologists [11, 25]. Hence, adding or using isolated MIE as an important histologic feature in staging system may yield more accuracy in identifying patients who are likely high-risk candidate for GC. Hence, staging system used in OLGA, which is based on atrophy changes may be improved by replacing it with a system using less controversial MIE, i.e. OLGIM (operative link on gastric intestinal metaplasia). Evidences have shown a correlation between the extent of atrophy with risk of development of gastric cancer [21–25]. Advancing gastritis stages express increasing extent of atrophy in histological studies in antral and corpus biopsies, however follow-up studies have shown that all patients who had exhibited stages III and IV type of mucosal atrophy do not develop GC [17–20].

References

1. Price AB. The Sydney system: histological division. J Gastroenterol Hepatol. 1991;6:209–22.
2. Stolte M, Meining A. The updated Sydney system: classification and grading of gastritis as the basis of diagnosis and treatment. Can J Gastroenterol. 2001;15:591–8.
3. International statistical classification of diseases and related health problems, 10th revision, Fifth edition, 2016.
4. Owen DA. Normal histology of the stomach. Am J Surg Pathol. 1986;10:48–61.
5. Correa P, Plazuelo MB. The gastric precancerous cascade. Jl Dig Dis. 2012;13:2–9.
6. Wong HH, Chu P. Immunohistochemical features of the gastrointestinal tract tumors. J Gastrointest Oncol. 2012;3:262–84.
7. Park JS, Yeom JS, Seo JH, et al. Immunohistochemical expressions of MUC2, MUC5AC, and MUC6 in Normal, *Helicobacter pylori* infected and metaplastic gastric mucosa of children and adolescents. Helicobacter. 2015;20:260–8.
8. Correa P, Haenszel W, Cuello C, et al. Gastric precancerous process in a high risk population: cohort follow-up. Cancer Res. 1990;50:4737–40.
9. Solcia E, Fiocca R, Villani L, et al. Hyperplastic, dysplastic, and neoplastic Enterochromaffin-like-cell proliferations of the gastric mucosa. Classification and Histogenesis. Am J Surg Pathol. 1995;19(Suppl 1):S1–7.
10. Misiewicz J, Tygat G, Goodwin C et al. The Sydney system: a new classification of gastritis. Working Party Reports 1990:1–10.
11. Dixon MF, Genta RM, Yardley JH, et al. Classification and grading of gastritis. The updated Sydney system. International workshop on the histopathology of gastritis, Houston 1994. Am J Surg Pathol. 1996;20:1161–81.
12. Zaitoun A, Record C. Application of quantitative techniques for the assessment of gastric atrophy. J Clin Pathol. 2001;54:161–2.
13. Crum CP. Symposium part 1: should the Bethesda system terminology be used in diagnostic surgical pathology? Int J Gynecol Pathol. 2003;22:5–12.
14. Rubio CA. My approach to reporting a gastric biopsy. J Clin Pathol. 2007;60:160–6.
15. Rugge M, Genta RM, OLGA-Group. Staging gastritis: an international proposal. Gastroenterology. 2005;129:1807–8.
16. Rugge M, Correa P, Di Mario F, et al. OLGA staging for gastritis: a tutorial. Digest Liver Dis. 2008;40:650–8.

17. Capelle LG, de Vries AC, Haringsma J, et al. The staging of gastritis with the OLGA system by using intestinal metaplasia as an accurate alternative for atrophic gastritis. Gastrointest Endosc. 2010;71:1150–8.
18. Rugge M, de Boni M, Pennelli G, et al. Gastritis OLGA-staging and gastric cancer risk: a twelve-year clinico-pathological follow-up study. Aliment Pharmacol Ther. 2010;31:1104–11.
19. Carrasco G, Diaz J, Valbuena JR, Ibanez P, et al. Overexpression of p73 as a tissue marker for high-risk gastritis. Clin Cancer Res. 2010;16:3253–9.
20. Rugge M, Fassan M, Pizzi M, et al. Operative link for gastritis assessment gastritis staging incorporates intestinal metaplasia subtyping. Hum Pathol. 2011;42:1539–44.
21. el-Zimaity HM, Graham DY, al-Assi MT, et al. Interobserver variation in the histopathological assessment of *Helicobacter pylori* gastritis. Hum Pathol. 1996;27:35–41.
22. Chen XY, van der Hulst RW, Bruno MJ, et al. Interobserver variation in the histopathological scoring of helicobacter pylori related gastritis. J Clin Pathol. 1999;52:612–5.
23. Offerhaus GJ, Price AB, Haot J, et al. Observer agreement on the grading of gastric atrophy. Histopathology. 1999;34:320–5.
24. de Vries AC, Haringsma J, Kuipers EJ. The detection, surveillance and treatment of premalignant gastric lesions related to *Helicobacter pylori* infection. Helicobacter. 2007;12:1–15.
25. Guarner J, Herrera-Goepfert R, Mohar A, et al. Interobserver variability in application of the revised Sydney classification for gastritis. Hum Pathol. 1999;30:1431–4.

5 Enterochromaffin-Like Cell and Associated Pathology

"Enterochromaffin-like (ECL) cells" are triangular-shaped small-sized cells located along the basal region of gastric pits of the stomach, in conjunction with the basement membrane of the gastric glands (Fig. 5.1). They are similar to enterochromaffin cells of the intestine, hence they have been named as enterochromaffin-like cell. They are located in between and also partly covered by the parietal cells. ECL cells normally are located mainly in the gastric body. These cells secrete histamine and are rich in gastrin receptors. ECL cells secrete histamine in response to gastrin released by G cells and adenylyl cyclase-activating peptide released by pituitary. The ultimate effect of histamine is in getting the parietal cells in releasing hydrochloric acid. In such a way, ECL cells play important role in regulating parietal cell function [1].

Gastrin executes its function through two mechanisms. First by acting directly on cholecystokinin B (CCKB) receptors present on basolateral membrane of the parietal cells. Second is by indirect mechanism by binding to ECL cells which respond by releasing histamine that binds to histamine 2 receptor present along basolateral aspect of the parietal cell resulting in acid secretion [2]. To be noted at this point is that this circuit ECL cell stimulation by gastrin is not activated by acetylcholine. Hence, this circuit cannot be blocked by acetylcholine antagonists as it will not result in inhibitory action in the pathway of vagal stimulation of G cells [3]. The pathway where ECL cells are activated directly by vagal nerve activation by releasing acetylcholine resulting in histamine release, will be inhibited by atropine [4]. G cells being endocrine cells secrete gastrin directly into blood stream exposing ECL cell. Gastrin acts synergistically with histamine as the important stimulator for parietal cells for production of gastric acid; these two in combination further stimulates pepsinogen secretion by the chief cells [3]. Somatostatin secreted by D cells present in gastric mucosa has inhibitory effect on ECL cell function. ECL cells produces many hormones including peptides and factors responsible for cellular growth and multiplication including pancreastatin [4].

ECL cells have been named as such due to its similarity with enterochromaffin cells though it is a different cell type and does not synthesize serotonin [1]. These cells are argyrophilic. They were recognized in early 1945 by Dawson [5] and was later characterized by Solcia and co-workers [6]. ECL cells were demonstrated by Sevier and Munger's silver impregnation technique [7]. Also, by immunostaining of general endocrine cell markers such as chromogranin A [8] (Fig. 5.1). No peptide product has been identified as yet in human ECL cells, although those of rodents are known to secrete histamine which can be demonstrated using specific antibodies or antibodies against the enzyme histidine decarboxylase. By electron microscope, ECL cells are easily distinguishable from EC cells as they contain

K. Vaiphei, *Interpretation of Endoscopic Biopsy - Gastritis, Gastropathies and Beyond*,
https://doi.org/10.1007/978-981-16-6026-9_5

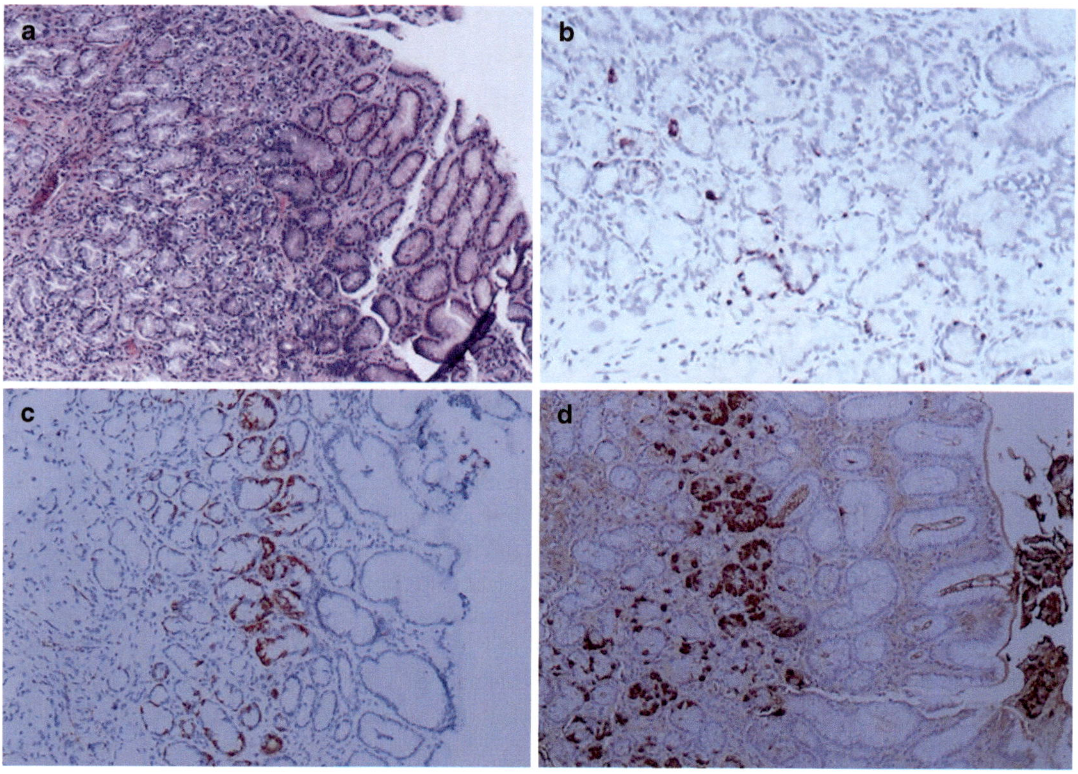

Fig. 5.1 **a**—A panel photomicrograph showing antral biopsy with mild lamina propria fibrosis and chronic inflammatory cell infiltration along with many ECL cells along the deeper portion of foveolae and the mucous glands (HE, x300). **b**—Immunohistochemistry using chromogranin A primary antibody carried out on the same section as in **a**, highlighting a few positively stained scattered cells indicated by the brown nuclear staining (Peroxidase anti-peroxidase, x300). **c**—Immunohistochemistry using gastrin primary antibody to highlight normal pattern and number of positively stained scattered cells indicated by the brown cytoplasmic staining (Peroxidase anti-peroxidase, x300). **d**—Immunohistochemistry using gastrin primary antibody to bring out increased number of positively stained cells indicating hyperplasia in cases of atrophic gastritis (Peroxidase anti-peroxidase, x300)

numerous, large vesicles within which a core of variable electron density is surrounded by a thin halo and membrane. ECL cells proliferation may be identified best using immunohistochemistry (IHC), ideally a panel of primary antibodies, i.e. chromogranin A, synaptophysin, CD56, neuron-specific enolase and gastrin, help to classify and identify their endocrine properties [9, 10] (Fig. 5.1). In stomach, synaptophysin, and chromogranin immunostainings though not specific, highlight adequately ECL cells and are helpful to detect any increased in their numbers or any undue increase. Their classic site of location is fundic mucosa and are relatively rare or absent in other gastric segments. However, presence of ECL cells may be highlighted using antibodies against histamine-forming enzyme histidine decarboxylase and CCKB receptor in any biopsy of the stomach exhibiting chronic inflammation, usually co-existing with loss of specialized glands and appearance of abnormal mucosa not native for the site of biopsy [10]. ECL cells are usually identified in the deeper mucosa in fundic mucosa, a few cells in neck area of the foveolae and none along lining epithelium [10].

ECL cell hyperplasia requires further grading to indicate extend and type of proliferation and tends to be multifocal. Hence all the mucosal fragments included in the biopsy requires critical examination for further management of the patient. Proliferative lesions and hyperplasia of gastrointestinal tract endocrine cells have been classified into simple hyperplasia, linear hyperplasia, micronodular hyperplasia, adenomatoid hyperplasia, dysplasia and intra-mucosal or invasive carcinoid to intramucosal invasive tumours [11, 12] (Figs. 5.2, 5.3, 5.4, 5.5, 5.6, 5.7 and 5.8). The basic concept behind grading should have prognostic and therapeutic implications so that the patient may be given appropriate treatment. ECL cells undergoes excessive proliferation in the background of hypergastrinemia (Figs. 5.9 and 5.10). Situations where there can be increased number of G cells associated with increased gastrin levels are—(i) atrophic gastritis of autoimmune and environmental aetiologies, (ii) primary G cell hyperplasia and hyperfunction, (iii) ulcers of stomach, (iv) multiple endocrine neoplasia type I, (v) Zollinger Ellison syndrome, (vi) injudicious use of H2 receptor blocker and proton pump inhibitors, (vii) acromegaly, (viii) gastric distention and outlet obstruction, (ix) Uraemia and hypercalcinosis, (x) gastric cancer, (xi) post-vagotomy and (xii) retained and excluded antrum [13]. Though these conditions result in ECL cell hyperplasia, they seldom result in frankly malignant neuroendocrine tumour and have indolent course [14]. Hence, there are three situations where gastric neuroendocrine pathology is clinically applicable. First one is the situation where an obvious neuroendocrine tumour (NET) is present, which can be visualized during the process endoscopy as a nodule or polypoidal lesion. The second situation is the one where

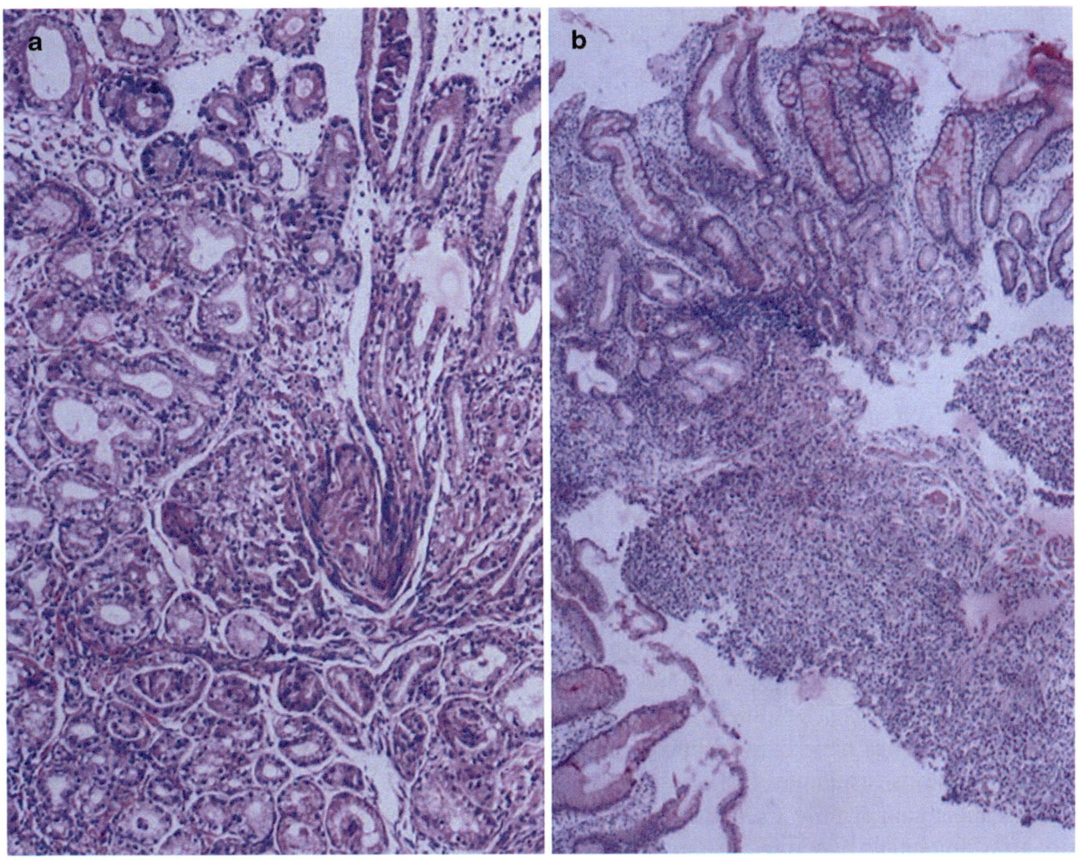

Fig. 5.2 **a**—Photomicrograph of an endoscopic biopsy form body/fundus showing near total loss of parietal cells, foveolar hyperplasia, extensive pyloric metaplasia, mild chronic inflammatory cell infiltration and clusters of shedded epithelial cells. **b**—Photomicrograph of the same biopsy of another tissue fragment showing similar mucosal atrophy changes with intestinal metaplasia and a large area of tumour cells in sheets at deeper portion of the mucosa (HE, x300)

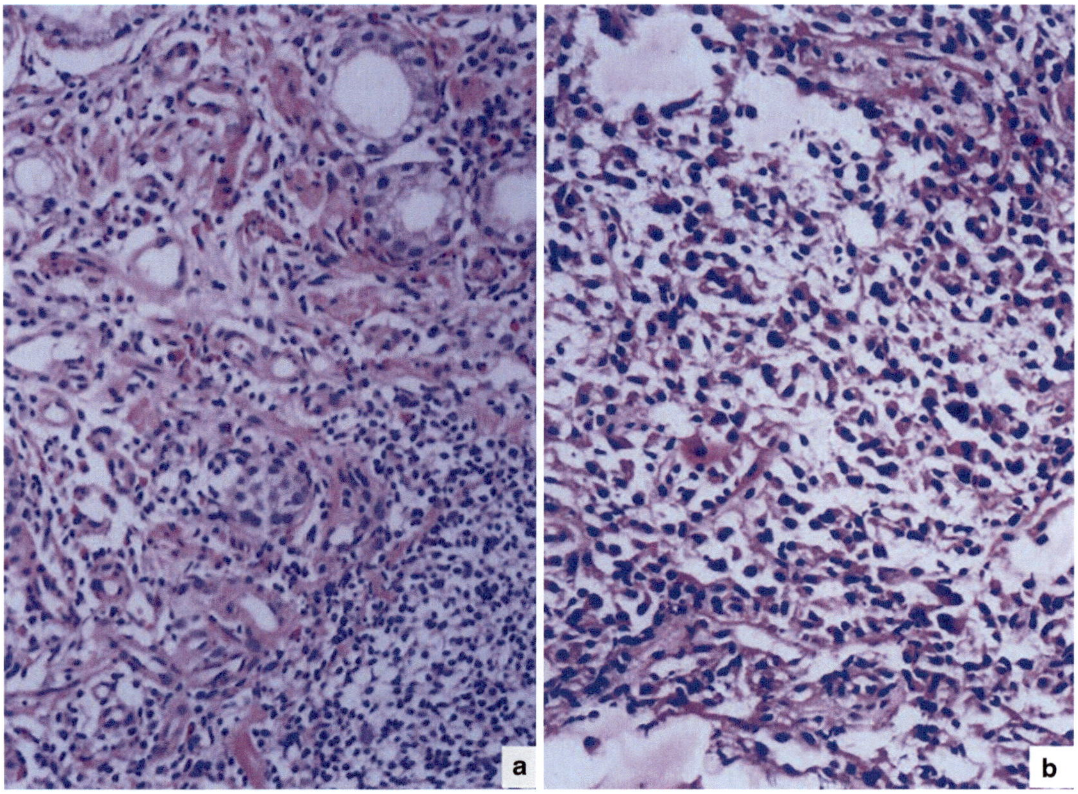

Fig. 5.3 High power view of the tumorous area showing **a**—tumour cells infiltrating in between benign mucous glands and fibres of muscularis mucosae singly and in small nest along with clusters of lymphoid cells. **b**—loose clusters of tumour cells exhibiting significant nuclear pleomorphism with scanty to moderate eosinophilic cytoplasm (HE, x500)

there is ECL cell undergoes proliferation, which may be of various grades ranging from simple hyperplasia to adenoma to dysplasia to lamina propria infiltration and all these different grades of ECL cell proliferation are seen in context to gastric atrophy. The third one is an iatrogenic situation due to excessive administration or intake of proton pump inhibitors resulting in iatrogenic hypergastrinemia [15].

ECL cell hyperplasia gradings carried out in endoscopic biopsies have its own limitations as limited tissue is available for interpretation. Though these studies have made efforts to classify and differentiate hyperplasia from more possibly aggressive lesions including stromal invasive lesions, the importance of histological examination lies in documenting the possible behaviour of the proliferating ECL cells. Hence, a nodular lesion of a few millimetre size with accompanied by breakage in basement membrane and infiltration of lamina propria with stromal reaction requires more aggressive management. Ki67 staining of these proliferating cells may also be of help, and Ki67 scoring may be carried out using WHO classification for neuroendocrine tumours where both mitotic count per 10 high power fields and Ki67 positivity expressed in percentages counted in hot spot area of at least 500 to 2000 cells [16, 17] (Figs. 5.11, 5.12, 5.13, 5.14, 5.15, 5.16, 5.17, 5.18, 5.19, 5.20, 5.21 and 5.22).

Histological gradings of NETs depend on the number of mitosis counted both in H&E stain sections and Ki67 immunohistochemistry stain sections. Grade 1 tumours are graded as the ones with less than 2 mitoses per ten high power fields,

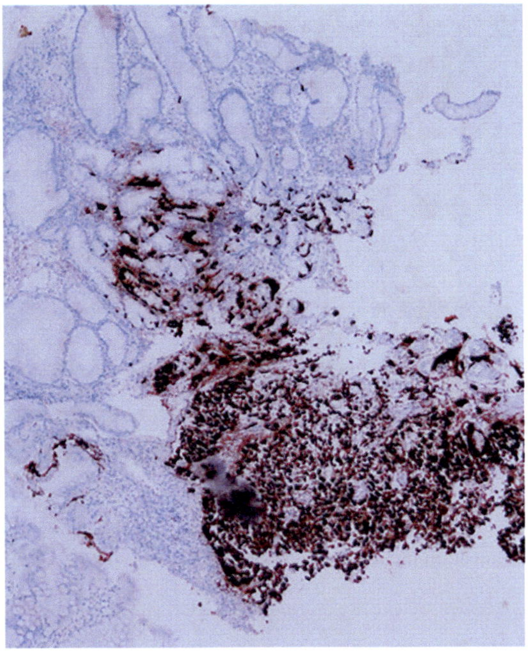

Fig. 5.4 Photomicrograph of an immunohistochemistry stain section using chromogranin A primary antibody highlighting all the tumour cells stained positively indicated by the brown staining (PAP, x200)

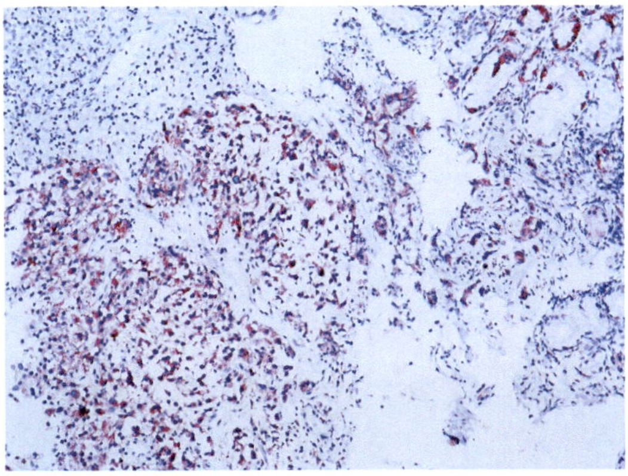

Fig. 5.5 Photomicrograph of an immunohistochemistry stain section using synaptophysin primary antibody highlighting a few scattered positively stained tumour cells (PAP, x200)

alternatively less than 3 percentage of Ki67 index. Mitosis count for grade 2 tumour is 2 to 20 mitoses per ten high power fields or 3 to 20 percentage of Ki67 index. And for grade 3 tumours, it is more than 20 mitoses per ten high power fields or more than 20 percentage of Ki67 index [18]. Gastric

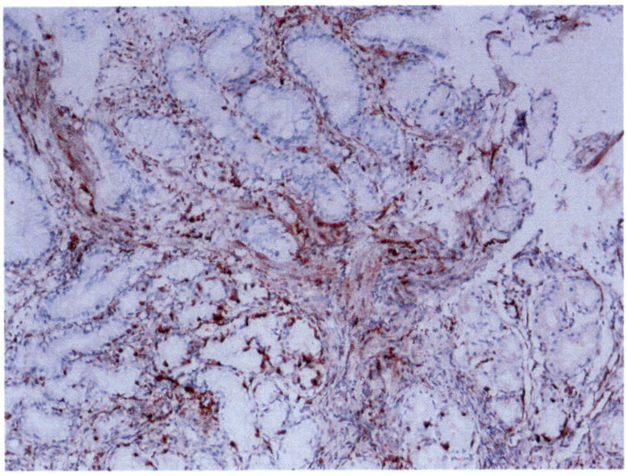

Fig. 5.6 Photomicrograph of an immunohistochemistry stain section using neuron-specific enolase primary antibody highlighting a few scattered positively stained tumour cells which are round and the spindle cells are likely to be nerve fibres (PAP, x200)

neck with foveolar cells may show a high Ki67 labelling index, this is to be differentiated from those positively stained proliferating ECL cells. It was Gosset and Masson who had documented carcinoid tumour as neuroendocrine tumour (NET) based on their properties of amine uptake and decarboxylation [19]. The term "carcinoid" for these tumours was introduced by Lubarsch [20]. Gastric NETs have been grouped under four types [21–23].

- Type I—Patients who are found to have features of chronic multifocal atrophic gastritis in their gastric mucosal biopsies in addition to the tumour, and clinically presenting with features of pernicious anaemia. This group is the commonest type constituting about 70–80% of all gastric NETs. These patients are also found to have an association with hypergastrinaemia, antral G cell and ECL cell hyperplasia; majority of the tumours show G1morphology and rarely G2. The patients usually have good survival outcome [24].
- Type II—These lesions are usually associated with gastrin-producing tumours and known as Zollinger-Ellison syndrome. They may have syndromic presentation with multiple endocrine neoplasia type I. Gastric mucosal biopsy tend to show parietal cell hyperplasia, multiple small nodular gastric mucosal lesions and

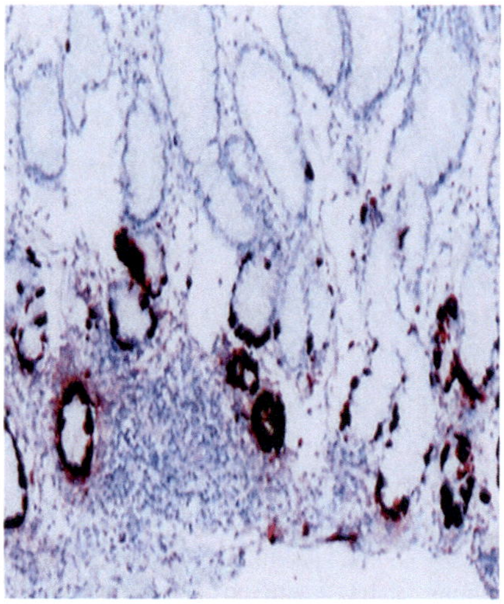

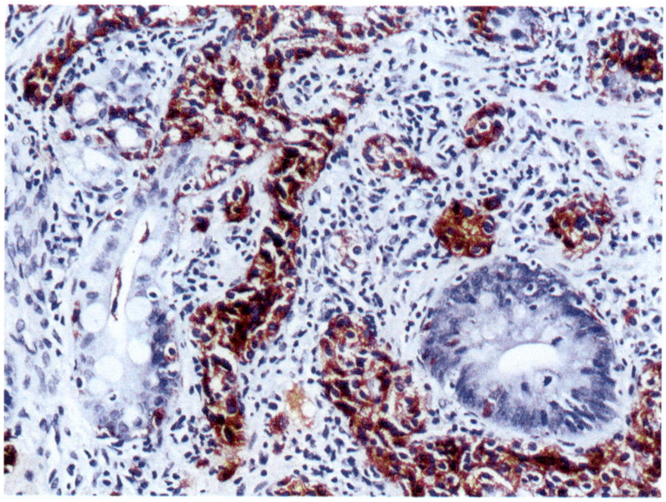

Figs. 5.7 and 5.8 Both IHC are of chromogranin A antibody. The first one highlights few positively stained cells along the base of the foveolae. The second one highlights the patterns of chromogranin A positive tumour cells arranged in interconnected cords and in nests (PAP, x300)

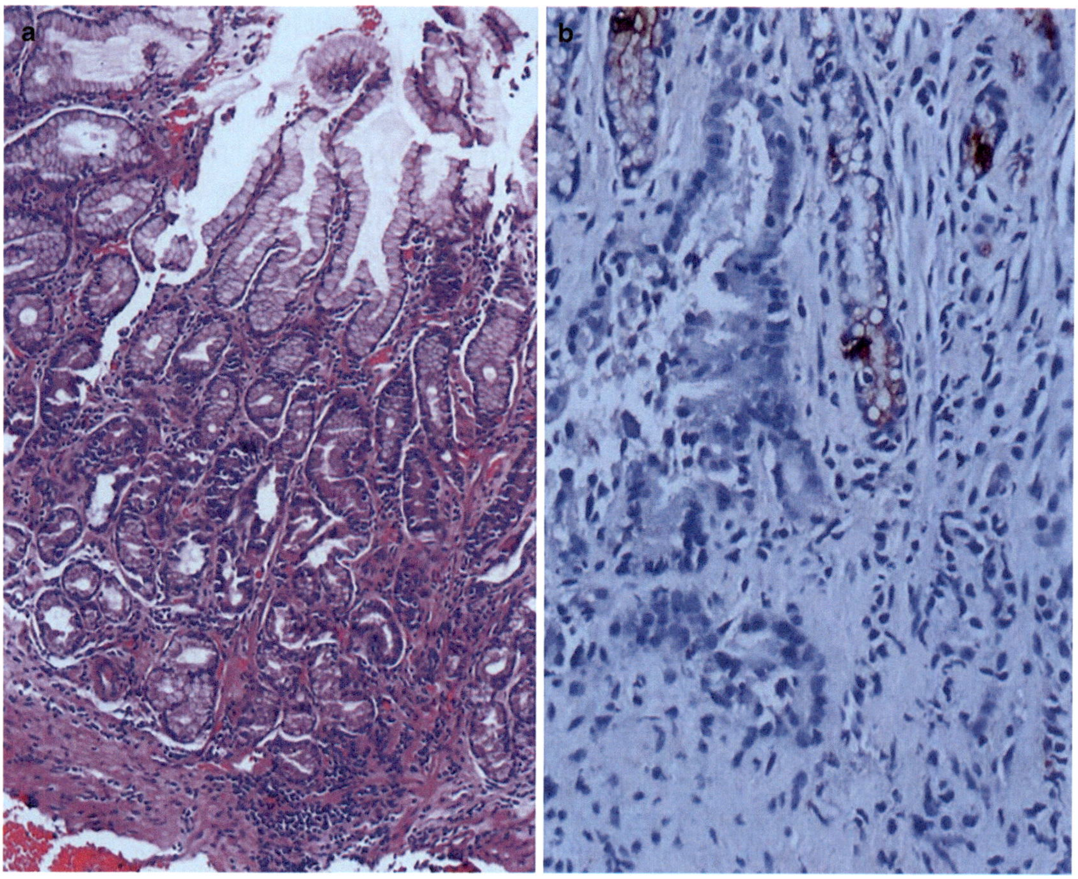

Fig. 5.9 **a**—A routine endoscopic biopsy of antral mucosa showing loss of mucous glands, mild chronic inflammatory cell infiltration and streaks of fine lamina propria fibrosis (HE, x300). **b**—IHC on the same section using gastrin to highlight normal number of gastrin secreting cells located at the depth of foveolae (PAP, x300)

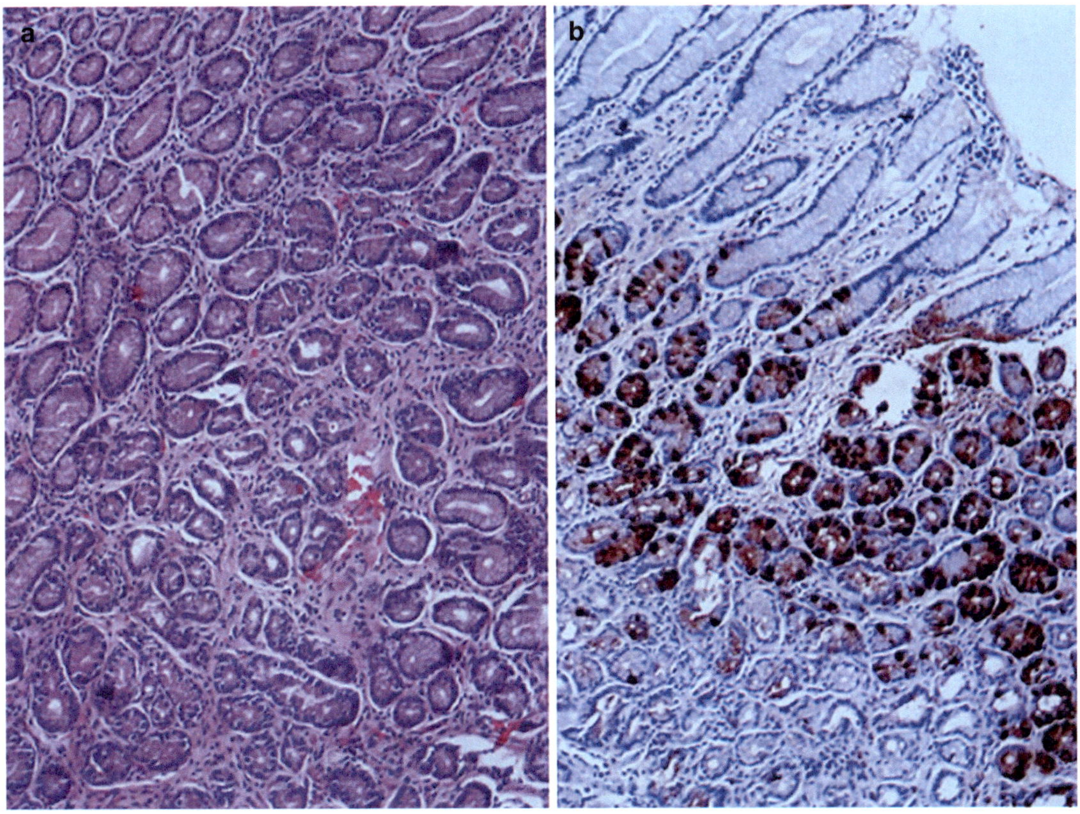

Fig. 5.10 **a**—A routine endoscopic biopsy of antral mucosa showing loss of mucous glands, mild chronic inflammatory cell infiltration and streaks of fine lamina propria fibrosis with proliferation of ECL cells as indicated by scattered cells with clear cytoplasm and small round hyperchromatic nuclei (HE, x300). **b**—IHC on the same section using gastrin to highlight grossly increased number of gastrin secreting cells corresponding to those cells seen as the ones with clear cytoplasm in HE section, located mainly at deeper half of the biopsy (PAP, x300)

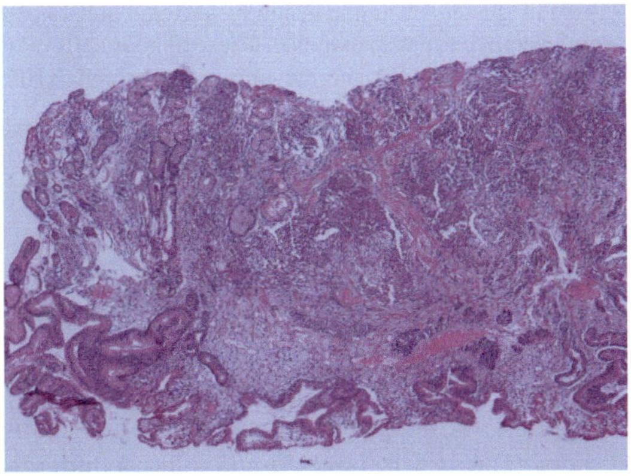

Fig. 5.11 Low power view of a gastric biopsy showing grossly atrophic mucosa with clusters of atypical cells present in the lamina propria and muscularis mucosae along with extensive mucinous degeneration of the stroma (HE, x100)

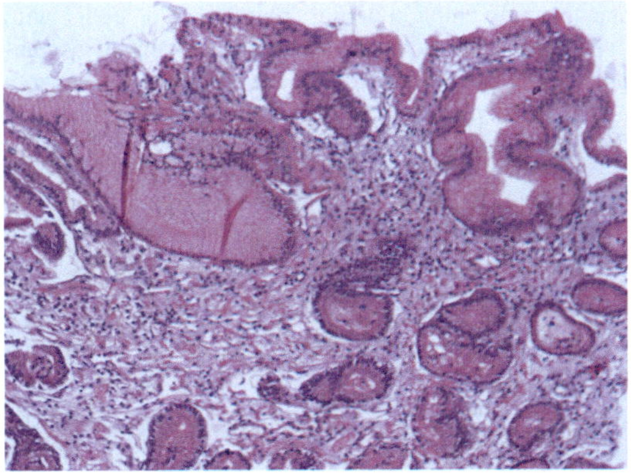

Fig. 5.12 Higher power view to shoe the grossly abnormal mucosa with no specialized glands, hyperplastic foveolae and loose myxomatous lamina propria along with sparse chronic inflammatory cells (HE, x400)

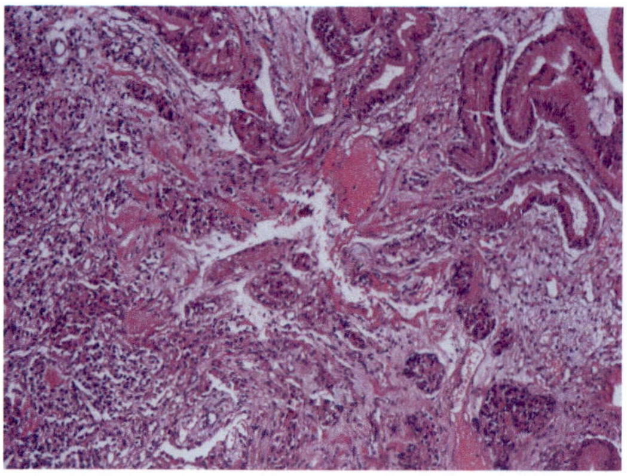

Fig. 5.13 Higher power view of the mucosal biopsy to show the monomorphic tumour cells present in lamina propria arranged in small clusters/nests and in diffuse sheets (HE, x200)

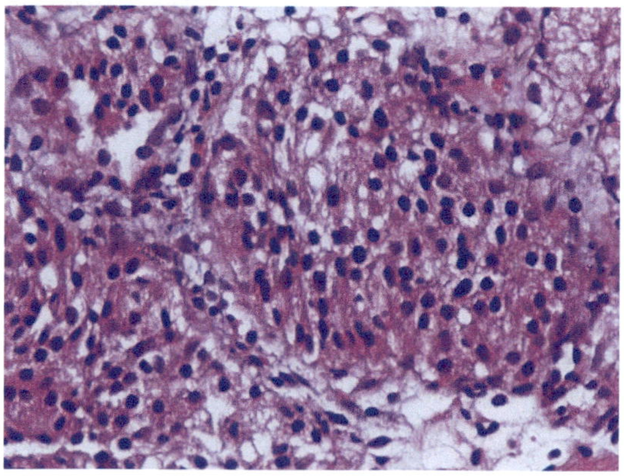

Fig. 5.14 Tumour cells on high power to highlight the characteristic monomorphic plasmacytoid cells with hyperchromatic nuclei and moderate amount of eosinophilic cytoplasm. Tumour cells are seen arranged in large nodule, no atypical mitosis or areas of necrosis visible in this photomicrograph (HE, x500)

constitutes about 5–7% of all gastric NETs. These cases serologically show hypergastrinaemia, high acid output and ECL cell proliferation. Majority of these tumours are G1 with good disease outcome.

- Type III—Refers to sporadic group of NETs of stomach constituting about 10–15%. These patients have normal gastric acid output. Mucosal biopsy does not show ECL cell proliferation or any specific mucosal pathology. Majority of these tumours are G2, rarely G1 or G3 associate with aggressive tumour behaviour and frequent liver metastasis.

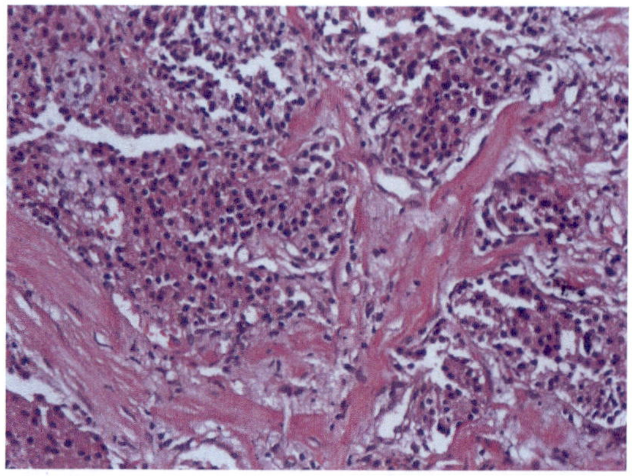

Fig. 5.15 Another area of the tumour to highlight the characteristic innocuous appearance of the monomorphic plasmacytoid cells intersecting in between fibres of muscularis mucosae (HE, x500)

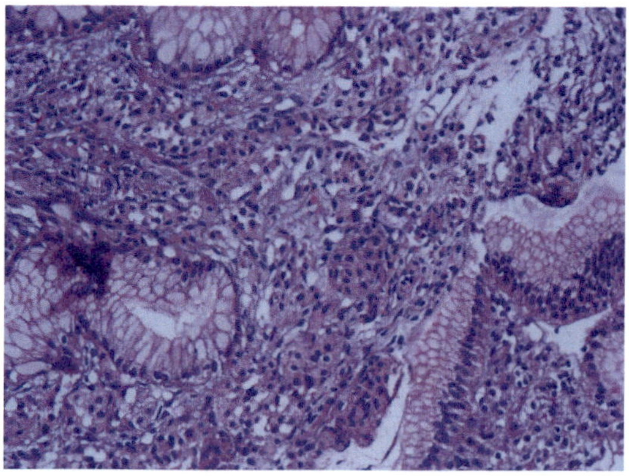

Fig. 5.16 Another area of tumour where tumour cells are present in clusters/nests and in singly scattered in between benign and hyperplastic foveolae. These tumour cells may be easily mistaken for chronic inflammatory cells (HE, x500)

- Type IV—There a few recent studies that had suggested a fourth type of gastric NET consisting of multiple small mucosal nodular lesions. Histologically these nodules show ECL cells proliferation exhibit linear as well as micronodules involving body mucosa. These tumours express chromogranin A and very small numbers express serotonin. Fundic glands undergo hyperplasia containing pinkish amorphous material. These distended glands contain huge size and grossly vacuolated cells bearing apical snouts and luminal cilia which are recognisable as parietal cells having hyperchromatic nuclei. At ultrastructure, these parietal cells

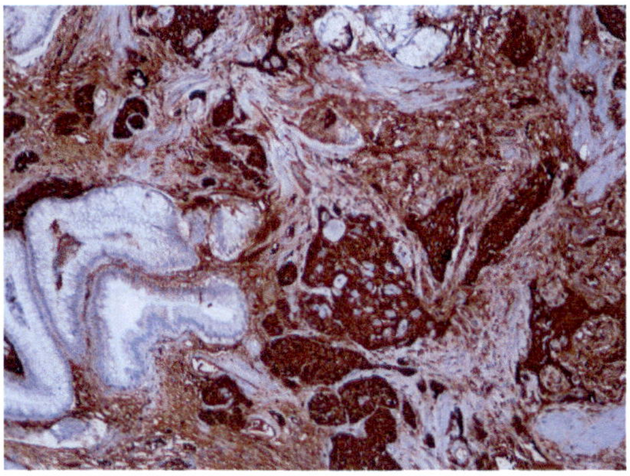

Fig. 5.17 A medium power photomicrograph of chromogranin A stained section to show the strongly positive tumour cells in small groups, nests, cord and in singly scattered (PAP, x300)

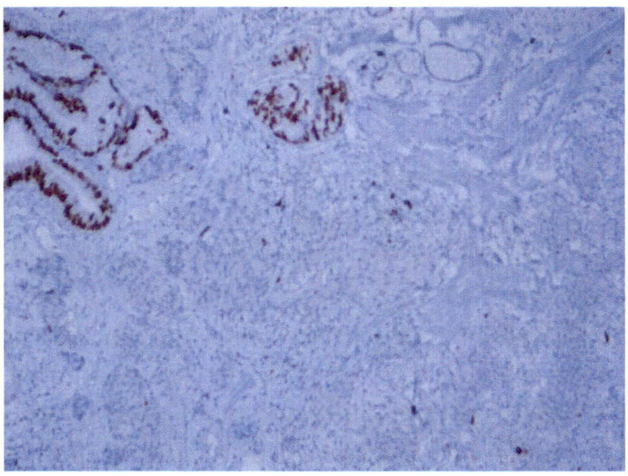

Fig. 5.18 A medium power photomicrograph of the biopsy in which Ki67 immunostaining had been carried out. Tumour cells present as solid sheets shows just a few scattered positively stained nuclei with one hot spot focus at the upper portion of the picture. The positive nuclei along the glandular structures on the left-hand side are the gastric foveolar cells showing active proliferation. This picture highlights the importance interpretation rightly understanding the cells to be interpreted (PAP, x300)

show poorly developed intracytoplasmic canaliculi with many mitochondria. These cases do not have any co-existing gastric or duodenal ulceration [25–27].

Gastric NETs have site-specific location, type I and II have predilection for gastric body, D and G cell-associated tumours in antrum; enterochromaffin (EC) cell NETs both in antrum, corpus/fundus and morphologically they look similar to

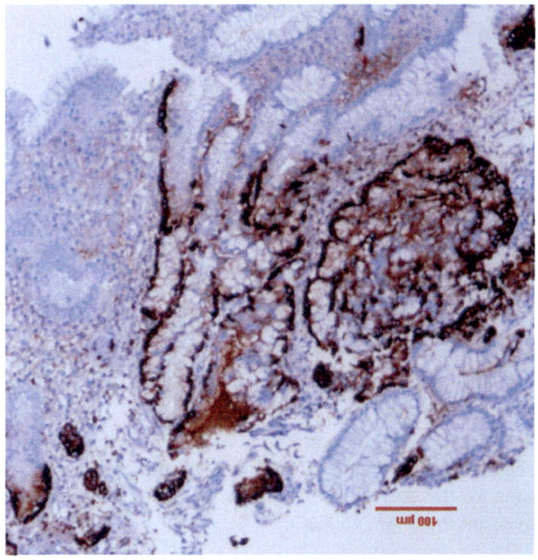

Fig. 5.19 Another focus of the tumour cells showing cribriform pattern and also in nests showing strong positivity for gastrin (IHC, x400)

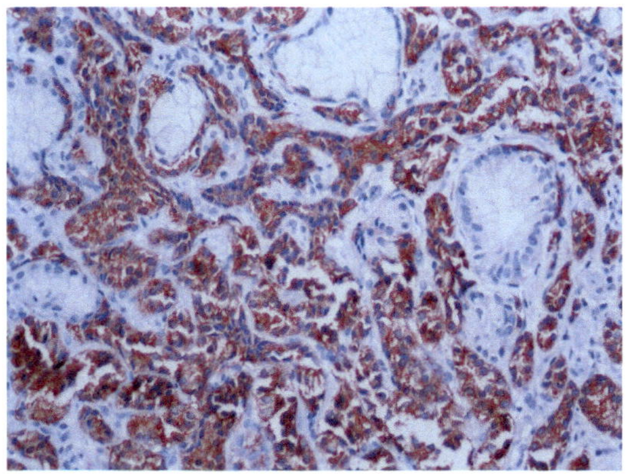

Fig. 5.20 Another photomicrograph of the tumour in Synaptophysin staining the varied patterns of positively stained tumour cells (IHC, x400)

ECL cell tumours. NETs and mixed neuroendocrine non-neuroendocrine tumours can be seen in any part of the stomach, usually in antrum and cardiac region of the stomach [28]. Gross features: Type I NETs are multiple in 60% of the cases and present as small polypoidal or nodular mucosa lesions smaller than 1 cm in size, mainly affecting the corpus and fundus, intervening gastric mucosa usually is atrophic. Type II NETs also have similar presentation involving the corpus and fundus with multiple nodules, the nod-

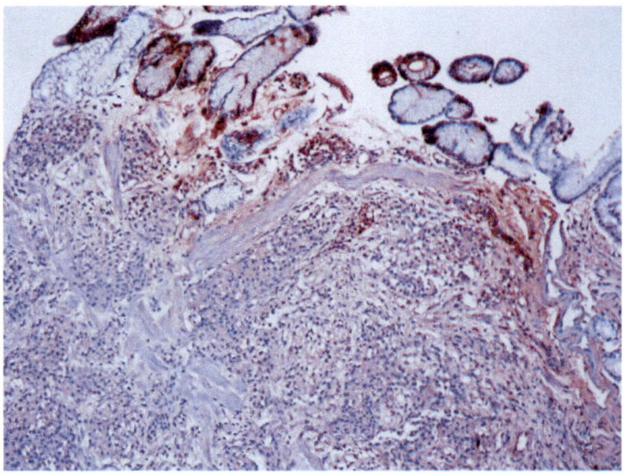

Fig. 5.21 A photomicrograph of the tumour to show negatively staining for gastrin in the tumour cells, whereas some of the overlying foveolar cells have taken up positive staining (PAP, x300)

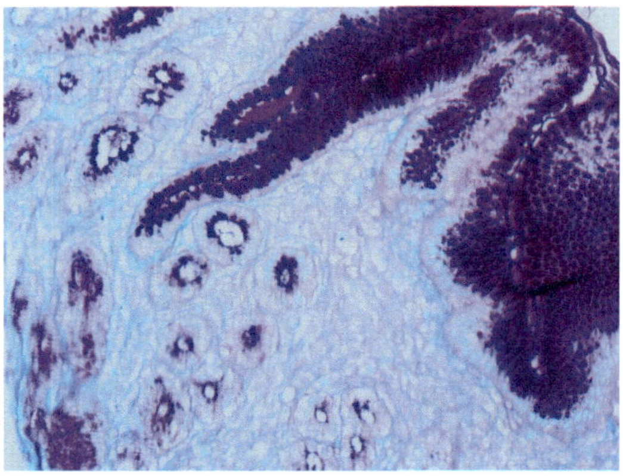

Fig. 5.22 Alcian blue PAS staining of the same biopsy to highlight the hyperplastic foveolar epithelial cells to exhibit incomplete metaplasia indicated by the purplish-blue colour of the cytoplasm and purple colour by the native mucinous cells (PAS AB, x300)

ules may be as large as 2 cm in size and the intervening gastric mucosa tends to be thickened due to associated hypertrophic hypersecretory gastropathy. In type III NETs, it tends to be single and large tumour which are more than 2 cm in size. The surrounding gastric mucosa may show changes of gastritis, otherwise there is no specific associated mucosa changes [29].

Histologically they are composed of discohesive monomorphic cells, plasmacytoid cells in appearance, intermediate size cells, the nuclei are eccentrically placed nuclei. These cells have basophilic to faintly eosinophilic compact cytoplasm with no perinuclear halo. These cells may show many stripped nuclei with finely disperse chromatin and nucleoli may be visible. These cells are arranged in one or two cell thick cords, in small groups or nests, larger islands and broader cell groups of trabeculae, insular and tubular patterns, acini, pseudo-rosettes separated and are separated by fine fibrovascular core (Figs. 5.8, 5.13, 5.14, 5.15, 5.16, 5.17, 5.19, 5.20). Usual conventional tumours do not show significant pleomorphism or mitosis, though more aggressive variants of NETs are well known (Fig. 5.3). WHO has three gradings depending upon the cellular morphology, mitotic count and Ki67 labelling indices [16, 17, 20]. Most type I and II tumours are G1 or G2 tumours with low mitosis and Ki67 scoring. Type III tumours tends to be either G2 or G3 tumours with more mitotically active and higher Ki67 scores [17, 20]. There may be frankly malignant variant with areas of tumour necrosis in higher grade tumour with more undifferentiated histology. Most gastric NETs do not produce any specific clinical symptomatology, they are detected during the endoscopic procedure for gastric-related problems. Majority are non-secretory tumours except when associated with syndromic presentations like Zollinger-Ellison syndrome. All ECL cell NETs may be producing histamine including type III tumours when the patient presents with liver and omental metastatic tumours with carcinoid syndrome. EC cell NET may be serotonin producing though very rare and non-functioning tumour, but rarely the patient may come with metastatic tumour and carcinoid syndrome. Gastrin producing G cell NET—again very situation and minority of these tumours may present with ZE syndrome. NETs are positively stained with chromogranin A and synaptophysin, and other immunomarkers that will be positive in gastric ECL cell tumours are somatostatin, gastrin, serotonin, alpha human chorionic gonadotrophin [23], vesicular monoamine transporter 2 [29], Ghrelin [30, 31], histidine decarboxylase [32] and somatostatin receptor type 2A [33].

Neuroendocrine carcinomas: Gastric neuroendocrine carcinomas (NEC) are tumours composed of large cells, poorly formed trabeculae or sheets of poorly differentiated cells (Figs. 5.2B, 5.3, 5.4). NEC may have pleomorphic cell morphology ranging from larger to smaller cell types [22, 34]. In large cell type, the cells have large pleomorphic nuclei having vesicular chromatin with prominent nucleoli and abundant pale to eosinophilic cytoplasm [34]. In small cell type, the cells are small, round to oval with nuclear hyperchromasia and arranged in nest, cords, trabeculae and islands. NECs have high mitotic count, more than 20 per10 high power fields and Ki67 count is usually more than 60 to 70%, higher Ki67 count is seen in small cell variant of NEC [22].

Mixed neuroendocrine and non-neuroendocrine neoplasms (Figs. 5.23, 5.24, 5.25, 5.26, 5.27 and 5.28). The term "mixed neuroendocrine-nonneuroendocrine neoplasm (MiNEN)" was propose din 2016 as an unifying concept to refer to heterogenous groups of neoplasms [35]. The strength of this terminology lies in the fact that it has a broad outlook bringing various terminologies resulting from combinations of different tumour types. A pathology report with the diagnosis of MiNEN requires specification and categorization of the different histological components of the tumour. The proposed entity had been scrutinized discussing the strength and also the possible shortcomings and a consensus opinion could be reached during the last meeting of World Health Organisation Editorial board at Lyon (26–28/04/2016) during 2017 World Health Organisation revised classification of endocrine tumours [36, 37]. Cordier had described the first mixed tumour of gastrointestinal tract composed of a neuroendocrine neoplasm intermixed with classic glandular component of a carcinoma [38]. Much later on Lewin suggested these mixed tumours to be classified into three groups as collision, combined and amphicrine [39]. Capella and co-workers in 2000 proposed for terms that might be used to prognosticate rather than just simply having mor-

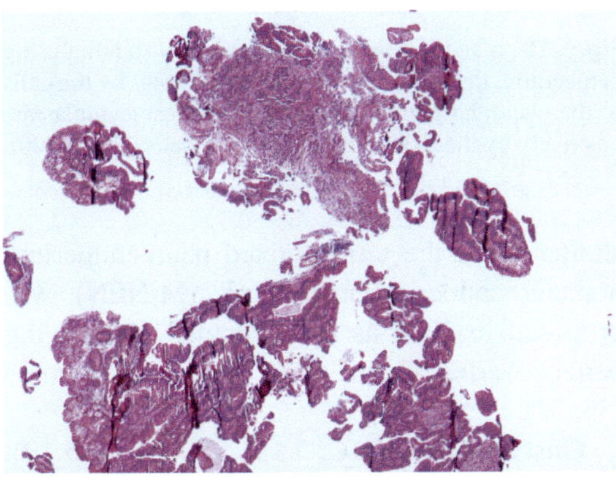

Fig. 5.23 A low power photomicrograph of an endoscopic biopsy from the body region showing tumour fragments of tumour tissue (HE, x150)

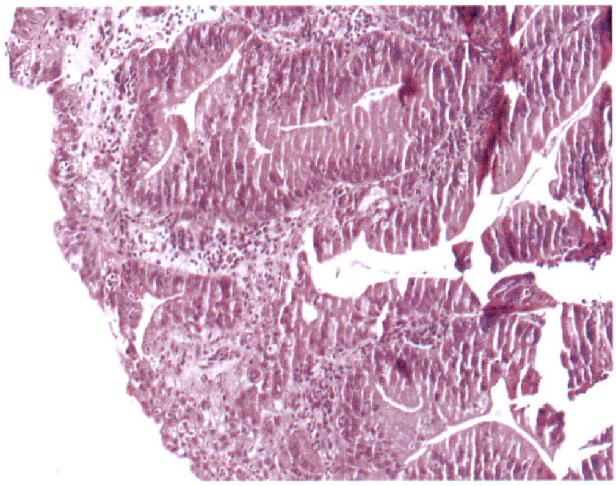

Fig. 5.24 A medium power photomicrograph of one of the tissue pieces to show a tumour with the features of a moderately differentiated adeno carcinoma (HE, x300)

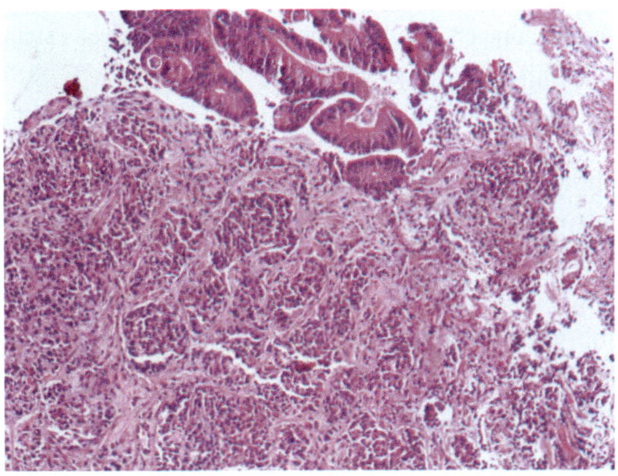

Fig. 5.25 In continuity with the adenocarcinomatous component, a large area of tumour tissue exhibiting a different looking morphology. The tumour cells are monomorphic in appearance and arranged in small groups, islands and in nests with minimal pleomorphism. Along the upper corner, there cells which are larger and showing features of adenocarcinoma (HE, x400)

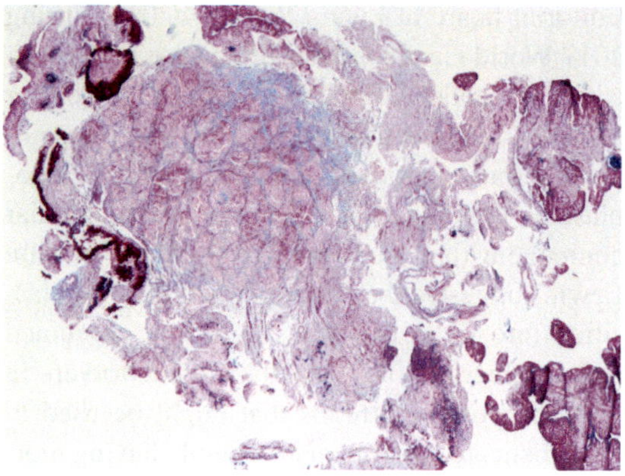

Fig. 5.26 These monomorphic population of tumour cells does not take up neither PAS nor alcian blue (PAS-AB, x300)

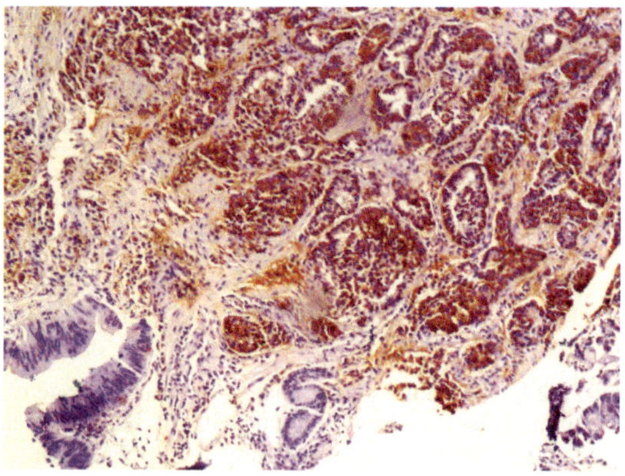

Fig. 5.27 On immunohistochemistry staining using chromogranin A, all the monomorphic tumour cells stain positively whereas carcinomatous component are negative for the stain (PAP, x300)

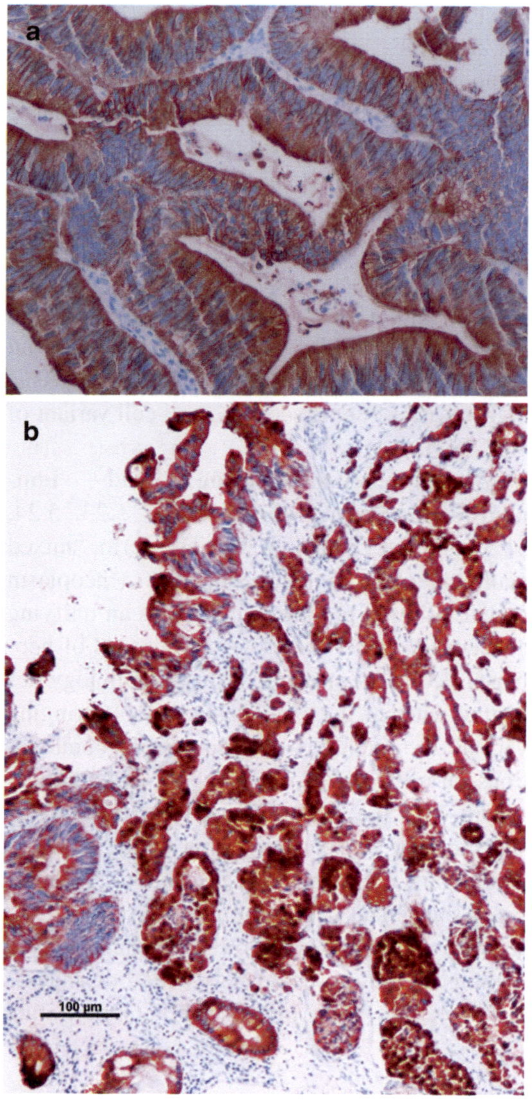

Fig. 5.28 **a** and **b**. Immunohistochemistry staining using cytokeratin, there was membranous positivity by the cells of the glandular component and also diffuse cytoplasmic positively by the monomorphic tumour cells (PAP, x300)

phological classification [40]. Same year WHO introduced the term "mixed exocrine-endocrine tumour" defining the morphological and functional components under the three morphological subtypes proposed by Lewin with an arbitrary cut-off of 30% for each type [41]. In 2010, WHO classification replaced the term mixed mix exocrine endocrine tumour by MANEC which stands for mixed adenoneuroendocrine carcinoma [42]. These terminologies have its own limitations as all the neuroendocrine components may not be frankly malignant, not qualifying for the term of neuroendocrine carcinoma but qualifying for the term of neuroendocrine tumour. Due to this shortcoming, the term "mixed neuroendocrine-nonneuroendocrine neoplasm" (MiNEN) was proposed in 2016 as a conceptual term having better covering of wide range of different tumours [35, 37].

Gastrinomas (5.1C, 5.1D, 5.9, 5.10B, 5.19), one of the functional neuroendocrine tumour associated with overt synthesis of gastrin hormone. These individuals usually present with recurrent peptic ulcer diseases, gastroesophageal reflux diseases, watery diarrhoea and abdominal pain. The syndromic condition is referred as Zollinger-Ellison syndrome (ZES) [43–46]. This rare tumour arises from gastrin hormone-secreting G cells which are located normally in duodenum, pancreas and less in numbers in stomach. Gastric acid hypersecretion by the parietal cells due to the hyperstimulation by the excess amount of gastrin associated with these tumours cause multiple ulcers in stomach and duodenum [44–46]. High level of acid results in hyperperistalsis and also has the property to inhibit pancreatic lipase resulting in severe watery diarrhoea. Almost 90% of gastrinomas are believed to be located within the well-known triangle known as Passaro's triangle. The landmark for this triangle is formed by joining the following three points: (i) superior-body of gallbladder (earlier it was identified as the confluence of the cystic and common bile duct), (ii) inferior-junction of the second and third portion of duodenum, and (iii) medial-junction of the neck and body of the pancreas [47, 48]. Type 1 and 2 gastric NETs develop in a clinical situation of hypergastrinaemia in an environment gastric mucosal exhibiting features of atrophic gastritis associated with achlorhydria and a gastrinoma. Type 3 is not associated with increased levels of gastrin and is a sporadic tumour [49, 50].

Patients with gastric gastrinomas have been found to be older than duodenal or pancreatic gastrinomas [51, 52]. They also tend to have higher serum gastrin level. Grossly they tend to be smaller in size in majority of the cases and are sub-centimetre mucosal nodular lesions, like any other ECL cell proliferation. Histologically they are G1 and G2 tumours in majority of the cases. Microscopic appearance does not have any specific feature and is similar to any other NETs. It is usually a well-differentiated NET having typical organoid pattern of arrangement of the tumour cells, also exhibit small and or larger clusters, trabeculae or intertwine cord patterns. Tumour cells may be oval or round or plasmacytoid having monomorphic nuclei with regular shape and sizes and bland nuclei chromatin, moderate amount of amphophilic cytoplasm containing large numbers of secretory granules. Tumour cells tend to show diffuse cytoplasmic expression for neuroendocrine markers. High grade or G3 tumour has large pleomorphic cells, arranged dominantly in broad trabeculae, or in sheets, irregular nuclei, pale eosinophilic cytoplasm containing lesser number of secretory granules expressing limited immunomarkers. Important features in the diagnosis of neuroendocrine tumours are expressions for immunomarkers like chromogranin A and synaptophysin. Tumour cells may be further tested for gastrin by IHC to confirm phenotypic character of the tumour. Gastrinoma may be densely positive for somatostatin and presence of high number of somatostatin receptor will make somatostatin scintigraphy effective to identify its location. Endoscopic mucosal resections have helped minimizing the need for medication but with frequent local recurrence. Gastric gastrinomas are relatively have indolent course with rare distant metastasis. Prognosis of gastric origin tumours are better than those located in other parts of GIT [51]. Gastrinoma is mostly sporadic but can be component of MEN 1 in 20 to 30% of cases. Unlike insulinoma, gastrinomas have more malignant (60% to 90%) course and at the time of first presentation, majority of the patients already had developed liver metastasized. Five-year survival rate range from 62% to 75% in patients with gastrinoma [53, 54].

References

1. Prinz C, Zanner R, Gerhard M, et al. The mechanism of histamine secretion from gastric enterochromaffin-like cells. Am J Phys. 1999;277:C845–55.
2. Zhao CM, Chen D. The ECL cell: relay station for gastric integrity. Curr Med Chem. 2012;19:98–108.
3. Beales IL. Regulation of gastric function by gastrin releasing peptide. Gut. 2002;50:897–8.
4. Tobin G, Giglio D, Lundgren O. Muscarinic receptor subtypes in the alimentary tract. J Physiol Pharmacol. 2009;60:3–21.
5. Dawson I. The endocrine cells of the gastrointestinal tract. Histochem J. 1970;2:527–49.
6. Capella C, Solcia E, Vassallo G. Identification of six types of endocrine cells in the gastrointestinal mucosa of the rabbit. Arch Histol Cytol. 1969;30:479–95.

7. Sevier AC, Munger BL. Technical note: a silver method for paraffin sections of neural tissue. J Neuropathol Exp Neurol. 1965;24:130–5.
8. Facer P, Bishop AE, Lloyd RV, et al. Chromogranin: a newly recognized marker for endocrine cells of the human gastrointestinal tract. Gastroenterology. 1985;89:1366–73.
9. Tanaka-Shintani M, Watanabe M. Immunohistochemical study of enterochromaffin-like cell in human gastric mucosa. Pathol Int. 2007;57:572–83.
10. Cockburn AN, Morgan CJ, Genta RM. Neuroendocrine proliferations of the stomach: a pragmatic approach for the perplexed pathologist. Adv Anat Pathol. 2013;20:148–57.
11. Müller J, Kirchner T, Müller-Hermelink HK. Gastric endocrine cell hyperplasia and carcinoid tumors in atrophic gastritis type a. Am J Surg Pathol. 1987;11:909–17.
12. Solcia E, Fiocca R, Villani L, et al. Hyperplastic, dysplastic, and neoplastic Enterochromaffin-like-cell proliferations of the gastric mucosa. Classification and histogenesis. Am J Surg Pathol. 1995;19(Suppl 1):S1–7.
13. Dayal Y. Hyperplastic proliferations of enteroendocrine cells. Endocr Pathol. 1994;5:4–26.
14. Modlin IM, Kidd M, Latich I, et al. Current status of gastrointestinal carcinoids. Gastroenterology. 2005;128:1717–51.
15. Graham DY, Genta RM. Long-term proton pump inhibitor use and gastrointestinal cancer. Curr Gastroenterol Rep. 2008;10:543–7.
16. De Caro MLDB, Guadagno E, Rosa GD (2018) Pathological classification: GEP, TNET, and rare forms in Colao A, Faggiano A, de Herder W edited Neuroendocrine tumors in real life from practice to knowledge. Springer Ed. pp. 29–50.
17. Bosman FT, Carneiro F, Hruban RH, et al. World Health Organization (WHO) classification of Tumours of the digestive system. 4th ed. Geneva, Switzerland: WHO Press; 2010.
18. Orditura M, Petrilloa A, Ventriglia J. Pancreatic neuroendocrine tumors: nosography, management and treatment. Int J Surg. 2016;28(Suppl 1):S156–62.
19. Masson P. Carcinoids (argentaffin-cell tumors) and nerve hyperplasia of appendicular mucosa. Am J Pathol. 1928;4:181–212.
20. Modlin IM, Lye KD, Kidd M. A 5-decade analysis of 13, 715 carcinoid tumors. Cancer. 2003;97:934–59.
21. Kulke MH, Anthony LB, Bushnell DL, et al. NANETS treatment guidelines: well-differentiated neuroendocrine tumors of the stomach and pancreas. Pancreas. 2010;39:735–52.
22. Klimstra DS, Klöppel G, La Rosa S, et al. Classification of neuroendocrine neoplasms of the digestive system. In: WHO Classification of Tumours Editorial Board, editor. WHO classification of tumours: digestive system tumours. 5th ed. IARC: Lyon; 2019. p. 105.
23. Abraham SC, Carney JA, Ooi A, et al. Achlorhydria, parietal cell hyperplasia, and multiple gastric carcinoids: a new disorder. Am J Surg Pathol. 2005;29:969–75.
24. Nakata K, Aishima S, Ichimiya H. Unusual multiple gastric carcinoids with hypergastrinemia report of a case. Surg Today. 2010;40:267–71.
25. Ooi A, Ota M, Katsuda S, et al. An unusual case of multiple gastric carcinoids associated with diffuse endocrine cell hyperplasia and parietal cell hypertrophy. Endocr Pathol. 1995;6:229–37.
26. La Rosa S, Vanoli A. Gastric neuroendocrine neoplasms and related precursor lesions. J Clin Pathol. 2014;67:938–48.
27. Rindi G, Bordi C, Rappel S, et al. Gastric carcinoids and neuroendocrine carcinomas: pathogenesis, pathology, and behaviour. World J Surg. 1996;20:168–72.
28. Rindi G, Luinetti O, Cornaggia M, et al. Three subtypes of gastric argyrophil carcinoid and the gastric neuroendocrine carcinoma: a clinicopathologic study. Gastroenterology. 1993;104:994–1006.
29. Rindi G, Paolotti D, Fiocca R, et al. Vesicular monoamine transporter 2 as a marker of gastric Enterochromaffin-like cell tumors. Virchows Arch. 2000;436:217–23.
30. Srivastava A, Kamath A, Barry SA, et al. Ghrelin expression in hyperplastic and neoplastic proliferations of the enterochromaffin-like (ECL) cells. Endocr Pathol. 2004;15:47–54.
31. Papotti M, Cassoni P, Volante M, et al. Ghrelin-producing endocrine tumors of the stomach and intestine. J Clin Endocrinol Metab. 2001;86:5052–9.
32. Tsolakis AV, Grimelius L, Granerus G, et al. Histidine decarboxylase and urinary methylimidazoleacetic acid in gastric neuroendocrine cells and tumours. World J Gastroenterol. 2015;21:13240–9.
33. Kimura N, Pilichowska M, Date F, et al. Immunohistochemical expression of somatostatin type 2A receptor in neuroendocrine tumors. Clin Cancer Res. 1999;5:3483–7.
34. Chetty R. Combined large cell neuroendocrine, small cell and squamous carcinomas of the lung with rhabdoid cells. Pathology. 2000;32:209–12.
35. La Rosa S, Sessa F, Uccella S. Mixed neuroendocrine-nonneuroendocrine neoplasms (MiNENs): unifying the concept of a heterogeneous group of neoplasms. Endocr Pathol. 2016;27:284–311.
36. Klimstra DS, Klöppel G, La Rosa S, et al. Classification of neuroendocrine neoplasms of the digestive system. In: WHO Classification of Tumours Editorial Board, editor. WHO classification of tumours: digestive system tumours. 5th ed. Lyon: IARC; 2019. p. 16–9.
37. Rosa SL, Uccell S Classification of neuroendocrine neoplasms: lights and shadows. Rev End Met Dis published online 9th Nov 2020. https://doi.org/10.1007/s11154-020-09612-2
38. Cordier R. Les cellules argentaffines dans les tumeurs intestinales. Arch Int Med Exp. 1924;1:5.

39. Lewin K. Carcinoid tumors and the mixed (composite) glandular-endocrine cell carcinomas. Am J Surg Pathol. 1987;11(Suppl 1):71–86.
40. Capella C, La Rosa S, Uccella S, et al. Mixed endocrine-exocrine tumors of the gastrointestinal tract. Semin Diagn Pathol. 2000;17:91–103.
41. Solcia E, Klöppel G, Sobin LH, et al. Histological typing of endocrine tumours. Heidelberg: Springer-Verlag; 2000.
42. Rindi G, Arnold R, Bosman FT, et al. Nomenclature and classification of neuroendocrine neoplasms of the digestive system. In: WHO classification of tumours of the digestive system. IARC: Lyon; 2010. p. 13–4.
43. Gong S, Li Z, Liu XB, et al. Gastrinoma in multiple endocrine neoplasia type 1 after total pancreatectomy. Medicine. 2019;98:e18275.
44. Ito T, Igarashi H, Jensen RT. Zollinger-Ellison syndrome: recent advances and controversies. Curr Opi Gastroenterol. 2013;29:650–61.
45. Roy PK, Venzon DJ, Shojamanesh H, et al. Zolinger-Ellison syndrome. Clinical presentation in 261 patients. Medicine (Baltimore). 2000;79:379–411.
46. Gibril F, Schumann M, Pace A, et al. Multiple endocrine neoplasia type 1 and Zollinger-Ellison syndrome: a prospective study of 107 cases and comparison with 1009 cases from the literature. Medicine. 2004;83:43–83.
47. Stabile BE, Morrow DJ, Passaro E Jr. The gastrinoma triangle: operative implications. Am J Surg. 1984 Jan;147(1):25–31.
48. Yagnik V (2018) Fundamentals of operative surgery. BI Publications Pvt Ltd. p. 170. ISBN 9788172253004.
49. Sundaresan S, Kang AJ, Merchant JL. Pathophysiology of gastric NETs: role of gastrin and Menin. Curr Gastroenterol Rep. 2017;19:32.
50. McCarthy DM. Proton pump inhibitor use, Hypergastrinemia, and gastric carcinoids-what is the relationship? Int J Mol Sci. 2020;21:662.
51. Huang SF, Kuo IM, Lee CW, et al. Comparison study of gastrinomas between gastric and non-gastric origins. World J Surg Oncol. 2015;13:202.
52. Jensen RT, Niederle B, Mitry E, et al. Gastrinoma (duodenal and pancreatic). Neuroendocrinology. 2006;84:173–82.
53. Yu R. Chapter 150—neuroendocrine tumor syndromes. In: Jameson JL, DeGroot LJ, editors. Endocrinology: adult and pediatric. 7th ed. Philadelphia: Elsevier Saunders; 2016. p. 2606–2614 (e4).
54. Kloppel G. Classification and pathology of gastroenteropancreatic neuroendocrine neoplasms. Endocr Relat Cancer. 2011;18:S1–S16.

6 Demonstration of *Helicobacter pylori* (HP) and Other Related Organisms

Helicobacter pylori (HP) is an organism that stains negatively with Grams stain and resides in the stomach. Prevalence of *H. pylori*-positive status varies according to age of individual and socio-economic status of the country [1]. Important route of transmission appears to be person to person and contaminated food materials and poor basic sanitation; infection has been documented in people living in the same household [2]. HP infection is believed to acquire in young children living in unsuitable environments [3]. Every individual infected with HP and also harbouring the organism in their gastric mucosa may remain asymptomatic. However, the individual infected with HP may develop certain diseases like duodenal ulcers and gastric malignancy which are believed to be short-term as well as long-term complications [4]. Documentation of HP infection may be done by various methods that may be both an invasive and a non-invasive technique, and development of a vaccine against HP infection has been ongoing effort of many scientists since the time its epidemiology has been understood [5]. Until the time that Warren and Marshall documented presence of HP (Fig. 6.1), gastric mucosa was considered to be a sterile environment because of its low pH [6]. HP has various pathogenic varieties depending upon the expression for the virulence factors exhibiting specific effects on host cells—(1) cytotoxin-associated antigen A (Cag A), (2) vacuolating cytotoxin (Vag A), (3) duodenal ulcer promoting gene A protein (Dup A), (4) outer inflammatory protein (OipA), and (5) gamma-glutamyl transpeptidase [7–11]. HP executes its pathogenic function through Th1 [12]. In order to remain colonized in the hostile gastric environment HP is equipped with special properties. Firstly, the motility of its flagella start as soon as HP reaches the acid medium of the gastric content, with the help of which it penetrates through the mucous layer to reach the surface lining epithelium and

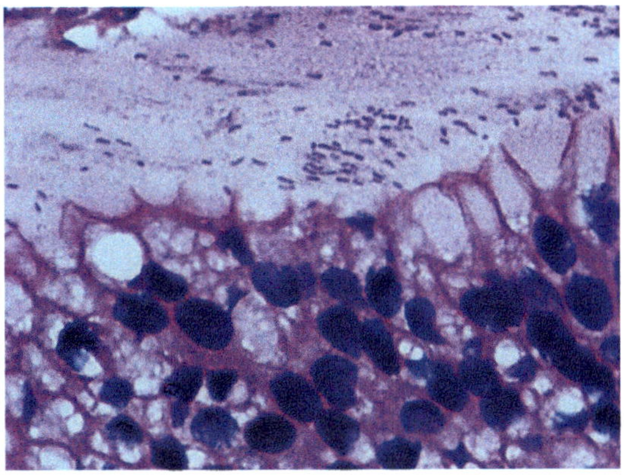

Figs. 6.1 Photomicrographs are of high-power oil immersion views taken along the mucosal surface of gastric biopsy. Within the thick mucus layer over the surface epithelium are many *H. pylori*, many are curved having inverted S shaped. The organisms are 5–8 microns in length and 2–3 microns in width, some are round to oval shape like other cocci but larger in size than the conventional cocci which are the coccoid form of *H. pylori* (HE, ×1000)

K. Vaiphei, *Interpretation of Endoscopic Biopsy - Gastritis, Gastropathies and Beyond*,
https://doi.org/10.1007/978-981-16-6026-9_6

remain to colonize along the surface [13], and the second type movement is by swimming and swarming of all the eight flagella that get spread out in all directions and this action of HP is best seen over the agar culture medium [14, 15]. The second property is the chemotactic action to many chemicals and molecules such as mucous, $NaHCO_3$, urea, NaCl, and various protein and amino acids [16, 17]. Thirdly, HP utilizes metals like Nickel as a cofactor for its enzymatic reactions, to maintain its normal physiological property by reducing oxidative stress and energy consumption to sustain itself [18]. Chemotactic properties of *H. pylori* are believed to control by at least 10 genes, which help in gastric colonization [19] and many other coupling proteins [20]. Nickel is an indispensable cofactor for urease and hydrogenase. Role of urease is in HP colonization by catalyzing the hydrolytic process of urea to CO_2 and NH_3. These end products act as buffering agents to control the gastric acid pH level [21]. An alternative pathway utilizes hydrogenase as the promoter enzyme to induce the cascade and HP utilizes hydrogen as an energy source [22]. HP surface antigens also interact with the gastric epithelial surface receptors [23, 24]. is a well-characterized molecule. Certain virulent HP strain expresses blood group antigen-binding adhesin A having specific binding site for Lewis H-1 antigen. This particular strain is considered to be more aggressive and associates with peptic ulcer and gastric cancer [25, 26]. Another adhesion molecule HP has been identified in the outer cell membrane that binds to host cell adhesion molecules that lead to initiation of cell signalling pathways and CagA translocation [27]. CagA protein can act as a modifier of epithelial cells by altering cell polarity and changes in cytoskeleton, which are believed to be associated with carcinogenesis [28]. HPs are also equipped with many non-CagA virulence factors. Namely VacA, a protein expressed by all to determine their pathogenicity. VacA protein produces host cell loss by producing injury to integrity of mitochondria, cytoplasmic membrane and many other cytoplasmic organelles [29]. This protein also results in activation of the host immune response and tolerance through activation of immune cells including dendritic cells [30]. DupA protein is associated with increase IL-8 production by gastric epithelial cells inducing epithelial cell injury and inflammation, thereby making HP to have survival benefits [9]. Similar to CagA, OipA has been associated with increased incidence of peptic ulcers and gastric cancer [10]. OipA functions by altering the signalling pathway for β-catenin, inducing epithelial proliferation and reducing intercellular junctional gaps [31]. Immune response to *H. pylori* infection is complex as both innate and adaptive mechanisms are activated through many lipid-based HP antigens, HSP-60 and Nap A interacts with epithelial Toll-like receptors [32, 33]. These interactions result in the release of proinflammatory cytokines [34]. The injured epithelial cells are infiltrated by inflammatory cells accompanied by accumulation of nitric oxide and ROS. The activated T cells are dominantly CD4 and CD8 with preferential activation of CD4 [35, 36].

Barry J. Marshall and Robin Warren, the joint winners of this year's Nobel Prize (2005) in Physiology or Medicine. Warren, a consultant pathologist now retired from Royal Perth Hospital in Australia, is a reserved man whose colleagues talk about his quiet persistence, thoughtfulness and careful observation. Marshall, a gastroenterologist 14 years his junior from the University of Western Australia, has described himself as brash. Others list his creativity, determination and entrepreneurial spirit [37]. These two Australian researchers discovered the bacterium *Helicobacter pylori* in the year 1982 [38] and confirmed it in 1990 to be the aetiological factor in the pathogenesis of gastritis and peptic ulcer disease [39]. This Gram-negative organism was observed to show characteristic gastric colonizing property was established to be aetiological factor for many gastric inflammatory conditions including gastric cancer [38, 40]. Clinical symptomatology related to HP infection is variable depending on host immune response. Antral predominant gastritis has a strong association with peptic ulcer disease, corpus dominant and multiple foci gastritis have an association with gastric ulcer, mucosal atrophy with or without metaplasia and dysplasia, and development of gastric cancer [41]. HP infected individual may present with a wide range of extra-intestinal clinical manifestations [42]. There are various diagnostic tests to detect *H. pylori* infection with their specific advantages and disadvantages. Histology is a technique consisting of observation of the typical bacteria accompanied by inflammation of the gastric biopsy. Histological method includes utilization of several special histochemical stains and immunostaining to highlight the infecting organism better [43]. Rapid urease test (RUT), an important diagnostic tool at the bedside. RUT is an indirect technique for HP based on the presence of urease in gastric mucosa and is usable only when mucosa is infected with the organism. It requires the infected mucosa or mucus to be added to the medium that may be a tube, gel or any other devices containing urea. Gastric urease breaks urea into ammonia and carbon dioxide. Different tests that may be used based on the component of the reaction include labelled CO_2 in serum or breath, breath ammonia. In RUT due to the change in pH induced by ammonia results in colour change of the solution which may also be detected using a pH meter. Originally phenol red had been used as colour indicator where there was colour change from yellow to pink or red with the increased pH [44, 45]. A positive RUT needs about 10^5 HP to be present in the mucosal fragment to produce the desired colour change in an agar-based test such as CLO test [46]. HP concentration is not an issue in routine practice as the sensitivity of the available RUT tests is high and reported to be between 80 and 100% with 97 and 99% specific [47, 48]. Another method to confirm presence of *H. pylori* is culturing a bit of the endoscopic biopsy tissue and is 100% specific. This method has a few drawbacks thereby precluding it from its widespread use. Firstly, it is less sensitive than other assays, secondly the biopsy needs to be put into the culture medium immediately as *H. pylori* are highly sensitive organism and cannot survive outside a suitable environment and an enriched medium is necessary. Thirdly HP is similar looking to *Campylobacter* group and cannot be distinguished morphologically. For all three techniques, endoscopic biopsy is the most important step to acquire the tissue to carry out the tests [49]. *H. pylori* can be detected by conventional molecular technique and in situ hybridization method, and are considered to be superior to simple RUT [42]. In spite of the fact that these techniques are sensitive and specific, there are certain groups of patients, where *H. pylori* may not be detectable [48–52]. These assays are also expensive and are not generally used for routine evaluation of patients.

With the advancement in technologies recently, non-invasive modes have become popular to be used as an alternative diagnostic method. Urea breath test (UBT) is a technology that has been preferred by many to document the presence of HP infection. The principle of this technology is based on capability of the organism to reduce 13C or 14C labelled urea compound into carbon dioxide. This is estimated with the help of mass or infra-red spectrometer of the exhaled air [53]. Stool antigen test (SAT) is a good alternative for the diagnosis of *H. pylori* infection. The principle of SAT utilizes enzymatic immunoassay against bacterial antigens and is a highly sensitive method in patients with active infection [54, 55] and SAT is not influenced by the administration of proton pump inhibitors [56]. A new detection of antibodies in urine is another upcoming technique and meta-analysis of 23 studies have shown that utilizing urine sample might be a good alternative non-invasive technique to diagnose *H. pylori* infection [57]. Serologic detection by ELISA method of hook-associated protein 2 homologue, i.e. FliD has been found to be highly specific (99%) and sensitive (97%) and is a simple and low-cost method [58].

Serologic test against HP is highly sensitive. In a seronegative individual, it is unlikely to find the bacterium in a biopsy and serology negativity amongst the general population in only 2% [59]. This test also has its own limitation as the antibodies will persist for a considerable period of time even after complete eradication. However, interpreting a positive serology depends on epidemiological factors and a positive serology is likely to be associated with an active infection in endemic zones were largely unavailable. Contrary to this, a serology positive individual in a non-endemic region has much lower chances of having HP infection and the geographic region also belongs to countries where antibiotic therapy is easily accessible [59].

There are various ways to bring out *H. pylori* (HP) better in section in light microscopy. In a well-stained H&E section, these organisms may be visible along the surface and gastric pits embedded within the mucous layer. HP is a curve organism measuring about the size of lymphocyte in length about 7–8 micron and a width of about 2 micrometer. A pathologist should be able to identify coccoid form of HP and measure about 4–5 micrometer in diameter. They may be easily differentiated from other common garden cocci as coccoid form of HP are larger in size. They are usually seen scattered along the surface and indicates the organism developing a cell wall to protect itself from the unfavourable environment. They are frequently co-present with the S-shaped form of the organism. In order to highlight HP better in a histological section, there are many histochemical stains that can be used. To name some of the stains that can be used for paraffin section in a Histopathology laboratory to highlight HP better than H7E stained sections are—half Gram, modified Giemsa, acridine orange, cresyl violet, Gimenez, Ziehl-Nielsen, Genta and modified Genta stain, *H. pylori* silver stain and Warthin Starry [60, 61] (Figs. 6.2 to 6.6). HP can also be demonstrated using a specific antibody, which is more sensitive and specific with lesser discrepancies amongst the pathologists compared to many other special stains [61, 62]. Amongst the various methods, the one that has been used for the first time in an endoscopic biopsy was Warthin-Starry, followed closely by Carbol-fuchsin [63, 64]. It was Marshall and Warren who had demonstrated HP with the help of Warthin-Starry silver staining in the process of discovery of HP in gastric mucosa. Later on, Rocha and colleagues adapted Carbol-Fuchsin technology for paraffinized tissue section. These two techniques have been replaced by other newer techniques which are easier to carry out. Carbol-Fuchsin method is a cheap technique and though it highlights the freely lying organism on the gastric mucosa, however, in a histological section, its utility becomes less useful [65]. Immunohistochemistry (peroxidase anti-peroxidase = PAP) for demonstration of HP was first used in 1988 to evaluate its efficacy to demonstrate its presence in antral mucosa of a dyspeptic patient [65–67]. This study was carried out to compare with HP cultures and was found to be 100% sensitive. IHC is highly specific with minimum variations amongst the observers. Due to the more expensive cost involved compared to other histochemical techniques, it has been used less frequently. IHC is reserved for cases exhibiting florid active gastritis in tissue biopsy with no demonstrable organism with the histochemistry techniques [67–69]. There are different opinions for routine reporting of gastritis associated with various conditions, some laboratories consider H&E staining to be adequate for initial step of assessment in routine gastric biopsies [70]. There are many studies which had carried out comparative analyses H&E with other special histochemical and IHC staining in demonstrating HP in tissue sections, H&E had been found to have a high index of positivity [71, 72].

A well-stained paraffin section by H&E will make detection of HP in routine biopsies across the histopathology labs easy in endoscopic biopsy samples of gastritis patients and the sensitivity may approach 100%. Utilization of basic special stains including IHC will definitely increase detection. IHC staining is specific for HP detection and is almost 100% sensitive and specific [59, 72, 73]. IHC technology is costlier than routine histochemical stains and is available for routinely used in more advanced and modernized laboratories only. For these reasons, there is still interest in the application of various histochemical stains to gastric mucosal biopsies for *H. pylori* detection [72]. *H. pylori* infection has become an old-world disease, it is important now to understand the situation where there can be different patterns of *H. pylori* positivity in routine gastric biopsies from different areas of the stomach. Before the era of freely available proton pump inhibitor for routine use, HP was mainly observed to colonize within the mucous layer on the gastric epithelium, more frequently involving the pyloric antral mucosa. This habit of HP

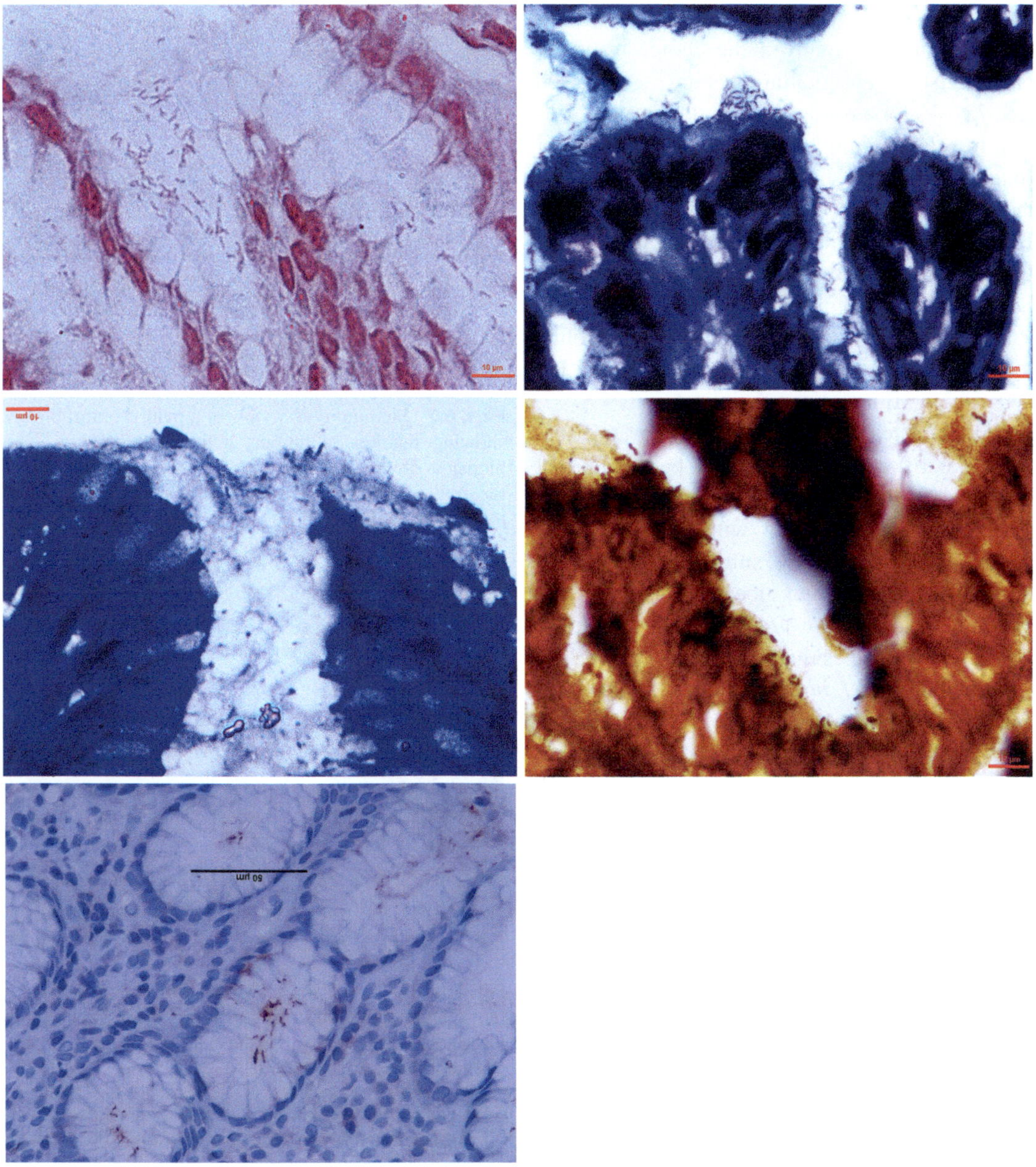

Figs. 6.2 to 6.6 Oil immersion photomicrographs taken along the surface of endoscopic gastric biopsies, similar to Fig. 6.1, in different special histochemical stains highlighting *H. pylori*. 6.2 is half Gram stain, 6.3 is Giemsa stain, 6.4 is toluidine stain, 6.5 is Warthin Starry silver impregnation stain and the last, i.e. 6.6 is immunohistochemistry staining using primary antibody against *H. pylori*. Organisms in all special stains appear similar (×1000)

infection of the gastric mucosa may still be true in many parts of the world. Following the random and frequent administration of proton pump inhibitors resulted in alteration in the way of HP colonization and are present in a lesser number. They tend to be located frequently in deeper gastric pits and glands. HP has shown a way of colonization more frequently in sites away from pylori antrum displaying coccoid forms, maybe an intracellular variety in a certain group of patients [59, 73]. Most histochemical stains and H&E have been found to have sensitivity in the range of 60–90% compared to IHC. IHC has been favour stain if given the choice by many pathologists if an ancillary testing is indicated [59, 72]. As for a routine diagnostic purpose, it is best to select a simple and economical stain for routine utilization. Half Gram staining is a simple technique and economical for routine use giving HP pinkish-red colour similar to the colour taken up by the nuclei of the epithelial cells, against the greyish mucus background. There are many more stains including Warthin Starry and immunohistochemistry that can be used to demonstrate HP better in paraffin sections.

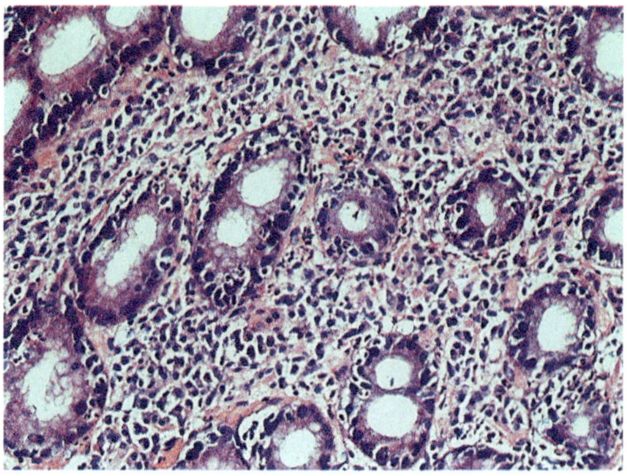

Figs. 6.7 Medium power view of a pyloric antral biopsy showing features of chronic active inflammation. The biopsy is of a patient who has *H. helmannii* infection and the mucosal inflammatory response is similar to that of *H. pylori* (HE, ×300)

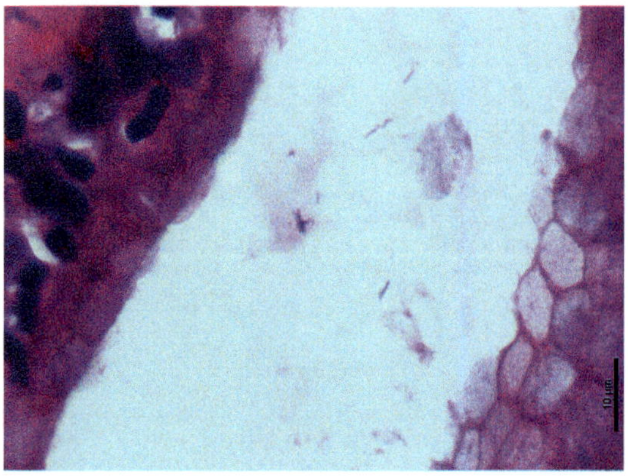

Fig. 6.8 Oil immersion view of the foveola to show the few scattered thin and fine spiral organisms, double the length of *H. pylori*, which is the characteristic appearance of *H. helmannii* (HE, ×1000)

***Helicobacter heilmannii* (HH)** (Figs. 6.7, 6.8, 6.9 and 6.10) is a Gram-negative bacterium that belonged to the species of *Helicobacter* genus [74]. Individuals infected with HH may have clinical symptomatology similar to those produced by HP, duodenum ulcers, stomach cancers including lymphomas [74–77]. Other non-HP *Helicobacter* species that may have similar clinical problems are *H. bizzozeronii*, *H. suis*, *H. felis* and *H. salomonis*, and all these organisms due to their similarity in morphology and clinical problems, they are often put together. The term *H. heilmannii* sensu lato and *H. heilmannii* s.s. designate the specific species within *H. heilmannii* group. "s.s" is appended for its characterization from other groups [77, 78]. HH is known to produce heavier mucosal inflammation and is zoonotic in origin. HH is more slender but longer and spiral measuring 10–14 microns in length [78]. HP which is commonly present in pyloric antrum, shifts its dominant localization to body and fundus regions in partially treated cases [79, 80]. HP infection is routinely assessed by histologic evaluation of the gastric biopsy samples. In the endoscopy room, HP infection may be documented immediately by carrying a rapid urase test. In addition to these, HP infection may be documented by a non-invasive testing with serology and time-consuming test like hydrogen breath test. Organism load may decrease with changing milieu of the environment like reduction in mucous production by gastric mucosa due to development of atrophic gastritis, as HP requires the thick mucus layer for its survival and protection from exposure to gastric acid content. Any serology-positive patient, who had never been treated for HP, should receive treatment, even if biopsies are negative [80].

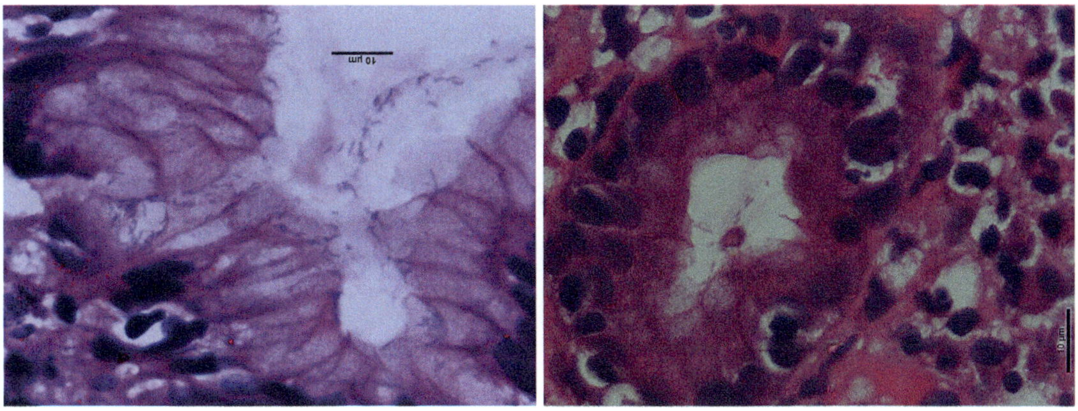

Figs. 6.9 and 6.10 Two oil immersion photomicrographs of two different patients of antral and body mucosal biopsies to highlight the presence of both *H. pylori* and *H. helmannii* within the surface mucus layer (HE, ×1000)

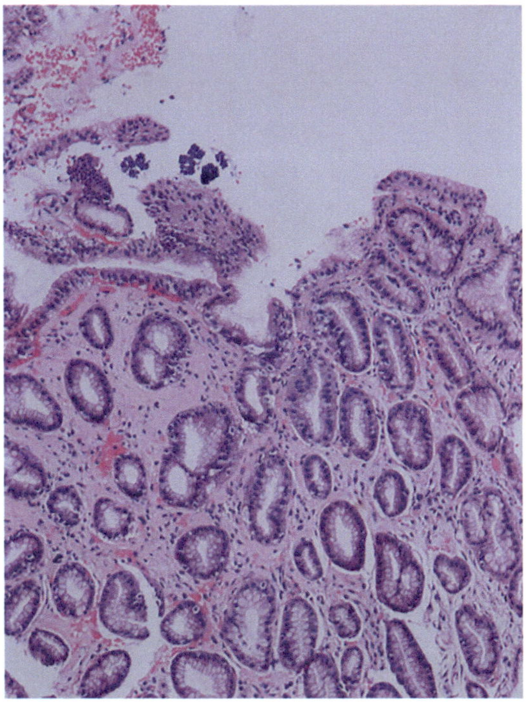

Figs. 6.11 A medium power view of a gastric body biopsy showing lamina propria fibrosis and loss of the specialized glands with a few strongly haematoxyphilic cuboid bodies over the surface (HE, ×300)

Another organism that may be observed in gastric biopsy in a patient who presents with gastric outlet obstruction or delayed gastric emptying is *Sarcina ventriculi* (Figs. 6.11, 6.12, 6.13, 6.14, and 6.15). *Sarcina* is a genus of Gram-positive cocci bacteria in the family Clostridiaceae. *Sarcina ventriculi* is a Gram-positive organism reportedly rare and has been implicated in the development of gastric ulcers, emphysematous gastritis and gastric perforation. *S. ventriculi* has characteristic morphological features—stains deeply basophilic on H&E section, cuboidal in shape measuring 1.8–3 micron in individually, arranged in packets approximately the size of a red blood cell having a tetrad pattern of arrangement. Casual look, it may mimic vegetable matter and generally is located along the mucosal surface within gastric mucus layer, rather than in gastric pits and are not invasive. Histologic features of gastric mucosa can vary ranging from being fairly normal looking to diffuse and haemorrhagic gastritis with ulceration. There can be concurrent presence of *H. pylori* and *S. ventriculi* in the same specimen [81–85].

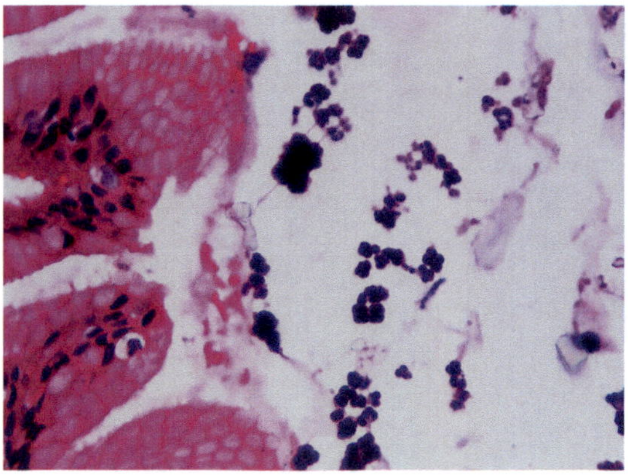

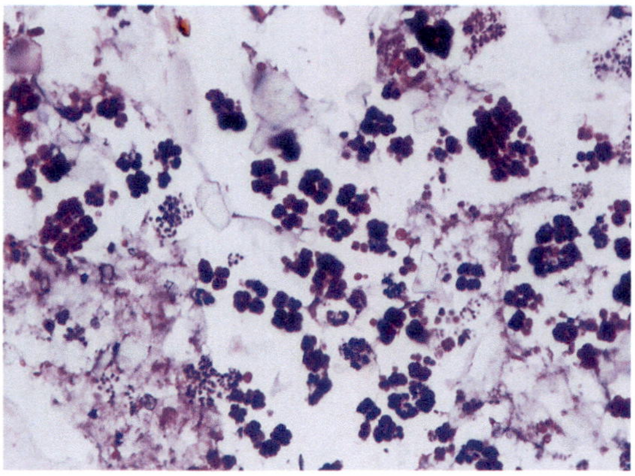

Figs. 6.12 and 6.13 Those organisms seen over the surface of the mucosa on high power view, having tetrad pattern of regular arrangement by the cuboid shape bodies intermixed with degenerated gastric content and mucus (HE, ×500)

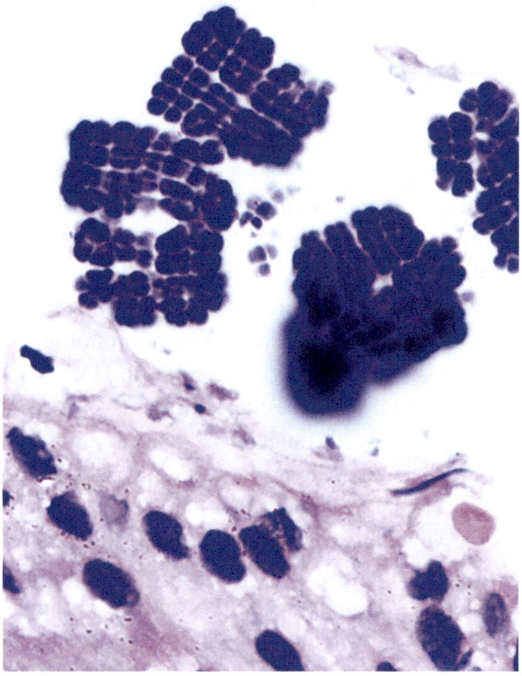

Fig. 6.14 The organism under oil immersion arranged regularly like matchboxes (HE, ×1000)

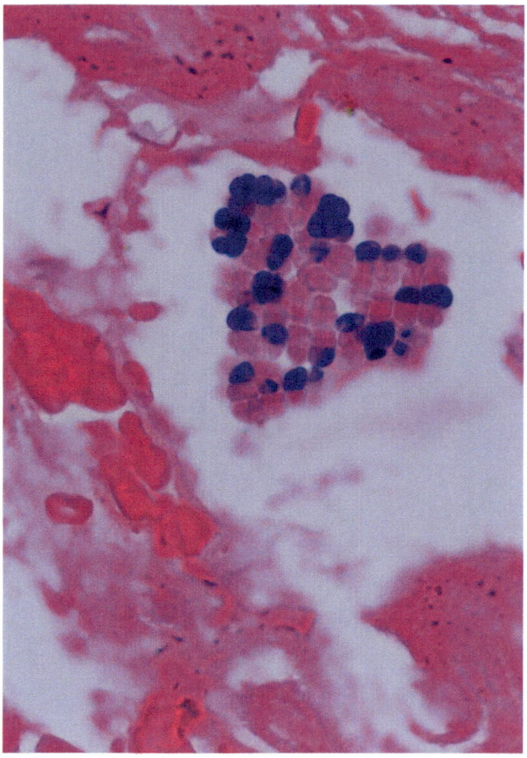

Fig. 6.15 The organisms showing Gram positivity (Gram stain, ×1000)

References

1. Peleteiro B, Bastos A, Ferro A, et al. Prevalence of helicobacter pylori infection worldwide: a systematic review of studies with national coverage. Dig Dis Sci. 2014;59:1698–709.
2. Urita Y, Watanabe T, Kawagoe N, et al. Role of infected grandmothers in transmission of helicobacter pylori to children in a Japanese rural town. J Paediatr Child Health. 2013;49:394–8.
3. Goh KL, Chan WK, Shiota S, et al. Epidemiology of helicobacter pylori infection and public health implications. Helicobacter. 2011;16(Suppl 1):1–9.
4. Malfertheiner P, Venerito M, Schulz C. Helicobacter pylori infection: new facts in clinical management. Curr Treat Options Gastroenterol. 2018;16:605–15.
5. Ogata SK, Kawakami EP, Patrício FRS, et al. Evaluation of invasive and non-invasive methods for the diagnosis of helicobacter pylori infection in symptomatic children and adolescents. Sao Paulo Med Jl. 2001;119:67–71.
6. Warren JR, Marshall B. Unidentified curved bacilli on gastric epithelium in active chronic gastritis. Lancet. 1983;1:1273–5.
7. Fischer W. Assembly and molecular mode of action of the helicobacter pylori cag type IV secretion apparatus. FEBS J. 2011;278:1203–12.
8. Boquet P, Ricci V. Intoxication strategy of helicobacter pylori VacA toxin. Trends Microbiol. 2012;20:165–74.
9. Lu H, Hsu PI, Graham DY, et al. Duodenal ulcer promoting gene of helicobacter pylori. Gastroenterol. 2005;128:833–48.
10. Yamaoka Y, Kwon DH, Graham DY. A M(r) 34,000 proinflammatory outer membrane protein (oipA) of helicobacter pylori. Proc Natl Acad Sci U S A. 2000;97:7533–8.
11. Shibayama K, Wachino J, Arakawa Y, et al. Metabolism of glutamine and glutathione via gamma-glutamyltranspeptidase and glutamate transport in helicobacter pylori: possible significance in the pathophysiology of the organism. Mol Microbiol. 2007;64:396–406.
12. Bamford KB, Fan X, Crowe SE, et al. Lymphocytes in the human gastric mucosa during helicobacter pylori have a T helper cell 1 phenotype. Gastroenterol. 1998;114:482–92.
13. Eaton KA, Morgan DR, Krakowka S. Motility as a factor in the colonisation of gnotobiotic piglets by *Helicobacter pylori*. J Med Microbiol. 1992;37:123–7.
14. Ottemann KM, Lowenthal AC. Helicobacter pylori uses motility for initial colonization and to attain robust infection. Infect Immunol. 2002;70:1984–90.
15. Gu H. Role of flagella in the pathogenesis of helicobacter pylori. Curr Microbiol. 2017;74:863–9.
16. Worku ML, Karim QN, Spencer J, et al. Chemotactic response of helicobacter pylori to human plasma and bile. J Med Microbiol. 2004;53:807–11.
17. Mizote T, Yoshiyama H, Nakazawa T. Urease-independent chemotactic responses of helicobacter pylori to urea, urease inhibitors, and sodium bicarbonate. Infect Immunol. 1997;65:1519–21.
18. Becker KW, Skaar EP. Metal limitation and toxicity at the interface between host and pathogen. FEMS Microbiol Rev. 2014;38:1235–49.
19. Alm RA, Ling LS, Moir DT, King BL, et al. Genomic-sequence comparison of two unrelated isolates of the human gastric pathogen helicobacter pylori. Nature. 1999;397:176–80.
20. Aizawa SI, Harwood CS, Kadner RJ. Signalling components in bacterial locomotion and sensory reception. J Bacteriol. 2000;182:1459–71.
21. Eaton KA, Brooks CL, Morgan DR, et al. Essential role of urease in pathogenesis of gastritis induced by helicobacter pylori in gnotobiotic piglets. Infect Immunol. 1991;59:2470–5.
22. Olson JW, Maier RJ. Molecular hydrogen as an energy source for helicobacter pylori. Science. 2002;298:1788–90.
23. Alm RA, Bina J, Andrews BM, et al. Comparative genomics of helicobacter pylori: analysis of the outer membrane protein families. Infect Immunol. 2000;68:4155–68.
24. Kalali B, Mejías-Luque R, Javaheri A, et al. H. Pylori virulence factors: influence on immune system and pathology. Mediators Inflammat. 2014;2014:426309.
25. Oliveira AG, Santos A, Guerra JB, et al. babA2- and cagA-positive helicobacter pylori strains are associated with duodenal ulcer and gastric carcinoma in Brazil. J Clin Microbiol. 2003;41:3964–6.
26. Björnham O, Bugaytsova J, Borén T, et al. Dynamic force spectroscopy of the *Helicobacter pylori* BabA-Lewis b binding. Biophys Chem. 2009;143:102–5.
27. Javaheri A, Kruse T, Moonens K, et al. Helicobacter pylori adhesin HopQ engages in a virulence-enhancing interaction with human CEACAMs. Nat Microbiol. 2016;2:16189.
28. Tsutsumi R, Higashi H, Higuchi M, et al. Attenuation of helicobacter pylori CagA x SHP-2 signalling by interaction between CagA and C-terminal Src kinase. J Biol Chem. 2003;278:3664–70.
29. Atherton JC, Peek RM, Tham KT, et al. Clinical and pathological importance of heterogeneity in vacA, the vacuolating cytotoxin gene of helicobacter pylori. Gastroenterol. 1997;112:92–9.
30. Djekic A, Müller A. The Immunomodulator VacA promotes immune tolerance and persistent heli-

cobacter pylori infection through its activities on T-cells and antigen-presenting cells. Toxins (Basel). 2016;8:E187.
31. Franco AT, Johnston E, Krishna U, et al. Regulation of gastric carcinogenesis by helicobacter pylori virulence factors. Cancer Res. 2008;68:379–87.
32. Nagashima H, Iwatani S, Cruz M, et al. Toll-like receptor 10 in helicobacter pylori infection. J Infect Dis. 2015;212:1666–76.
33. Smith SM. Role of toll-like receptors in helicobacter pylori infection and immunity. World J Gastrointest Pathophysiol. 2014;5:133–46.
34. Smith MF, Mitchell A, Li G, et al. Toll-like receptor (TLR) 2 and TLR5, but not TLR4, are required for helicobacter pylori-induced NF-kappa B activation and chemokine expression by epithelial cells. J Biol Chem. 2003;278:32552–60.
35. Wilson KT, Ramanujam KS, Mobley HL, et al. Helicobacter pylori stimulates inducible nitric oxide synthase expression and activity in a murine macrophage cell line. Gastroenterol. 1996;111:1524–33.
36. Lundgren A, Suri-Payer E, Enarsson K, et al. Helicobacter pylori-specific CD4+ CD25high regulatory T cells suppress memory T-cell responses to H. pylori in infected individuals. Infect Immunol. 2003;71:1755–62.
37. Pincock S. Nobel prize winners Robin Warren and Barry Marshall. Lancet. 2005;366(9495):1429.
38. Marshall BJ, Warren RM. Unidentified curved bacilli in the stomach of patients with gastritis and peptic ulceration. Lancet. 1984;16:1311–5.
39. Marshall BJ. One hundred years of discovery and rediscovery of helicobacter pylori and its association with peptic ulcer disease. In: Mobley HLT, Mendz GL, Hazell SL, editors. Helicobacter pylori: physiology and genetics. Washington, DC: ASM Press; 2001; Chapter 3.
40. Marshall BJ, Armstrong JA, McGechie DB, et al. Glancy RJ. Attempt to fulfill Koch's postulates for pyloric campylobacter. Medical J Australia. 1985;142:436–9.
41. Malfertheiner P, Megraud F, O'Morain CA, et al. European helicobacter study group. Management of Helicobacter pylori infection—the Maastricht IV. Florence Consensus Report Gut. 2012;61:646–64.
42. Gravina AG, Zagari RM, De Musis C, et al. Helicobacter pylori and extragastric diseases: a review. World J Gastroenterol. 2018;24:3204–21.
43. Patel SK, Pratap CB, Jain AK, et al. Diagnosis of helicobacter pylori: what should be the gold standard? World J Gastroenterol. 2014;20:12847–59.
44. Hazell SL, Borody TJ, Gal A, et al. Campylobacter pyloridis gastritis I: detection of urease as a marker of bacterial colonization and gastritis. Am J Gastroenterol. 1987;82:292–6.
45. Wang YK, Kuo FC, Liu CJ, et al. Diagnosis of helicobacter pylori infection: current options and developments. World J Gastroenterol. 2015;21:11221–35.
46. Mégraud F, Bessède E, Lehours P. Current methods used for the diagnosis of helicobacter pylori infection. In: Buzás GM. Eds. Helicobacter pylori - a worldwide perspective 2014. Oak Park: Bentham Science. 2014;2014:234–58.
47. Calvet X, Sánchez-Delgado J, Montserrat A, et al. Accuracy of diagnostic tests for helicobacter pylori: a reappraisal. Clin Infect Dis. 2009;48:1385–91.
48. Redéen S, Petersson F, Törnkrantz E, et al. Reliability of diagnostic tests for helicobacter pylori infection. Gastroenterol Res Pract. 2011;2011:940650.
49. Blanchard TG, Nedrud JG. Laboratory maintenance of Helicobacter species. Curr Protoc Microbiol Feb. 2012;Chapter 8:Unit8B.1.
50. Costamagna G, Zullo A, Bizzotto A, et al. Real-time diagnosis of H. pylori infection during endoscopy: accuracy of an innovative tool (EndoFaster). United European Gastroenterol J. 2016;4:339–42.
51. Ricci C, Holton J, Vaira D. Diagnosis of helicobacter pylori: invasive and non-invasive tests. Best Pract Res Clin Gastroenterol. 2007;21:299–313.
52. Cutler AF, Prasad VM. Long-term follow-up of helicobacter pylori serology after successful eradication. Am J Gastroenterol. 1996;91:85–8.
53. Coelho LG, Sant'Ana CR, Oliveira RB, et al. Performance of the 13C-urea breath test for the diagnosis of H. pylori infection using a substrate synthesized in Brazil: a preliminary study. Clinics (Sao Paulo). 2018;73:e16553.
54. Weingart V, Russmann H, Koletzko S, et al. Sensitivity of a novel stool antigen test for detection of *Helicobacter pylori* in adult outpatients before and after eradication therapy. J Clin Microbiol. 2004;42:1319–21.
55. Shimoyama T. Stool antigen tests for the management of helicobacter pylori infection. World J Gastroenterol. 2013;19:8188–91.
56. Kodama M, Murakami K, Okimoto T, et al. Influence of proton pump inhibitor treatment on helicobacter pylori stool antigen test. World J Gastroenterol. 2012;18:44–8.
57. Gong Y, Li Q, Yuan Y. Accuracy of testing for anti-helicobacter pylori IgG in urine for H. pylori infection diagnosis: a systematic review and meta-analysis. BMJ Open. 2017;7:e013248.
58. Khalifeh Gholi M, Kalali B, Formichella L, et al. Helicobacter pylori FliD protein is a highly sensitive and specific marker for serologic diagnosis of H. pylori infection. Int J Med Microbiol. 2013;303: 618–23.
59. Shukla S, Pujani M, Agarwal A, et al. Correlation of serology with morphological changes in gastric biopsy in helicobacter pylori infection and evaluation of immunohistochemistry for H. pylori identification. Saudi J Gastroenterol. 2012;18:369–74.
60. Batts KP, Ketover S, Kakar S, et al. Appropriate use of special stains for identifying helicobacter pylori. Recommendations from the Rodger C. Haggitt gastrointestinal pathology society. Am J Surg Path. 2013;37:e12–22.
61. Riba AK, Ingeneri TJ, Strand CL. Improved histologic identification of helicobacter pylori by immu-

nohistochemistry using a new Novocastra monoclonal antibody. Lab Med. 2011;42:35–9.
62. Mégraud F, Lehours P. Helicobacter pylori detection and antimicrobial susceptibility testing. Clin Microbiol Rev. 2007;20:280–322.
63. Marshall BJ, Warren JR. Unidentified curved bacilli in the stomach of patients with gastritis and peptic ulceration. Lancet. 1984;1(8390):1311–5.
64. Rocha GA, Queiroz DM, Mendes EN, et al. Simple carbolfuchsin staining for showing C pylori and other spiral bacteria in gastric mucosa. J Clin Path. 1989;42:1004–5.
65. Barbosa AJA, Queiroz DM, Mendes EN, et al. Immunocytochemical identification of campylobacter pylori in gastritis and correlation with culture. Arch Path Lab Med. 1988;112:523–5.
66. Wang XI, Zhang S, Abreo F, et al. The role of routine immunohistochemistry for helicobacter pylori in gastric biopsy. Ann Diag Path. 2010;14:256–9.
67. Jonkers D, Stobberingh E, de Bruine A, et al. Evaluation of immunohistochemistry for the detection of helicobacter pylori in gastric mucosal biopsies. J Infection. 1997;35:149–54.
68. Anim JT, Al-Sobkie N, Prasad A, et al. Assessment of different methods for staining helicobacter pylori in endoscopic gastric biopsies. Acta Histochem. 2000;102:129–37.
69. Hartman DJ, Owens SR. Are routine ancillary stains required to diagnose helicobacter infection in gastric biopsy specimens? An institutional quality assurance review. Am J Clin Pathol. 2012;137:255–60.
70. Sepulveda AR, Patil M. Practical approach to the pathologic diagnosis of gastritis. Arch Pathol Lab Med. 2008;132:1586–93.
71. Boldt MS, Pereira RD, Barbosa AJ. Histological identification of H. pylori stained by hematoxylin-eosin and Giemsa: review for quality control. J Bras Patol Med Lab. 2015;51:108–12.
72. Tajalli R, Nobakht M, Mohammadi-Barzelighi H, et al. The immunohistochemistry and toluidine blue roles for helicobacter pylori detection in patients with gastritis. Iranian Biomed J. 2013;17:36–41.
73. Graham DY, Genta R, Evans DG, et al. Helicobacter pylori does not migrate from the antrum to the corpus in response to omeprazole. Am J Gastroenterol. 1996;91:2120–4.
74. Debongnie JC, Donnay M, Mairesse J, et al. Gastric ulcers and helicobacter heilmannii. Eur J Gastroenterol Hepatol. 1998;10:251–4.
75. Bento-Miranda M, Figueiredo C. Helicobacter heilmannii sensu lato: an overview of the infection in humans. World J Gastroenterol. 2014;20:17779–87.
76. Iwanczak B, Biernat M, Iwanczak F, et al. The clinical aspects of helicobacter heilmannii infection in children with dyspeptic symptoms. J Physiol Pharmacol. 2012;63:133–6.
77. Kubota-Aizawa S, Ohno K, Fukushima K, et al. Epidemiological study of gastric helicobacter spp. in dogs with gastrointestinal disease in Japan and diversity of helicobacter heilmannii sensu stricto. Veterinary J (London, England). 2017;225:56–62.
78. Simmons J, Gibson S. Nonhuman primates in biomedical research, 2nd ed. Chap. 2 in Bacterial and mycotic diseases of nonhuman primates, 2nd ed., Elsevier. Diseases. American College of Laboratory Animal Medicine; 2012. p. 105–172.
79. Amieva MR, El-Omar EM. Host-bacterial interactions in helicobacter pylori infection. Gastroenterol. 2008;134:306–23.
80. Schreiber S, Konradt M, Groll C, et al. The spatial orientation of helicobacter pylori in the gastric mucus. Proc Natl Acad Sci U S A. 2004;101:5024–9.
81. Petersen AM, Krogfelt KA. Helicobacter pylori: an invading microorganism? A review. FEMS Immunol Med Microbiol (Review). 2003;36:117–26.
82. Lowe SE, Pankratz HS, Zeikus JG. Influence of pH extremes on sporulation and ultrastructure of Sarcina ventriculi. J Bacteriol. 1989;171:3775–81.
83. Goodsir J. XXIII: history of a case in which a fluid periodically ejected from the stomach contained vegetable organisms of an undescribed form. J Nat Hist. 1843;11:125–6.
84. Péré-Védrenne C, Flahou B, Loke MF, et al. Other Helicobacters, gastric and gut microbiota. Helicobacter. 2017;22(Suppl 1):e12407.
85. Al Rasheed MRH, Senseng CG. Sarcina ventriculi: review of the literature. Arch Pathol Lab Med. 2016;140:1441–5.

7 Gastritis: Acute, Erosive, Haemorrhagic, Eosinophilic and Phlegmonous Types

Normal number of inflammatory cells present in normal human gastric mucosa is minimum, just a few scattered ones. Defining the number of inflammatory cells present in normal gastric biopsy has been a matter of controversy. Defining precisely the exact number of mononuclear cells present in gastric mucosa is hampered by lack of a universal consensus opinion. Normal number can be influenced by individual's permanent location and the community and observer's impression. Hence, it may be more practical to interpret as the expected number of inflammatory cells to define a normal gastric mucosa [1]. Despite these limitations in defining normal number of inflammatory cells in normal gastric mucosa, the normal number in lamina propria has been described as not more than 2 to 5 lymphocytes with plasma cells and histiocytes per high-power field and in simplified form 2 or 3 lymphocytes or plasma cells in lamina propria between two adjacent foveolae. Plasma cells are sparse or usually do not form a component of the cells visible in normal individual. Presence of plasma cell may be taken as a component of chronic inflammatory process (Fig. 7.1 A and B). Occasionally there may be a few scattered intra-epithelial lymphocytes in normal gastric mucosa, may be up to 5 per 100 epithelial cells [1]. Lymphoid follicle may appear in the deeper mucosa as age-related changes (Fig. 7.2).

Any inflammation of the stomach mucosa is characterized by increased number of inflammatory cells in lamina propria which may be isolatedly only lymphomononuclear cells, i.e. chronic inflammatory cells with or without polymorphonuclear neutrophils. In gastric erosions that may be seen in various situations, there is absence of the surface lining with minimum inflammatory cells and oedema of the lamina propria (Fig. 7.3). The term gastritis is non-specific referring to broad histopathological and topographical spectra of morphological changes that lead to gastric mucosal disease conditions with characterized terminologies. A wide range of terminologies are used for similar looking, morphologically defined mucosal inflammatory changes by different groups of histopathologists worldwide, that have resulted in considerable confusion and misunderstanding [1]. Most common aetiology for gastritis is related to *H. pylori*. The tissue inflammatory response for HP infection is considered to be related to the different strain of the infecting organism. An inflamed mucosal biopsy may reveal variable degree of activity. Presence of activity in a biopsy is indicated by the presence of neutrophils, usually infiltrating lamina propria and epithelial cells of foveolae and the glands (Fig. 7.4 A). Neutrophils are the cells accompanying the destruction of the epithelial cells in HP infection. However, these infiltrating cells may not only be neutrophils but may also be eosinophils and lymphocytes associated with the active destruction of the epithelial cells (Fig. 7.4 B). Usually, the inflammatory cells infiltrating the

K. Vaiphei, *Interpretation of Endoscopic Biopsy - Gastritis, Gastropathies and Beyond*,
https://doi.org/10.1007/978-981-16-6026-9_7

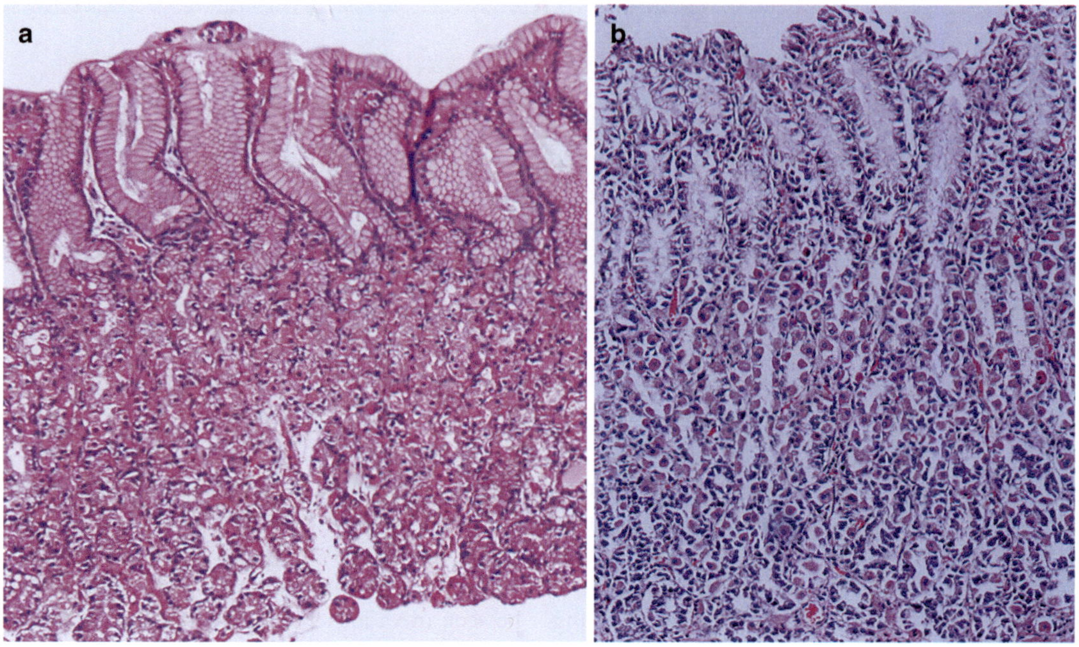

Fig. 7.1 A and B Both the photomicrographs show normal gastric fundic mucosa in HE staining in different magnification

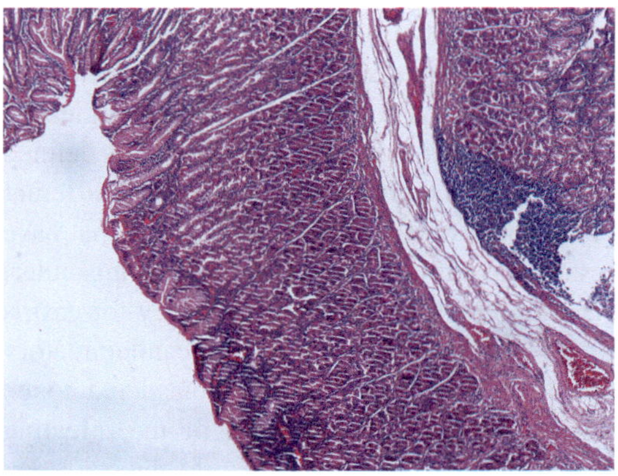

Fig. 7.2 Low-power photomicrograph of gastric mucosa showing the normal mucosal fold covered by the mucosa all around with lymphoid follicle on the deeper aspect of the mucosa (HE, x100)

epithelium and lamina propria are combinations of lymphoplasmacytic mononuclear cells and neutrophils with variable degree of eosinophils (Fig. 7.5 A and B). Histiocytic component is usually sparse. The heavy acute inflammatory cells comprising mainly of neutrophils tends to be associated with neutrophil accumulation forming micro-abscesses within glands and foveolae. The

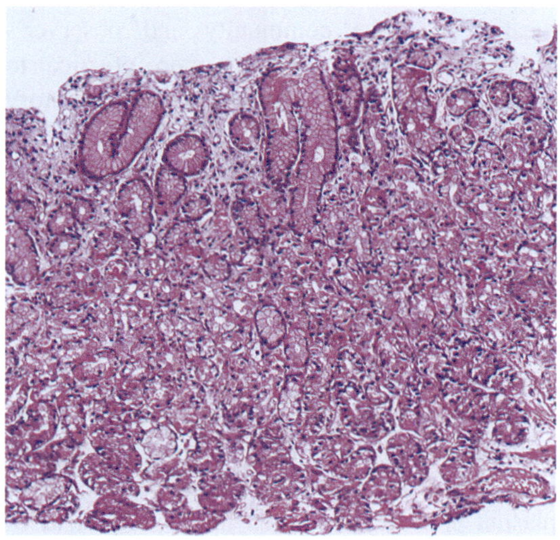

Fig. 7.3 Medium-power photomicrograph of an endoscopic biopsy to show denuded surface lining epithelium of the gastric mucosa, oedematous lamina propria with mild inflammation (HE, x200)

characteristic feature of HP associated longstanding chronic gastritis is indicated by the presence of lymphoid follicles, sometimes with a reactive germinal centre [2] (Fig. 7.6 A and B).

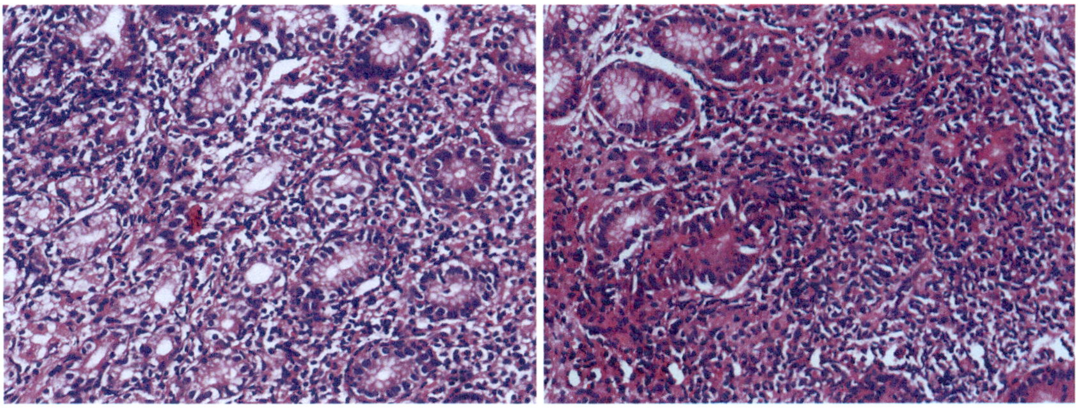

Fig. 7.4 A and B High-power photomicrographs showing gastric mucosa with heavy inflammatory cell infiltration comprising mainly of neutrophils with destruction of gastric glands and epithelial cells (HE, x500)

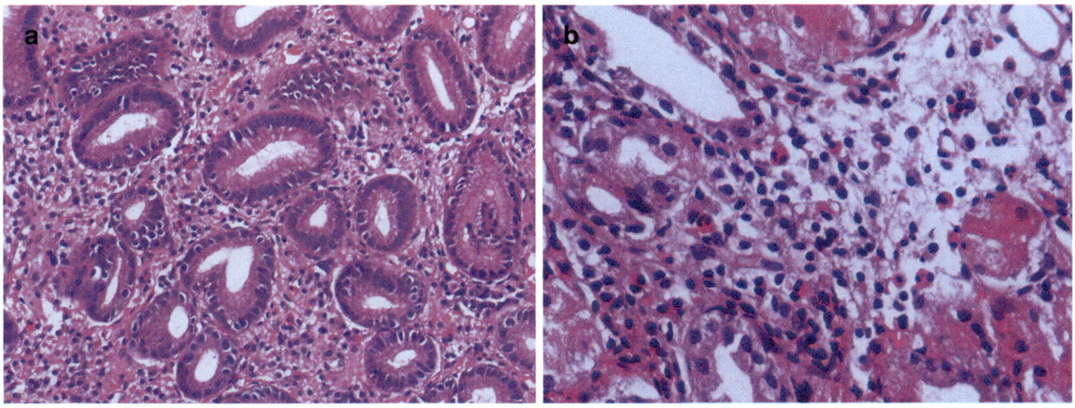

Fig. 7.5 A and B Photomicrographs showing mixed inflammatory cells in lamina propria and glandular epithelium with scattered eosinophils (HE, x500)

Both adaptive and innate types of immune response are stimulated by HP infection. If immunodeficient mice are being infected with *H. felis*, it results in an innate inflammatory cell response independent of the host immune response. This observation suggests that Helicobacters may cause low level of inflammation as such with no immune system activation. The direct effect of HP infection on tissue may play important role in further upregulation of the adaptive immune response [3]. Mononuclear cell infiltration mostly by lymphocytes associates with HP infection in human, accompanied by production of cytokines like interleukin-1b, tumour necrosis factor alpha and interferon gamma [4, 5]. Under certain circumstances the Th1-type response can be changed to a Th2 allergic or anti-inflammatory type with expression of cytokines IL-4 and IL-5. In experimental animals this immunological shift can be achieved with administration of anti-IFN gamma antibodies [6]. In human, *H. pylori* co-infection with intestinal worms has resulted in increased levels of IgE in the blood, and resulted in Th2-mediated IgG1 response [7]. Another group had observed in a group of patients in Colombia had increased eosinophil infiltration in gastric mucosa with *H. pylori* infection related to lesser incidence of malignancy of the stomach but these group of patients had revealed prevalence of intestinal worm infestations [8]. Hence, presence of eosinophils in HP associated mucosal eosinophilia in

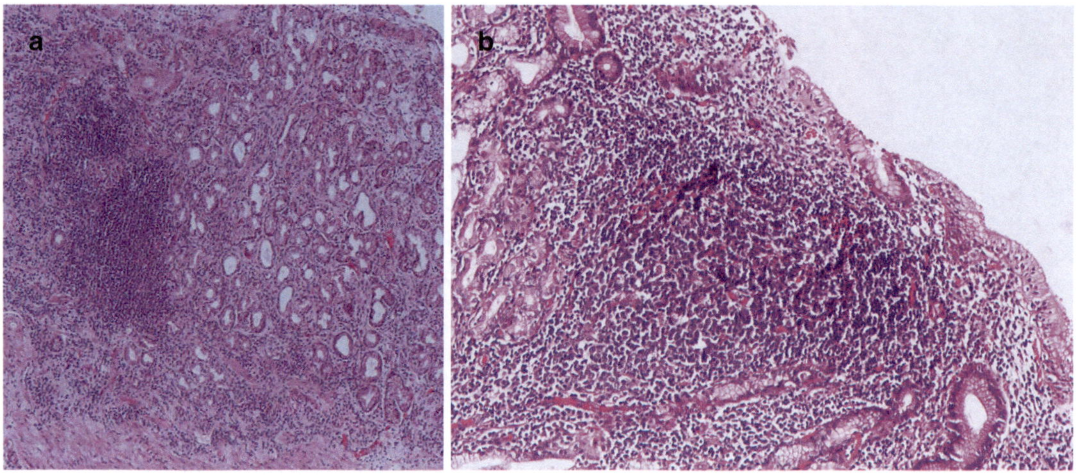

Fig. 7.6 A and B. Photomicrographs showing chronic gastritis with expansion of lamina propria dominantly by lymphoplasmacytic cells with lymphoid follicles indicating long-standing chronic gastritis (HE, x250)

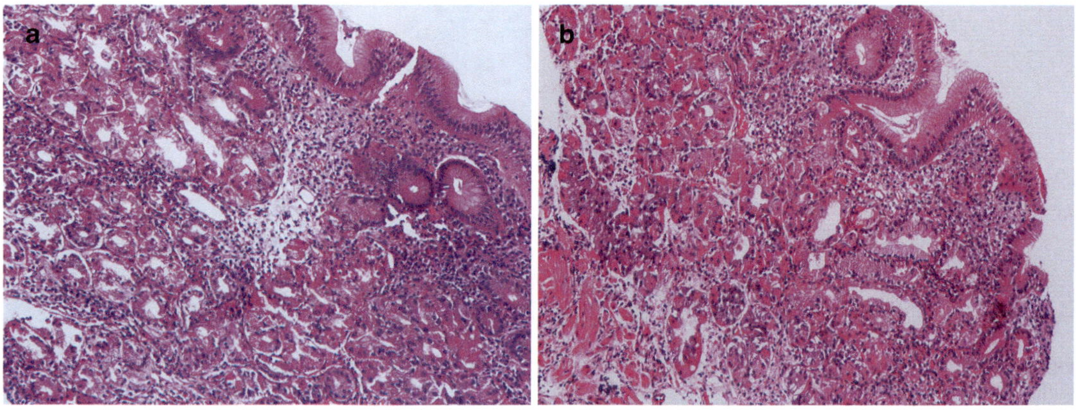

Fig. 7.7 A and B Medium-power photomicrographs of gastric biopsy to show focal aggregates of inflammatory cell collections indicating a focally enhanced inflammation along with lamina propria oedema. However, there is no destruction or loss of glands initial or an early stage of active gastritis (HE, x500)

stomach mucosa may influence T helper cell biasness to produce a protective role in reducing gastric epithelial cell irritation, thereby decreasing cancer development [9].

Mucosal inflammation has been observed to show a decreasing pattern as the infection by HP persists and the initial stage of infection, the virulent organisms target the normal mucosa of the stomach with well-maintained glandular components [10]. The initial stage by definition is an inflamed mucosa with no loss of the glandular component (Fig. 7.7 A and B). The process of progression of gastritis has been documented in a study conducted to analyse the epidemiological model and observed to be influenced by the interplay of three factors, i.e. the causative factor, i.e. infection, the susceptibility depending on the genetic constitution of the host and the epigenetic factors of the surrounding environment [11]. Hence, early-stage gastritis is curable by controlling the causative factor like the HP infection. The exact sequence followed by the inflamed gastric mucosa to the development of atrophic gastritis is not clearly explainable still so far, it may persist as gastritis as such (Fig. 7.8 A and B), or it may evolve into progressively more severe

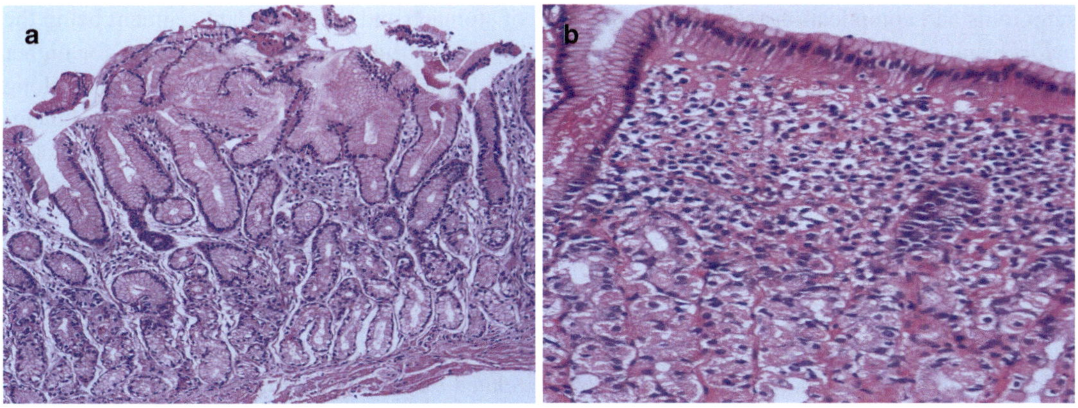

Fig. 7.8 A and B. Mucosal biopsies to show presence of chronic inflammatory cells in lamina propria along with foveolar hyperplasia indicating chronic gastritis with minimal fibrosis or glandular loss (HE, x500)

mucosal pathology associated with destruction of the glandular component resulting in the development of atrophic gastritis. The known determinant factor is the virulent factors of HP. Vac A s1m1 strain of the cag positive organism results in development of precancerous lesion, and persistent of non-atrophic gastritis has been associated with cag negative vac A s2m2 [12]. Individuals who develop duodenal ulcer classically has antral predominant non-atrophic gastritis last for decades. However, these groups of patients do not have increased risk for gastric cancer despite being infected with virulent strains of *H. pylori* [13].

7.1 Acute Gastritis

Acute gastritis covers various entities that induce gastric mucosal inflammation having similar clinical presentation [14]. The inflammation may be diffused involving the entire stomach, e.g. pangastritis, or mainly involving the pyloric antrum. This can have two morphological features—erosive and non-erosive. Erosive may be superficial or deep, or haemorrhagic. Acute gastritis may be associated with both infective and non-infective factors. To name some of the factors are NSAIDs and many other drugs, ethyl alcohol, bile, any condition related to mental stress and shock including traumatic injury, hypotension and ischemic perfusion, radiation, food allergy and poisoning, and infective agents like bacteria, viruses and fungus [15, 16]. Gastritis is believed to be result of imbalance between the factor producing irritation or ischaemia and the gastric mucosal protective factor. These patients present with epigastric discomfort that may be associated with pain, nausea and vomiting. Clinically the patient usually presents with acute sudden onset epigastric pain and the symptomatology may not co-relate with histological findings of endoscopic biopsies. Many patients with histological evidence of erosive gastritis may not have symptom relating to stomach. Greater curvature tends to get the brunt of many ingested agents possibly because of gravity, it gets accumulated and stay long along the dependent portion of the stomach. This explains why irritant induced acute gastritis is frequently observed along the pyloric antrum. One of the known factors responsible in the development of NSAID related gastritis is reduction in prostaglandin synthesis, which is the factor responsible for gastric mucosal protection. Long-standing intake of substances that produces gastric mucosal irritation, inflammation, and destruction of gastric glands, resulting in gastric mucosal atrophy, lamina propria fibrosis, and stricture formation along the gastric outlet passage [16–18].

Bacteria are common aetiological agent for acute gastritis. The common bacteria associated with acute gastritis being the S-shape Gram-negative bacterium *H. pylori*. Various clinical symptoms and complications associated with *H. pylori* result from long-standing persistent infection [19]. Prevalence of HP infection in healthy individual varies widely and is influenced by age of the individual, economic status and part of the world where the individual resides. The infection is usually acquired in childhood. In the Western world, the number of people infected with *H. pylori* increases with age [20–22].

In accordance to Sydney criteria, normal gastric mucosa is pink, smooth and shiny and the pyloric antral part, mucosa becomes flat with one or two roof shaped folds. Regularly arranged parallelly placed mucosal fold diameter in gastric corpus does not exceed 5 mm. These folds get flattened under insufflation with air during endoscopic process. Endoscopic features of mucosal inflammation include oedema, reddening in diffused spots or in red streaks, mucosa becomes friable with slightest injury evokes spot bleeding and mucosa looking mat, there may be spots of exudate or larger in macular shapes, which tends to remain adherent to gastric mucosa during lavage, there may be flat and raised varioliform erosions, mucosal folds may look swollen and thicker or may get flatten due to surrounding oedema, there will be increased vasculature with intramural extravasations, mucosal structure may have areas of nodularity [23].

Erosive gastritis (EG): It is clinical symptomatology that may be attributable to an acute event that can result from exposure to varieties of factors due to damage to mucosal defence mechanism. It is an acute insult that may manifest with upper GI bleed. It may have a milder form of clinical manifestation as a subacute or chronic symptom, usually with a few or no clinical symptom. The diagnosis is established during endoscopic examination of the stomach. Some of the well-known important agents that can produce EG include NSAIDs, alcoholic drinks, cocaine abuse, stress, radiation, bile reflux, infections by microorganisms and viruses, and ischaemia, of which NSAIDs are known to be the commonest aetiological agent. EG may be observed following oral as well as systemic administration [24–26]. NSAIDs effect is associated with the shape of stomach and the redundant segment being the pyloric antrum explaining the reason for higher incidence of involvement of distal stomach along greater curvature, and role of reduced prostaglandin synthesis by NSAIDs cannot be overlooked in EG. Prostaglandins play important role in protection of gastric mucosa from injurious effects of gastric acid [27]. In endoscopic examination, there may be superficial erosions, multiple punctate haemorrhages, ulcer and sometimes perforations [28–30]. The likely mechanism in NSAID related EG will be the resulting from a relatively irritated mucosa having weaken resistance to acid resulting in gastritis, superficial erosion, multiple varying size and depth ulcers, some of which may be bleeding which may led on to perforation [31]. These patients may present with dyspepsia, nausea and vomiting [32]. No co-relationship has been found between the clinical symptomatology and amount and duration of drug intake and endoscopic severity of mucosal damage. Hence, one needs to be aware of the seriousness of random use of NSAIDs to prevent un-expected gastric complications [25].

The morphological changes are visible after about 12 hours of exposure to the inciting agent. Erosion has been defined as mucosal defects having significant depth of at least 3 mm and less than 3 mm, respectively. Histologically erosions may be observed in acute injury and also in chronic mucosal inflammation. In acute erosive gastritis, there is denudation or absence of gastric mucosal lining epithelium, which may be diffuse involving the whole surface area of a particular biopsy fragment or may be patchy and multiple foci involving multiple mucosal fragments in a given biopsy. These features of erosive gastritis may be observed in association with bile reflux gastritis [33–36]. There mucosal lesions usually have lesser amount of inflammatory cell response, varying degree of mucosal oedema and prominence of the mucosal small blood vessels which may appear as telangiectatic area in endoscopic examination (Fig. 7.9 A and B). In addition, under the microscope, there may be foveolar hyperplasia and increased number of smooth muscle fibres splaying into the mucosa in between

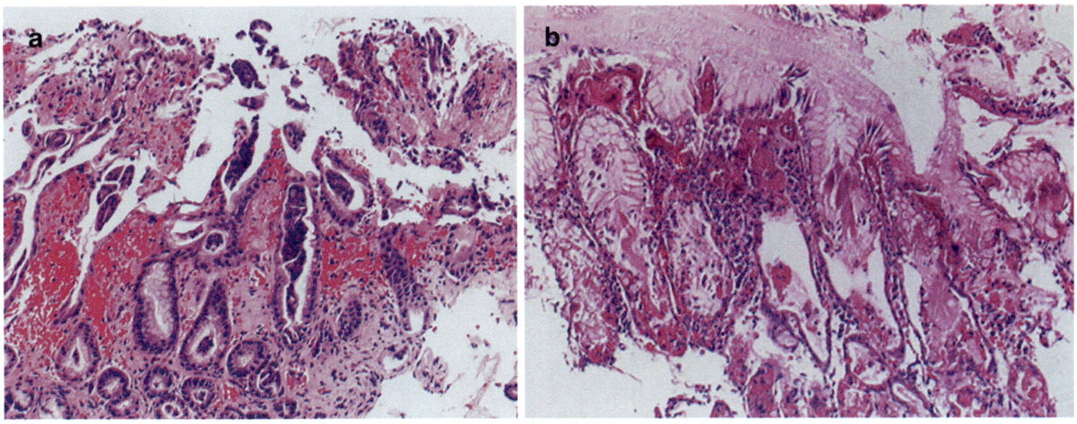

Fig. 7.9 A and B. Photomicrographs of gastric biopsies sampled from mucosal haemorrhagic areas showing mucosal erosions, shedding off epithelial cells, lamina propria haemorrhages oedema and fibrin deposition with sparse inflammatory cell response. In addition, Fig. 7.9 B shows mucodepleted and degenerated glandular lining epithelial cells and excess amount of mucous along the surface (HE, x300)

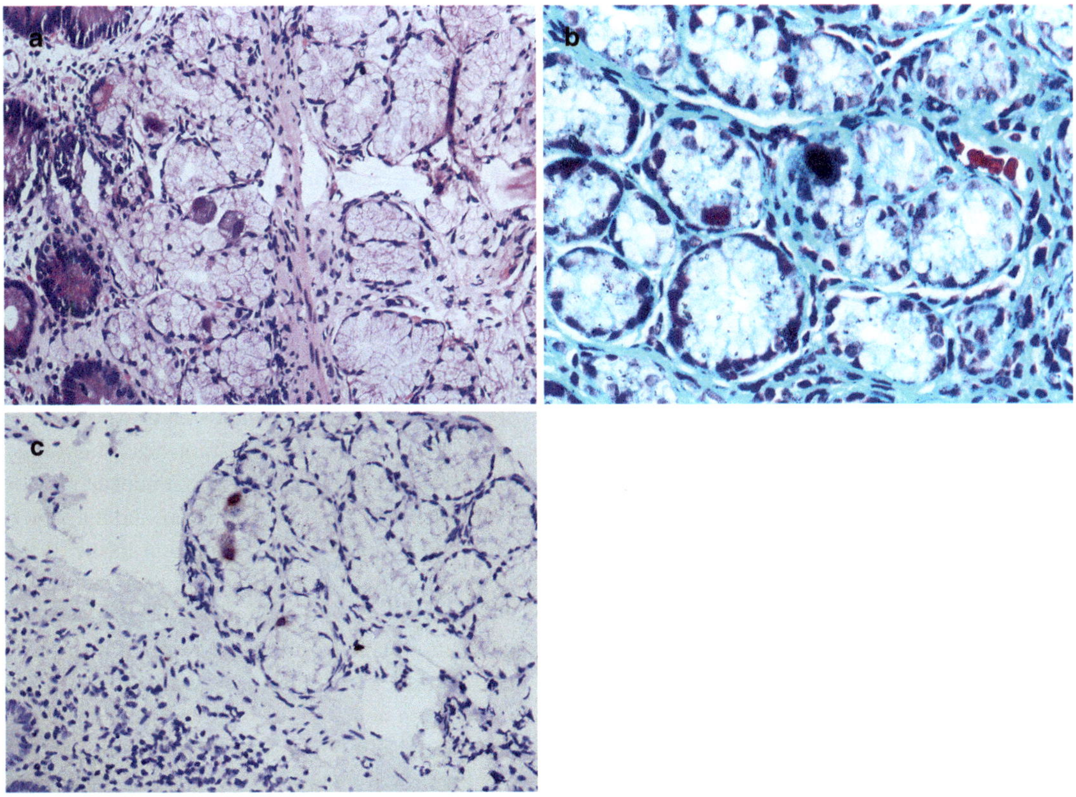

Fig. 7.10 A, B, and C. High-power micrograph of pyloric antral biopsy to show cytomegaly changes in the infected epithelial cells of the mucus glands along with nucleomegaly in different stainings—HE, Masson's trichrome and immunohistochemistry using primary antibody against Cytomegalovirus

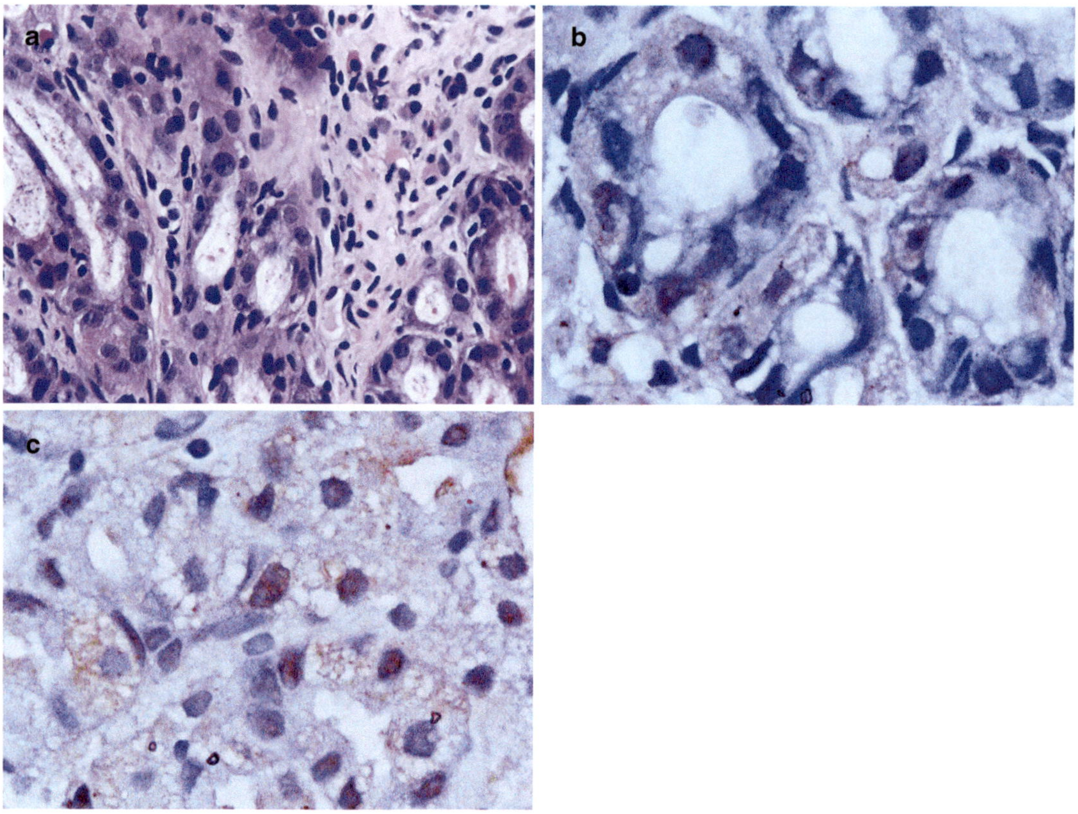

Fig. 7.11 A: High-power photomicrographs of gastric body biopsy showing mucosa inflammation and lamina propria fine fibrosis and epithelial cells showing enlarge smudgy and hyperchromatic nuclei (HE, x300). B and C: high-power photomicrographs of immunostained sections using primary antibodies against herpes simplex virus type 1 and 2 respectively, showing positively stained nuclei in both the pictures (peroxidase anti-peroxidase, x300)

the hyperplastic foveolae especially in chronic cases. Inflammatory cell response may be variable, almost negligible to mild to moderate inflammatory cells usually neutrophils, occasional scattered eosinophil, depending on the injurious agent. There may be a thin layer of neutrophilic exudate overlying the denuded area. Depending upon the time gap between the event of injury and time of biopsy, epithelial cells along the surface and foveolae may start showing features of regeneration. Erosions in chronic inflammatory condition, erosion site will be formed by chronic inflammatory cells with or without lamina propria fibrosis. Erosions in such situation possibly are related to tissue handling as an inflamed mucosa will be more friable than a normal mucosa. As the result of trauma induced by the endoscopic procedure, there may be fresh lamina propria haemorrhages. Artefactual fragmentation of the gastric glands and foveolae may also be identified on routine biopsies. In contrast to erosions, ulcers are deeper mucosal gap or dehiscence with definite fibrinous exudate, which may be associated with granulation tissue along the ulcer bed. An interesting study carried out by El-Zimaity et al. who observed NSAIDs induced gastric injuries to be patchy and similar in appearances to infective and reflux gastritis [37, 38].

The term acute gastritis should be selectively used for those biopsies where there is no associated features for chronic gastritis and should be distinguished from a biopsy exhibiting active inflammation in the background of chronic gastritis (Figs. 7.4 A, B and 7.7 A, B). It may be a localized disease involving the pyloric antrum or body and fundus, or a pangastritis or diffuse erosive gastritis. Amount and extent of inflammation may be variable, associated with destruction of epithelial cells and gastric glands which may also be referred as apoptotic bodies, affecting dominantly superficial mucosa with congestion and oedema associated with extravasated red blood cells. These changes are to be differentiated from paucity of glands in atrophic gastritis. Bacterial infection can also result in acute gastritis, HP being the most common one. Detection rate of HP in such mucosa varies grossly across the globe, depends on various epidemiological factors and demographic location. Infection is usually acquired in childhood in endemic countries. *H. pylori* gastritis usually involves the stomach as an acute gastritis localizing to antrum to begin with, which may extend to more proximal compartment. An early-stage infection may be clinically silent. In long-standing cases, a biopsy may show features of chronic gastritis. *H. pylori* remains entangled in mucus layer and protects itself from exposing to the acid content of the stomach. HP produces large amount of urease which is enough to catalyse urea to alkaline ammonia and carbon dioxide. This flagellate organism moves by penetrating the mucus layer coming in contact with gastric surface epithelium and remains adherent by means of its adhesion molecules. This whole process incites inflammation producing cytokines and other inflammatory mediators resulting in accumulation of neutrophils and lymphocytes causing acute gastritis. Infection is established within a few days to weeks. Extent and severity of gastritis in HP infection is determined by its virulence [1, 16, 17, 21, 22].

Acute erosive gastritis may also be the result of viral infections. Viruses that may be observed are—Cytomegalovirus (Fig. 7.7 A-C), Herpes group of viruses (Fig. 7.9 A-C), Adenoviruses or Epstein–Barr virus [39–41]. These viruses tend to infect the gastric epithelial cells. In HE stain section, one may be able to identify or suspect the possibility of infection by one of these viruses from the nuclear and cytoplasmic appearances. In presence of an ulcerating lesion, endothelial cells and proliferating myofibroblast may show evidence of viral inclusion. Type of virus may be further confirmed by immunohistochemistry. These infections are frequently identified in immunocompromised individuals like post-transplant individuals, AIDs, cancer patients. Gastric involvement may be localized or systematic, may be associated with mucosal erosions and ulcerations [39–41].

Fungi that may produce gastritis include *Candida albicans* and histoplasmosis. Mucormycosis tends to involve the mucosa with infarction and necrosis. With the morphological changes of gastritis if mucormycosis is identified in routine endoscopic biopsy, it may be a superadded infection (Fig. 7.12 A and B). Otherwise

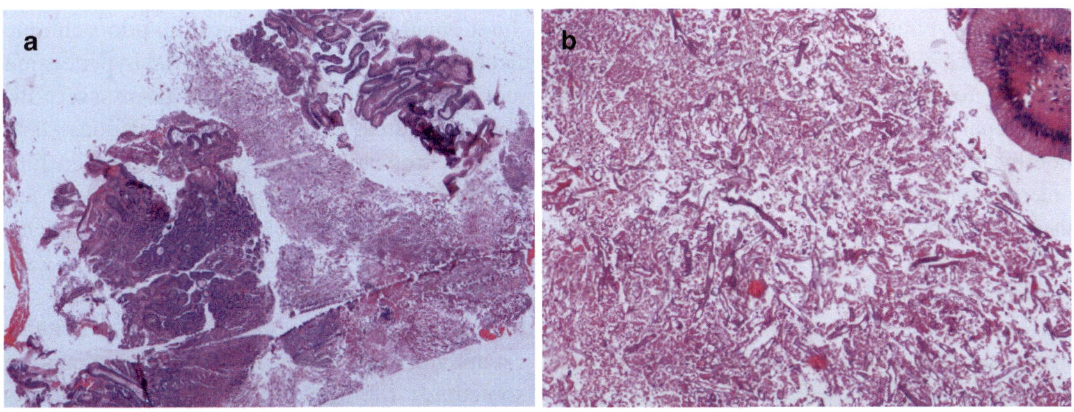

Fig. 7.12 A: Photomicrographs of gastric biopsy taken from grossly discoloured and thicken mucosal folds show changes of hyperplastic gastric mucosal fragments with a lightly stained fragment of tissue (HE, x250)' B: on higher power, the lighter fragment is comprising of necrotic material along with varying sized broad dominantly aseptate and right angled branched fungal profile conforming to the morphology of mucormycosis (HE, x500)

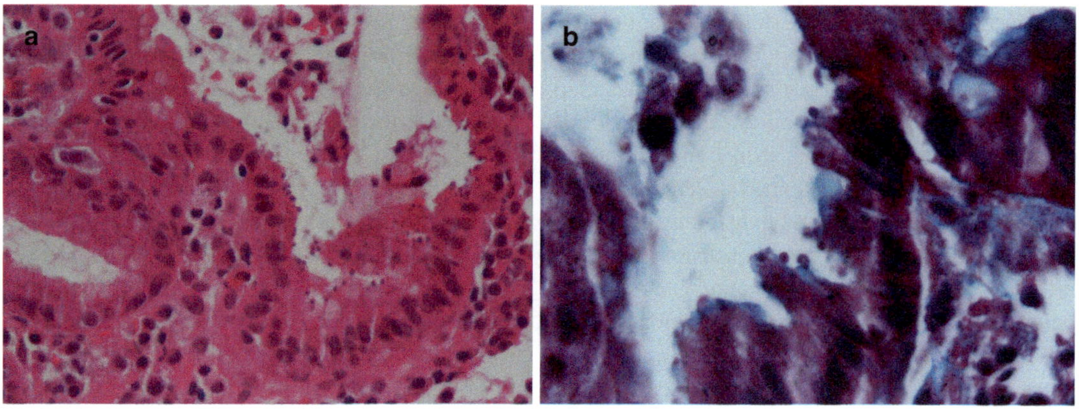

Fig. 7.13 A: high-power photomicrograph of an endoscopic gastric mucosal piece showing features of chronic gastritis with many round lightly basophilic bodies (size of 3 to 5 micron) attached along the surface epithelium (HE, x1000); B: these bodies are highlighted better in MT staining seen as intracellular however extra-cytoplasmic (MT, x1000)

mucormycosis along with Aspergillus are angioinvasive, produce mucosal or transmural infarction and necrosis, and are a part of disseminated disease [42, 43]. Disseminated histoplasmosis can involve the gastrointestinal tract, however, mainly involving the small and large intestine in an immunocompromised setting [44]. These patients' common presenting symptoms were related to gastric erosions and ulcers, that may be associated with upper GL bleed. Primary fungal infection is seldom encountered, majority of the cases are terminally ill patients or immunocompromised individuals. Similarly, parasitic infestation rarely causes gastritis. In Anisakidosis, the nematode remains entrapped within gastric mucosa involving the dependent portion of the stomach. This infection is a result of consuming infected food and raw fish resulting in severe abdominal pain. Like any other organisms, infection by this nematode also results in oedema of mucosal fold, erosion and ulcer [45, 46]. Rarely, there could be infection by cryptosporidium as well, which can be the primary aetiology for the gastritis or can be a superadded infection in a primary gastric lymphoma or an opportunistic infection in an immunocompromised individual. The one present within the cell membrane but extra-cytoplasm are trophozoite form which does not have the property of acid fastness, the cyst form which are usually freely present within the lumen of GIT are the ones with the property of acid fastness. In routine practice, they can be easily identifiable in HE as well as in Masson's trichrome staining (Fig. 7.13 A, and B).

7.2 Acute Haemorrhagic Gastritis

In individuals who presents with upper gastrointestinal bleeding, endoscopic studies have documented the common underlying aetiology to be acute haemorrhagic gastritis [47, 48]. Most of these patients who presents with upper GI bleed usually give history of intake of painkillers of any duration, impulsive alcohol consumption, chronic liver disease with evidence of portal hypertension and undue stress like suffering from severe illness or trauma. Endoscopic examinations show multiple petechial haemorrhages mostly in fundus and body that may appear as beefy red mucosa due to diffuse mucosal haemorrhages. The endoscopic appearances are similar to gastric mucosal injury associated with intake of painkillers and other gastric mucosal irritants except for the location. This condition may be sometimes life-threatening requiring an emergency gastrectomy [49, 50]. The close differential diagnosis will be Phlegmonous gastritis. Acute haemorrhagic gastritis is characterized by many endoscopic and gross features involving the gastric mucosa which may range from hyperaemia and oedema to erosions and ulcers, and all these lesions may be associated with variable degree of active mucosal bleeding [51]. Histologically this condition may have similar features to acute erosive gastritis with large areas of haemorrhages and congestion with tissue necrosis. Depending upon the time of the biopsy observed under the microscope, there may be variable amounts of inflammatory cells dominantly neutrophils. Surface erosions or ulceration with fibrin rich exudate may also be present [52–54] (Fig. 7.9 A and B).

7.3 Eosinophil Rich Acute Gastritis

An endoscopic gastric biopsy in a patient who presented with clinical features of acute gastritis may show excess of eosinophils in the gastric biopsy. Hence, evidence of eosinophilic gastritis or excess of eosinophils in lamina propria in an endoscopic gastric biopsy may not be an uncommon observation [54]. This condition may also be seen in infants and children. This may also be a part of systemic disorder like eosinophilic gastroenteritis and more commonly it may have underlying disorders of collagen vascular diseases, intolerance to certain dietary component like milk and other proteins, parasitic infestations, many drugs and *H. pylori* infections. In collagen vascular disorder, there may be small vessel vasculitis involving capillaries and venules located within the muscularis mucosae (Fig. 7.13 A – C). Sometimes, an adult worm or egg of a parasite may be present in the mucosal biopsy. In a limited sample like in an endoscopic biopsy, a diagnosis of eosinophilic gastroenteritis may be a difficult diagnosis as it is a disease which tends to involve full thickness of the gut wall. Furthermore, number of eosinophils present in the lamina propria, within and outside the gastric glands may not be the soul criteria to make the diagnosis, though in eosinophilic gastroenteritis, infiltrate may be heavier, it may also be mixed with variable components of lymphomononuclear cells and activity in the form of infiltration of the gastric glands resulting in degenerative changes in epithelial cells [53–55]. But all said and done, an eosinophil rich gastric biopsy, possibility of *H. pylori* infection or drug-induced gastritis or remotely possibility of parasitic infestation need to be excluded first before entertaining a diagnosis of eosinophilic gastroenteritis [51, 53, 54].

Eosinophilic gastritis is a condition in which there are predominant eosinophils amongst the inflammatory cells infiltrating the gastric mucosa and the muscular wall without any definite known underlying aetiological condition [55, 56]. An isolated involvement of the stomach is rarely observed in clinical practice; it is frequently seen along with similar cellular infiltration of immediate adjacent organs like duodenum, oesophagus and any portion of the intestine. When there is involvement of the various segments of the GIT, the term used to refer this condition is eosinophilic gastroenteritis [55–57]. In day-to-day routine practice, variable number of eosinophils is usually seen to be present along with the other inflammatory cells and a diagnosis of eosinophilic gastritis supposedly not suitable to offer in such situation. There are numerous studies where different numbers of eosinophils have been proposed to qualify for the diagnosis of eosinophilic gastroenteritis. Lwin et al. in 2011 [55] studied number of eosinophils in normal gastric mucosal biopsies including conditions where there is increase in tissue eosinophils in the biopsies sampled from stomach. Depending upon the observations made by them, diagnostic criteria had been proposed as follows, i.e. any individual having an average of >127 eosinophils per mm2 (or $\geq$ 30 eosinophils per HPF in microscopes with wide ocular lens) having no known underlying aetiology for eosinophilia [55]. Normally except oesophagus, scattered eosinophils are identifiable in routine biopsies [58]. Three years later in the year 2014, Collins [59] made another proposal: i) stomach: greater than or equal to 30 eosinophils per high-power field in 5 HPF; ii) duodenum: greater than or equal to 30 eosinophils; iii) ileum: more than 56 per HPF in the ileum; iv) right colon: more than 100 per HPF; v) transverse and descending colon: more than 84 per HPF and vi) rectosigmoid colon: more than 64 per HPF. These studies were carried out in attempts to bring out uniformity in the biopsy interpretation of the endoscopic mucosal biopsies of the gastrointestinal tract [57–60]. Interpretation of the involvement will depend upon extent of involvement of segment of GIT and extent of involvement of the layers of the gut wall, i.e. mucosal, submucosal, mural and transmural. In stomach, it has been observed that limited involvement of the mucosa possibly is most frequent, and involvement of the muscular and serosal layers is less frequently documented [60]. Patient clinical presentation is usually related to the site, level and extent of involvement. Gastric mucosal involvement may present like any other condition that give rise to gastritis and the non-specific symptoms may include upper GI haemorrhage, dyspeptic symptoms, whereas if there is infiltrative involvement of the gastric wall, patient may have features of outlet obstruction with mural thickening. When the infiltration extends to serosal layer, there may be ascites rich in eosinophils. The underlying aetiology for this condition is still undefined, possibly may be related to an underlying allergic condition. Frequently these individuals give history of atopy and may be with the involvement of eotaxin-1 [58–60]. Reduction in the disease symptomatology has been sometimes associated with changing in the components of food. These patients have also been found to have mast cell degranulation in tissue specimens, blood eosinophilia and family history of atopy [57, 58]. Some patients have also been found to have high serum IgE levels [59–61].

7.4 Phlegmonous Gastritis or Acute Bacterial Gastritis

Phlegmonous gastritis (PG) is an uncommon condition where there is recent onset bacterial infection involving primarily submucosa, though may extend to involve gastric muscular wall, rarely mucosa may also be involved. In spite of the disease being primarily a non-mucosal condition, the term gastritis still holds true for this particular condition. It is a difficult diagnosis to entertain in endoscopic biopsy; however, a suggestion may be put forward. It is a condition that progresses aggressively and clinical this condition is seldom considered in one of the differentials, and the diagnosis is confirmed at laparotomy or at autopsy. It possibly might have been more common in the past or in the pre-antibiotic era. This condition was first described by Cruveilhier' in 1862 [62]. Many years later, Sundberg in 1919 wrote a review article based on 215 cases [63]. Since then, there has been single case reports continued approximately one per year. The term phlegmonous has been continued to use and it refers to a condition where there is rapid and progressive extension of the inflammatory condition from stomach transmurally to adjoining other soft tissue structures. It is a fatal condition if left untreated [64]. Hence, a prompt diagnosis is important for the effective management. This condition usually occurs in middle-aged population with male predominance. Though exact underlying aetiology is still unknown, it has been seen in patients with prolonged illness like malignancy, post chemotherapy with neutropenia, acquired immunodeficiency syndrome, alcoholism with chronic alcoholic liver disease [65, 66]. This is exceedingly rare and most of the reported cases were diagnosed post-mortem. Common organisms that have been associated with this fatal condition are both Gram-positive and Gram-negative organisms [64, 65].

Grossly, the stomach has very characteristic bogy appearance with thicken gastric wall, mucosa may appear normal, pale or nodular with discolouration. Mucosal ulceration and perforation, though may be present, are relatively uncommon. This may involve the whole stomach or may dominantly involve a segment, may appear grossly discoloured giving an appearance of ischaemic aetiology. Clinical diagnosis may be established in vivo during the process of emergency laparotomy as these patients have severe pain in abdomen associated with bloodstained vomitus [66]. If left unattended with no emergency treatment, the patient may develop peritonitis and septicaemia [67]. In a chronically ill patient, the serosa tends to be slimy due to mucinous degeneration of serosal fat which may be seen as fat necrosis in histology. Cutting through the wall, which may be discoloured and congested, the submucosal collection may be seen better or there may be purulent exudate, flowing out through the cut end [68, 69]. On histological examination, the inflammatory process will be dominantly seen involving the submucosa, involvement of mucosa and muscle layer will be variable. There will be extensive necrotizing inflammation, necrosis of the collagen, muscle, blood vessels and fat with neutrophilic infiltration [66–70] (Fig. 7.14 A–C). In untreated virgin patient, bacterial colony may be identified. If identified, further special staining to be carried out to subtype the organism. It is essential to exclude presence of fungal profile as well. To be noted at this point is that though the condition is seen in a neutropenic individual, the inflammatory exudate tends to be rich in neutrophils mixed with fibrin. Due to involvement of the submucosal blood vessels, haemorrhagic component may sometimes be a prominent feature overshadowing the inflammatory component simulating an ischaemic aetiology. The involved blood vessels may contain fibrin thrombi and inflammatory cell infiltration of the vessel wall mimicking a diagnosis of vasculitis. In such situation, best practice will be a vigilant approach beginning from tissue sampling, making efforts to have multiple site sampling including the less involved areas and examining critically all the sections so that a definitive diagnosis of PG be established by differentiating from other close differential diagnosis. The gross finding of the specimen and also

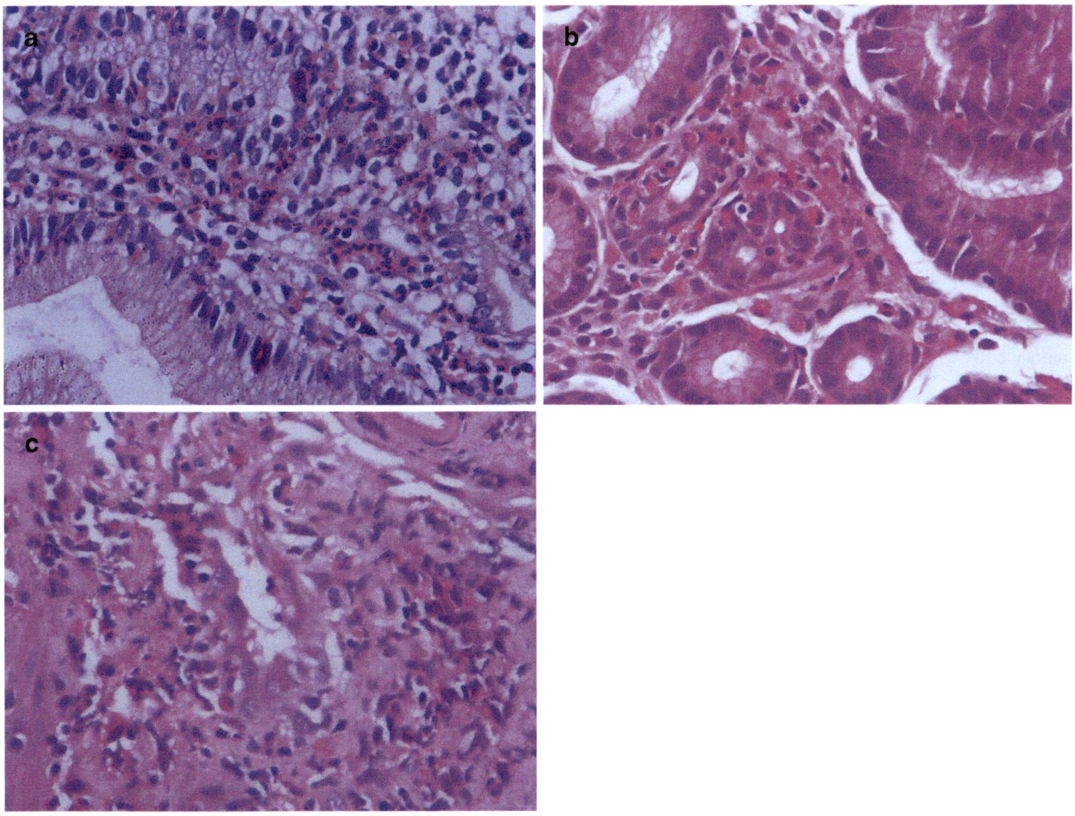

Fig. 7.14 A + B: high-power photomicrographs of gastric biopsy mucosal fragments showing moderate to heavy lamina propria inflammatory cells including many eosinophils in small aggregates and infiltrating and destroying the epithelial cells (HE, x500); C: a high-power photomicrograph of an endoscopic biopsy of stomach from mucosal ulcer showing evidence small vessel vasculitis as indicated by swollen endothelial cells and infiltration by inflammatory cells including many eosinophils (HE, x500)

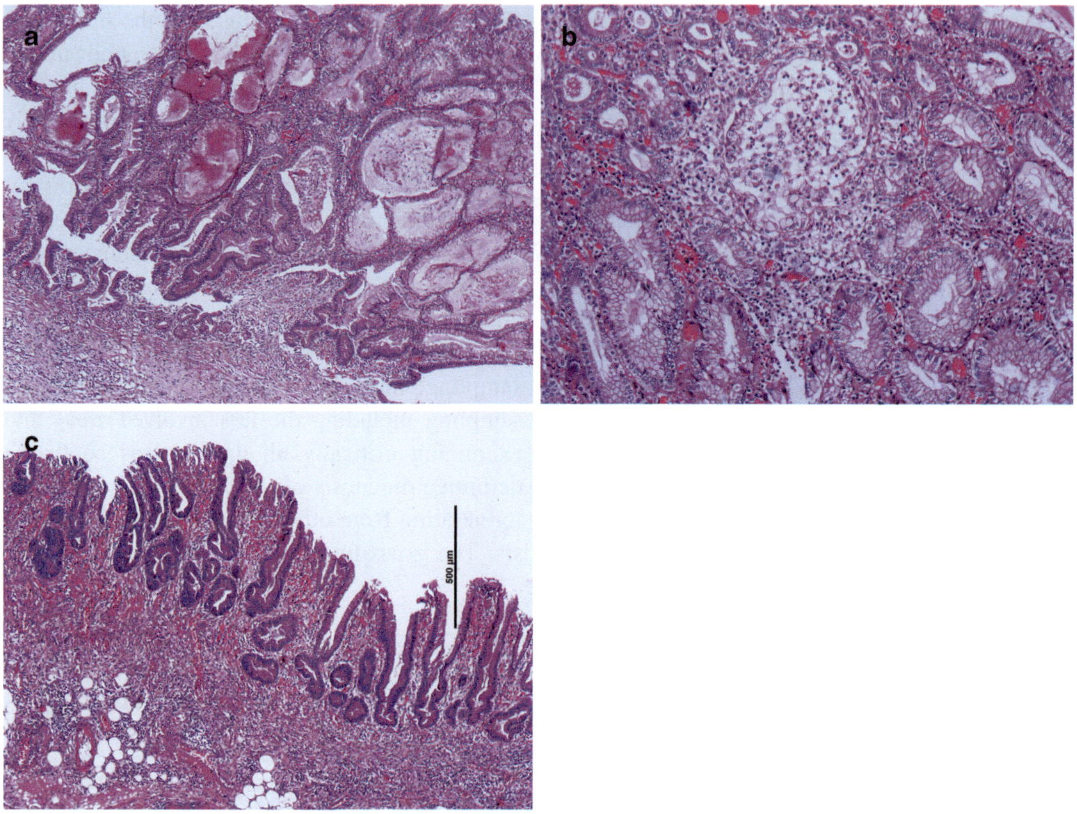

Fig. 7.15 A: a low-power view of grossly hyperplastic gastric mucosa with marked foveolar hyperplasia and heavy neutrophil infiltration in the mucosa with features qualify for crypt abscesses (HE, x250); B: The same are shown in A in high power to bring out the type of inflammatory cells which are mainly of neutrophils (HE, x500); C – a view of the adjoining area where mucosa is largely friable as indicated by friability and mucodepleted epithelial cells due to inflammation and regeneration, and heavy inflammatory cells in lamina propria and submucosa (HE, x500)

the clinical background should be taken into consideration. In addition to the above-mentioned situations where PG may be observed, it may also occur following a direct injury to the gastric mucosa by trauma, primary gastric cancer or following endoscopic interventions, which may be the primary aetiology for the direct microbial invasion. Sometimes, it may also be the result of infections present in the neighbouring organs such as infected pancreatic pseudocyst, liver abscess or fulminant acute cholecystitis [67–72].

The real practical challenge to establish a diagnosis of PG is in endoscopic biopsies with limited or non-specific endoscopic description [67]. The pathologist may casually written off the report with the diagnosis of a non-specific inflammation of gastric biopsy, similar to any other active/acute or chronic active gastritis, mentioning no *H. pylori* seen. However, it is important to pay attention to the extent and location of the inflammation. In multiple fragment endoscopic biopsy, it is essential to examine every bit. In PG, though there be areas of mucosal ulceration covered by exudates, but the inflammation will be located more in the deeper aspect of the mucosa, which may be associated with variable degree of lamina propria fibrosis, oedema, haemorrhages and rarely vascular changes [68] (Fig. 7.15 A-C). There will be definitely oddities for a diagnosis of conventional gastritis. Best is to suggest the possibility and to correlate with other investigations and clinical profiles. Clinical symptomatology is non-specific. In order to establish a diagnosis of PG in patients who are already sick and immunocompromised might be a difficult challenge clinically, however awareness and high index of suspicion may help to establish the diagnosis [70]. Patient's dominant clinical presentation localized to epigastric region may be a helpful clue associated with recent onset fever, nausea and vomiting. Less common symptoms are diarrhoea and Haematemesis. PG may be considered in the differential diagnosis if the radiology reveals grossly thicken gastric wall accompanied by low-intensity areas, and sometimes in a few cases, it may be associated with gas accumulation within the thickened gastric wall [69].

References

1. Dixon MF, Genta R, Yardley J, et al. Classification and grading of gastritis: the updated Sydney system. Am J Surg Pathol. 1996;20:1161–81.
2. Correa P, Piazuelo MB. The gastric precancerous cascade. J Dig Dis. 2012;13:2–9.
3. Blanchard TG, Czinn SJ, Nedrud JG, et al. Redline RW. Helicobacter-associated gastritis in SCID mice. Infect Immunol. 1995;63:1113–5.
4. Blanchard TG, Czinn SJ. Review article: immunological determinants that may affect the helicobacter pylori cancer risk. Alim Pharmacol Ther. 1998;12(Suppl 1):83–90.
5. Chmiela M, Kupcinskas J. Review: pathogenesis of helicobacter pylori infection. Helicobacter. 2019;24(Suppl. 1):e12638.
6. Reinfein Z, Cheng G, Liuhua W, et al. Involvement of aryl hydrocarbon receptor and aryl hydrocarbon receptor repressor in helicobacter pylori-related gastric pathogenesis. J Cancer. 2018;9:2757–64.
7. Whary MT, Sundina N, Bravo LE, et al. Intestinal helminthiasis in Colombian children promotes a Th2 response to helicobacter pylori: possible implications for gastric carcinogenesis. Cancer Epidemiol Biomark Prev. 2005;14:1464–9.
8. Piazuelo MB, Camargo MC, Mera RM, et al. Eosinophils and mast cells in chronic gastritis: possible implications in carcinogenesis. Hum Pathol. 2008;39:1360–9.
9. Makristathis A, Hirschl AM, Mégraud F et al (2019) Review: diagnosis of helicobacter pylori infection. Helicobacter 24 (Suppl 1):e12641.
10. Lehours P, Ferrero RL. Review: helicobacter: inflammation, immunology, and vaccines. Helicobacter. 2019;24(Suppl1):e12644.
11. Wroblewski LE, Peek RM Jr, Wilson KT. Helicobacter pylori and gastric cancer: factors that modulate disease risk. Clin Microbiol Rev. 2010;23:713–39.
12. Camargo MC, Figueiredo C, Machado JC. Review: gastric malignancies: basic aspects. Helicobacter. 2019;24(Suppl 1):e12642.
13. Uemura N, Okamoto S, Yamamoto S, et al. Helicobacter pylori infection and the development of gastric cancer. N Engl J Med. 2001;345:784–9.
14. Andersen LP. Colonization and infection by helicobacter pylori in humans. Helicobacter. 2007;12(Suppl 2):12–5.
15. Ali Khan M, Howden CW. The role of proton pump inhibitors in the management of upper gastrointestinal disorders. Gastroenterol Hepatol (N Y). 2018;14:169–75.
16. Frezza M, Gorji N, Melato M. The histopathology of non-steroidal anti-inflammatory drug induced gastroduodenal damage: correlation with helicobacter pylori, ulcers, and haemorrhagic events. J Clin Pathol. 2001;54:521–5.
17. Haber MM, Lopez I. Gastric histologic findings in patients with nonsteroidal anti-inflammatory drug-associated gastric ulcer. Mod Pathol. 1999;12:592–8.
18. Srivastava A, Lauwers GY. Pathology of non-infective gastritis. Histopathol. 2007;50:15–29.
19. Boltin D, Niv Y, Schütte K, Schulz C. Review: helicobacter pylori and non-malignant upper gastrointestinal diseases. Helicobacter. 2019;24(Suppl1):e12637.
20. Chmiela M, Kupcinskas J. Review: pathogenesis of helicobacter pylori infection. Helicobacter. 2019;24(Suppl 1):e12638.
21. Andersen LP. Colonization and infection by helicobacter pylori in humans. Helicobacter. 2007;12(Suppl 2):12–5.
22. Suerbaum S, Michetti P. Helicobacter pylori infection. N Engl J Med. 2002;347:1175–85.
23. Misiewicz JJ, Tytgat GNJ, Goodwin CS et al (1990) The Sydney System: a new classification of gastritis. Working Party Reports, Sydney: Ninth World Congress of Gastroenterology. pp 1–10.
24. Graumlich JF. Preventing gastrointestinal complications of NSAIDs. Postgrad Med. 2001;109(117–120):123–8.
25. Byrd DC. NSAID-induced gastropathy: prevention and treatment strategies. Pharm Times. 1999;65:44–50.
26. Wolfe MM, Lichtenstein DR, Singh G. Gastrointestinal toxicity of nonsteroidal anti-inflammatory drugs. N Engl J Med. 1999;340:1889–99.
27. Schoen RT, Vender RJ. Mechanisms of nonsteroidal anti-inflammatory drug- induced gastric damage. Am J Med. 1989;86:449–58.
28. McCarthy DM. Nonsteroid anti-inflammatory drugs - the clinical dilemmas. Scand J Gastroenterol. 1992;192(suppl):9–16.
29. Mohammed S, Croom DW II. Gastropathy due to celecoxib, a cyclooxygenase-2 inhibitor. N Engl J Med. 2006;340:2005–6.

30. Henry D, Lim LL-Y, Rodríguez LA, et al. Variability in risk of gastrointestinal complications with individual non-steroidal anti-inflammatory drugs: results of a collaborative meta-analysis. BMJ. 1996;312: 1563–6.
31. U.S. Department of Health and Human Services (1992) Harmful effects of medicines on the adult digestive system. NIH Publication No. 97–3421.
32. Fuller SH, McKenzie C (1992) Gastropathy. US Pharmacist 17:35–36,41-42,47-48,53-55,87.
33. Taha AS, Nakshabendi I, Lee FD, et al. Chemical gastritis and helicobacter pylori related gastritis in patients receiving non-steroidal anti-inflammatory drugs: comparison and correlation with peptic ulceration. J Clin Pathol. 1992;45:135–9.
34. Dixon MF, O'Connor HJ, Axon ATR, et al. Reflux gastritis: distinct histopathological entity? J Clin Pathol. 1986;39:524–30.
35. Ouinn M, Bjarnason I, Price AB. Gastritis in patients on nonsteroidal anti-inflammatory drugs. Histopathol. 1993;23:341–8.
36. Sobala GM, King RFG, Axon ATR, et al. Reflux gastritis in the intact stomach. J Clin Pathol. 1990;43:303–6.
37. El-Zimaity HMT, Genta RM, Graham DY. Histological features do not define NSAID induced gastritis. Hum Pathol. 1996;27:1348–54.
38. Varbanova M, Frauenschläger K, Malfertheiner P. Chronic gastritis - an update. Best Pract Res Clin Gastroenterol. 2014;28:1031–42.
39. Yamamoto S, Sakai Y. Acute gastritis caused by concurrent infection with Epstein-Barr virus and cytomegalovirus in an immunocompetent adult. Clin J Gastroenterol. 2019;12:274–8.
40. Bravender T. Epstein-Barr virus, cytomegalovirus, and infectious mononucleosis. Adolesc Med State Art Rev. 2010;21:251–64.
41. Olson D, Huntington MK. Co-infection with cytomegalovirus and Epstein-Barr virus in mononucleosis: case report and review of literature. S D Med. 2009;62(349):351–3.
42. Jung JH, Choi HJ, Yoo J, et al. Emphysematous gastritis associated with invasive gastric mucormycosis: a case report. J Korean Med Sci. 2007;22:923–7.
43. Yang D, Cho SH, Kim SH, et al. Imaging features of gastric invasive aspergillosis: a report of two cases. J Korean Soc Radiol. 2012;66:463–7.
44. Suh KN, Anekthananon T, Mariuz PR. Gastrointestinal histoplasmosis in patients with AIDS: case report and review. Clin Inf Dis. 2001;32:483–91.
45. Oshiro T, Tomisato K, Nakamatsu G, et al. Gastric anisakidosis: an unfavorable taste of sushi. Pol Arch Int Med. 2019;129:e00515.
46. Ugenti I, De Ceglie A, Ferrarese F, et al. L'anisakidosi gastrica: esperienza personale [Gastric anisakidosis: personal experience]. Chir Ital. 2004;56:301–5.
47. Jankelson OM, Jankelson IR, Zamcheck N. Hemorrhagic (erosive) gastritis. Am J Dig Dis. 1959;4:603–27.
48. Chamberlain CE. Acute hemorrhagic gastritis. Gastroenterol Clin N Am. 1993;22:843–73.
49. Weisenberg E (2021) Erosive gastritis. PathologyOutlines.com website. https://www.pathologyoutlines.com/topic/stomacherosive.html. Accessed Feb 8, 2021.
50. Sugawa C, Lucas CE, Rosenberg BF, et al. Differential topography of acute erosive gastritis due to trauma or sepsis, ethanol and aspirin. Gastrointest Endosc. 1973;19:127.
51. Lauwers GY, Fujita H, Nagata K, et al. Pathology of non-helicobacter pylori gastritis: extending the histopathologic horizons. J Gastroenterol. 2010;45:131–45.
52. Mihály E, Micsik T, Juhász M, et al. Gastritis and gastropathy. Orv Hetil. 2014;155:43–61.
53. Baldaia H. Eosinophilic gastritis. In: Carneiro F, Chaves P, Ensari A, editors. Pathology of the gastrointestinal tract. Encyclopedia of pathology. Cham: Springer; 2017.
54. Lash RH, Lawuers GY, Odze RD, et al. Inflammatory disorders of the stomach. In: Odze R, Goldblum J, editors. Surgical pathology of the GI tract, liver, biliary tract and pancreas. Philadelphia: Saunders; 2009.
55. Lwin T, Melton SD, Genta RM. Eosinophilic gastritis: histopathological characterization and quantification of the normal gastric eosinophil content. Mod Pathol. 2011;24:556–63.
56. Memon RJ, Savliwala MN (2020) Eosinophilic Gastroenteritis. [Updated 2020 Jun 28]. In: StatPearls [Internet]. Treasure Island (FL): StatPearls Publishing; Jan-. Available from: https://www.ncbi.nlm.nih.gov/books/NBK547729/
57. Rothenberg ME. Eosinophilic gastrointestinal disorders (EGID). J Allergy Clin Immunol. 2004;113:11–28.
58. Silva J, Canão P, Espinheira MC, et al. Eosinophils in the gastrointestinal tract: how much is normal? Virchows Arch. 2018;473:313–20.
59. Collins MH. Histopathologic features of eosinophilic esophagitis and eosinophilic gastrointestinal diseases. Gastroenterol Clin N Am. 2014;43:257–68.
60. Holroyd DJ, Banerjee S, Chaudhary KS, et al. Transmural eosinophilic gastritis with gastric outlet obstruction: case report and review of the literature. Ann Royal College Surg Eng. 2010;92:W18–20.
61. Robert ME. Inflammatory disorders of the small intestine. In: Odze R, Goldblum J, editors. Surgical pathology of the GI tract, liver, biliary tract and pancreas. Philadelphia: Saunders; 2009.
62. Cruveilhier J. Traite d'Anatomie Pathologique Generale, vol. 4. Paris: Masson et Cie; 1862. p. 485.
63. Sundberg HH. Ueber gastric phlegmone. Nord Med Arkiv. 1919;II:303–468.

64. Miller AI, Smith B, Rogers AI. Phlegmonous gastritis. Gastroenterol. 1975;68:231–8.
65. Kim GY, Ward J, Henessey B, et al. Phlegmonous gastritis: case report and review. Gastrointest Endosc. 2005;61:168–74.
66. Rada-Palomino A, Muñoz-Duyos A, Pérez-Romero N, et al. Phlegmonous gastritis: a rare entity as a differential diagnostic of an acute abdomen. Description of a case and a bibliographic review. Rev Esp Enferm Dig. 2014;106:418–24.
67. Yang H, Yan Z, Chen J, et al. Diagnosis and treatment of acute phlegmonous gastritis: a case report. Medicine (Baltimore). 2018;97:e0629.
68. Kobus C, van den Broek JJ, Richir MC. Acute gastric necrosis caused by a β-hemolytic streptococcus infection: a case report and review of the literature. Acta Chir Belg. 2020;120:53–6.
69. Ramphal W, Mus M, Nuytinck HKS et al (2018) Sepsis caused by acute phlegmonous gastritis based on a group A Streptococcus. J Surg Case Rep 2018: rjy188.
70. Zazzo JF, Troché G, Millat B, et al. Phlegmonous gastritis associated with HIV-1 seroconversion. Endoscopic and microscopic evolution. Dig Dis Sci. 1992;37:1454–9.
71. Nevin NC, Eakins D, Clarke SD, et al. Acute phlegmonous gastritis. Br Jl Surg. 1969;56:268–70.
72. Park CW, Kim A, Cha SW, et al. A case of phlegmonous gastritis associated with marked gastric distension. Gut liver. 2010;4:415–8.

8 Chronic Gastritis: Infectious, Non-infectious (Autoimmune, Chemical, Granulomatous), Chronic Superficial and Diffuse Antral Gastritis

It is one of the most common clinical conditions that may have clinical symptoms while the asymptomatic individuals may have this condition lifelong. More than half of the world population may have this disease and is an underrated condition clinically [1]. It is considered as the precursor lesion in the development of peptic ulcer disease and gastric malignancy [2–6]. Georg Ernst Stahl, a German Physician, in 1728 had used the term gastritis to describe inflammation of gastric mucosa [7] (Fig. 8.1 A to C). Initially gastritis was not considered to be a disease condition till the time *Helicobacter pylori* was documented to be the aetiological factor for gastritis by Robin Warren and Barry Marshall in 1982 [8]. Chronic gastritis has complex aetiological background as it may get exposed to varieties of substances ranging from diets and other ingested materials, gastric acid content, duodenal juice, and injury may be related to circulating autoantibodies. Gastric mucosa response to injurious agents may vary – it may range from minimal negligible mucosal injury in the form of mild edema to much more severe injury like erosions and ulceration accompanied by a variable degree of inflammatory cell response. All these changes may completely resolve and the mucosa may regain its normal contour. Sometimes, when the injury persists, inflammatory changes persist along with cellular reparation and replication processes. An important factor to determine the tissue response to an injurious agent is the individual's susceptibility. With concept of such complex aetiological background for chronic gastritis, it is not surprising that our understanding is far from complete. It was for the first time that Cruveilhier associated it with gastric ulcer in 1862 [9] and Fenwick with pernicious anaemia in 1870 [10]. Kupfer in 1883 described the intestinal metaplasia as a heterotopic tissue which is now recognized as a spectrum of chronic or atrophic gastritis [11] (Fig. 8.1 A to C). This view was challenged by Schmidt in 1896 but is now accepted as a metaplastic tissue [12]. Bonne et al. in 1938 noted a strong relationship between chronic gastritis with goblet cell metaplasia and gastric cancer amongst the Chinese immigrants than native Malays [13]. Around this time, it was also noted chronic gastritis associated with pernicious anaemia had different topographical distribution than the one associated with gastric ulcer [14]. The heterogenous morphological changes in chronic gastritis was first observed by Motteram in 1951 and Rao et al. in 1975 pointed out the differences in the level of infiltration by inflammatory cells and patients who also had associated loss of gastric glandular component with mucosal atrophy [15, 16]. Gastric mucosal morphological features observed under the microscope in biopsies from patients with chronic gastritis were subdivided into (i) superficial gastritis with minimal glandular loss (Fig. 8.2 A), (ii) gastric mucosal atrophy associated with moderate or severe loss of the gastric glandular compo-

K. Vaiphei, *Interpretation of Endoscopic Biopsy - Gastritis, Gastropathies and Beyond*,
https://doi.org/10.1007/978-981-16-6026-9_8

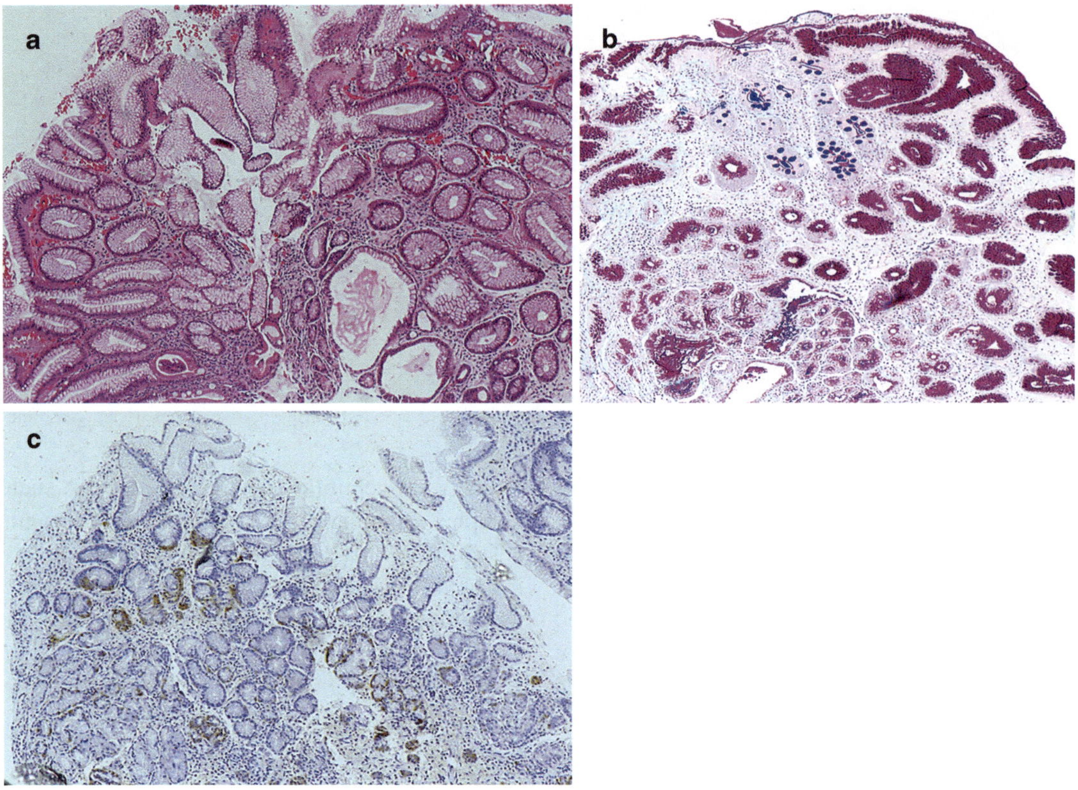

Fig. 8.1 A. Photomicrograph showing grossly hyperplastic gastric mucosa with near total loss of specialized gastric glands and mark foveolar hyperplasia. Chronic inflammatory cells are mild, few cystically dilated glands and along the lower half, there are few scattered goblet cell metaplasia (HE, x250). B. The same biopsy at another level in alcian blue PAS staining highlighting the goblet cell metaplasia (AB-PAS, x250). C. The same biopsy subjected to immunohistochemistry using chromogranin A primary antibody to highlight the number of ECL cells in an atrophic gastritis (PAP, x250)

nents (Fig. 8.2 B) and (iii) those biopsies which showed near or total loss of the gastric glands and gross thinning of the gastric mucosa [15, 16] (Fig. 8.2 C). Joske, Finkh and Wood (1955) have formulated almost similar with little modifications in the terms in reference to the features exhibited by the biopsies in cases of chronic gastritis as slight, moderate or severe, superficial gastritis, superficial gastritis with atrophy, atrophic gastritis, severe atrophic gastritis and gastric atrophy [16, 17]. In 1970s, it was learnt that diffuse corporal gastritis was associated with autoantibodies against parietal cells and intrinsic factor, characterized by hypergastrinaemia, hypochlorhydria and hypopepsinogenaemia [18] and antral gastritis to be associated with duodenal ulcer, excessive secretion of acid and pepsin. Multifocal gastritis was less well defined mostly because pathophysiological parameters appeared to change with the disease progress [19–21]. Later on, Strickland and Mackay combined morphological and physio-pathological parameters and proposed Type A gastritis for corporal lesions associated with pernicious anaemia and Type B gastritis for those associated with duodenal ulcer and multifocal gastritis [22]. In the process of establishing extend of involvement of the stomach as a pangastritis/autoimmune, or multifocal, or antral gastritis, it is essential to have biopsies from different areas of the stomach and each biopsy site be labeled.

Subsequent to this, there was proposal to keep uniformity for gastritis known as the Sydney system of classification and grading of gastritis in

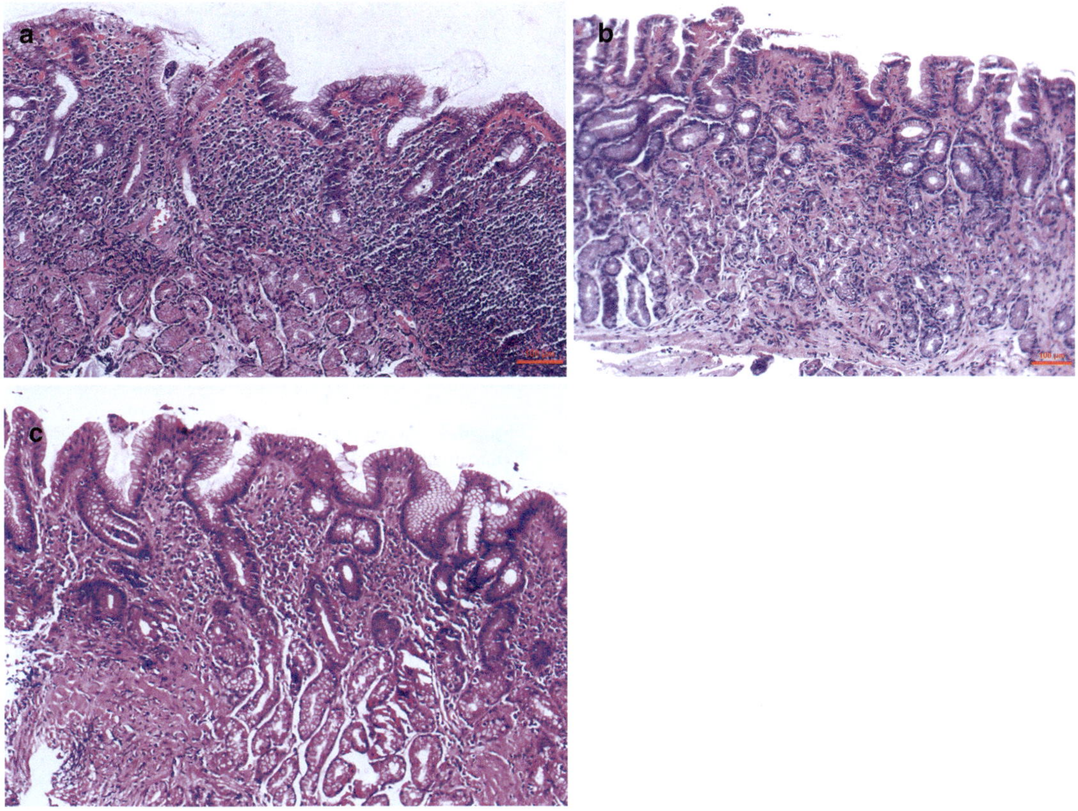

Fig. 8.2 A—a picture of chronic superficial gastritis with minimal glandular loss heavy mucosal inflammation with lymphoid follicles. B—gastric mucosal atrophy associated with moderate loss of the gastric glandular components. C—a near total loss of gastric glands. (HE, x250)

1991, which got modified in 2001 which takes into account the endoscopic and histological information and adds a prefix to indicate the aetiological and pathogenic associations [23]. This system does have shortcomings as it clearly does not clearly describe a separate nosological entity [24]. Correa had proposed simplified classification with attempts to reconcile morphology, pathophysiology, aetiology and the clinical setting in which it occurs. It recognizes five basic types of gastritis, two of which are atrophic and three are non-atrophic. Four of them represent well-defined clinical entity and the fifth one, i.e. superficial gastritis probably represents initial stage in many cases [25, 26]. It may present either as non-atrophic or atrophic form. Gastritis has been known since the early decades of twentieth century and more attention had been given only after Warren and Marshall made the first publication on the role of HP in gastritis [27]. Since than it has been understood that chronic gastritis is a curable disease by eradicating of HP infection [28–30]. Chronic gastritis is an indolent but advancing mucosal inflammation that begins in childhood as an acute or superficial gastritis or both co-existing together [31]. Acquisition of *H. pylori* infection takes place within the first five years of life [32]. Almost more than half of the population infected with *H. pylori* are asymptomatic [32, 33]. A wide range of infection, i.e. 1.2 to 12.2%, has been reported in more advanced countries and in developing countries, and it has been found to be commonest aetiology for infection [34–36]. Chronic gastritis is indicated by mononuclear cell infiltration restricting to superficial part of the gastric mucosa with focal neutrophilic infiltration or purely only acute inflammatory cell infiltration presenting as acute gastritis [37]. In developing countries, prevalence of atrophic and non-atrophic gastritis is influenced by individual's age and other age-related specific factors [38, 39]. Destruction of the normal mucosal glands by the inflammatory process gets replaced with formation of new glands and the regenerating epithelial cells may undergo either intestinal and/or pyloric type without the G cell [23, 40–42] (Fig. 8.3). HP associated tends to localize in antrum which is believed to be due to accumulation of HP in pyloric antrum due to gravity, hence it is antral dominant gastritis [38, 43]. The term superficial gastritis refers to when the mononuclear inflammatory cells and plasma cells occupies upper half of the mucosa. When the chronic inflammation is intermixed with neutrophils, it is believed to be due to dependent on cytotoxicity of HP strain [44, 45]. Chronic gastritis is known to progress from stage to the next stage of premalignant mucosal lesions as indicated by the presence of intestinal metaplasia and dysplasia (Fig. 8.4). Number of cases that undergoes such transformation is believed to be about 2–3% on average [46, 47]. Almost half the patients with chronic gastritis harbouring HP will develop atrophic gastritis during their lifetime and 5% will have severe degree atrophic gastritis [48]. Pure antral type of HP gastritis can evolve to corpus and fundus dominant types having diffuse, multifocal or corpus dominant types [49, 50].

A severe and extensive atrophy involving gastric mucosa usually has functional disorders causing particularly hypochlorhydria and failure to secrete intrinsic factor and gastrin by G cell in antral atrophy [39, 40] (Fig. 8.5). Isolated severe antral atrophic gastritis is obviously quite rare whereas involvement of both antrum and corpus together is relatively frequently observed [39, 40]. In long-term follow-up studies have suggested that along with gradual corporal extension by chronic gastritis by HP infection, antral mucosa may undergo healing [37, 38]. With the progression of non-atrophic gastritis to atrophic phenotype, there will be many other pathogenetic processes may be going on including even triggering of carcinogenesis pathway thereby linking the chronic gastritis with gastric cancer accord-

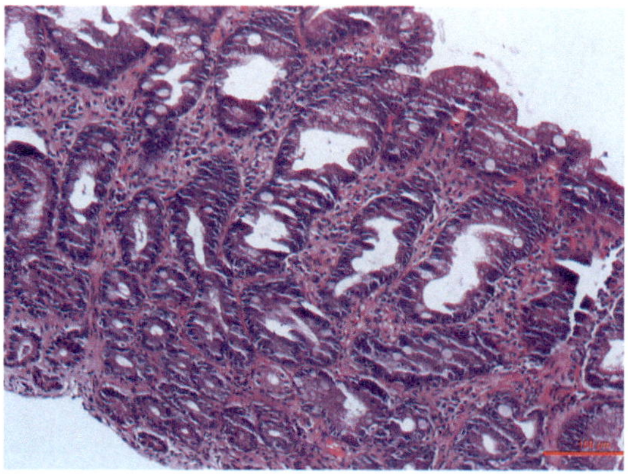

Fig. 8.3 Medium-power photomicrograph showing replacement of the normal mucosal glands by new glands and regenerating epithelial cells with intestinal metaplasia and lamina propria with fine fibrosis. Inflammatory cell component is minimal in this atrophic mucosa (HE, x300)

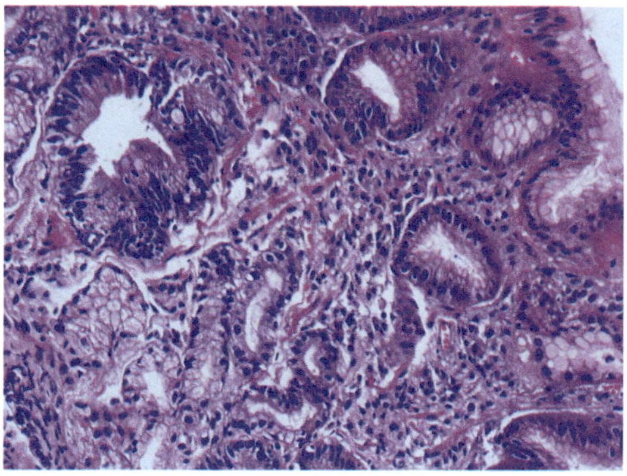

Fig. 8.4 Picture showing features of chronic gastritis with a focus of low-grade dysplasia and intestinal metaplasia (HE, x300)

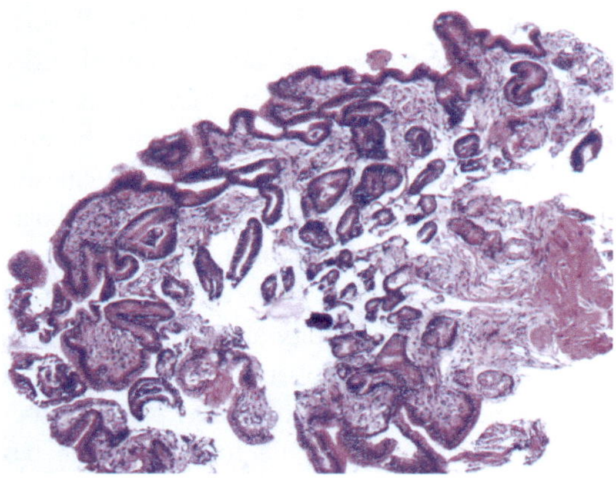

Fig. 8.5 Photomicrograph showing a biopsy of gastric body mucosa with severe and extensive atrophy and total lamina propria replacement fibrosis (HE, x300)

ing to the phenomenon described in Correa cascade [51, 52].

8.1 Chronic Gastritis May Be Infectious or Non-infectious [39–41, 53, 54]

Infectious gastritis can be produced by one or more of the following organisms, i.e. *H. pylori* infection which is the most common cause of chronic gastritis, *Helicobacter heilmannii*, granulomatous gastritis associated with infection by mycobacteriosis, syphilis, histoplasmosis, mucormycosis, South American blastomycosis, anisakiasis, or anisakidosis, parasitic infections—strongyloides species, schistosomiasis, or *Diphyllobothrium latum* and viruses like CMV, EBV and herpes [39–41, 53, 54].

Conditions that are associated with non-infectious gastritis: i) autoimmune gastritis, ii) reactive gastropathy which is also known as chemical gastritis as it is associated with various chemicals like chronic bile reflux, administration of NSAID and aspirin, cocaine, etc., iii) chronic or acute renal failure related gastropathy. Gastric mucosal histological profile is usually non-specific and tends to be associated with vascular ectasia, loss of specialized glands, lamina propria fibrosis and variable grades and types of inflammatory cell infiltration, iv) granulomatous gastritis seen with various conditions usually forming compact non-caseating epithelioid cell granulomas—Crohn's disease, sarcoidosis, Wegener's granulomatosis, foreign body granuloma, ingestion of cocaine, idiopathic granulomatous gastritis, chronic granulomatous disease of childhood, eosinophilic granuloma, allergic granulomatosis and vasculitis, plasma cell granulomas, rheumatoid nodules, tumoural amyloidosis and granulomas associated with gastric malignancies like carcinoma, lymphoma and Langerhans cell histiocytosis, v) lymphocytic gastritis including gastritis associated with celiac disease and collagenous gastritis. A significant number of children (~ 15-20%) with wheat or gliadin intolerance may also show evidence of lymphocytic gastritis where there will be significantly increase in intra-epithelial lymphocytes along with epithelial cell degeneration and lamina propria mononuclear cell infiltration and this will show a good respond to gluten-free diet. In coeliac disease related inflammatory cell response, there may be significant number of scatter eosinophils in the biopsy as the immune response is allergic reaction to gluten. Significant number of 10 to 35% of idiopathic ulcerative colitis patients may also have lymphocytic gastritis, morphologically indistinguishable from other conditions with similar morphology, on histology. However, no association has been observed between lymphocytic gastritis and *H. pylori* infection, vi) eosinophilic gastritis, vii) radiation induced gastritis, viii) graft versus host disease (GVHD), ix) ischaemic gastritis and other vascular associated gastropathies and x) systemic illnesses and post-operative stress [40, 41, 55, 56].

Autoimmune gastritis can be spoken in two terms—firstly as the one associated with anti-parietal cell antibody (Fig. 8.6 A); second one will be the one that may be seen in association with systemic collagen vascular disorders or in isolation involving the stomach with basement membrane thickening and predominant lymphocytic and plasma cell infiltration, morphologically will be similar to other gastritis including chronic *H. pylori* infection. Gastritis associated with systemic autoimmune disorders, the mucosal inflammation dominantly involves deeper mucosa sparing surface epithelium. Intra-epithelial lymphocytes will dominantly be involving foveolae and specialized gastric glands of both body and pyloric antrum which help to differentiate from autoimmune disorder of anti-parietal cell type. However, occasionally, extension to pyloric antral mucosa has been seen in anti-parietal cell associated autoimmune gastritis. When there is superadded *H. pylori* infection, it is a difficult situation to comment on presence of autoimmune component (Fig. 8.6 B and C). When such situation arises, the patient may be first treated for the infective aetiology and to be re-assessed again once the treatment for infection is completed. Vasculitis is an important morphological component of systemic autoimmune disorders.

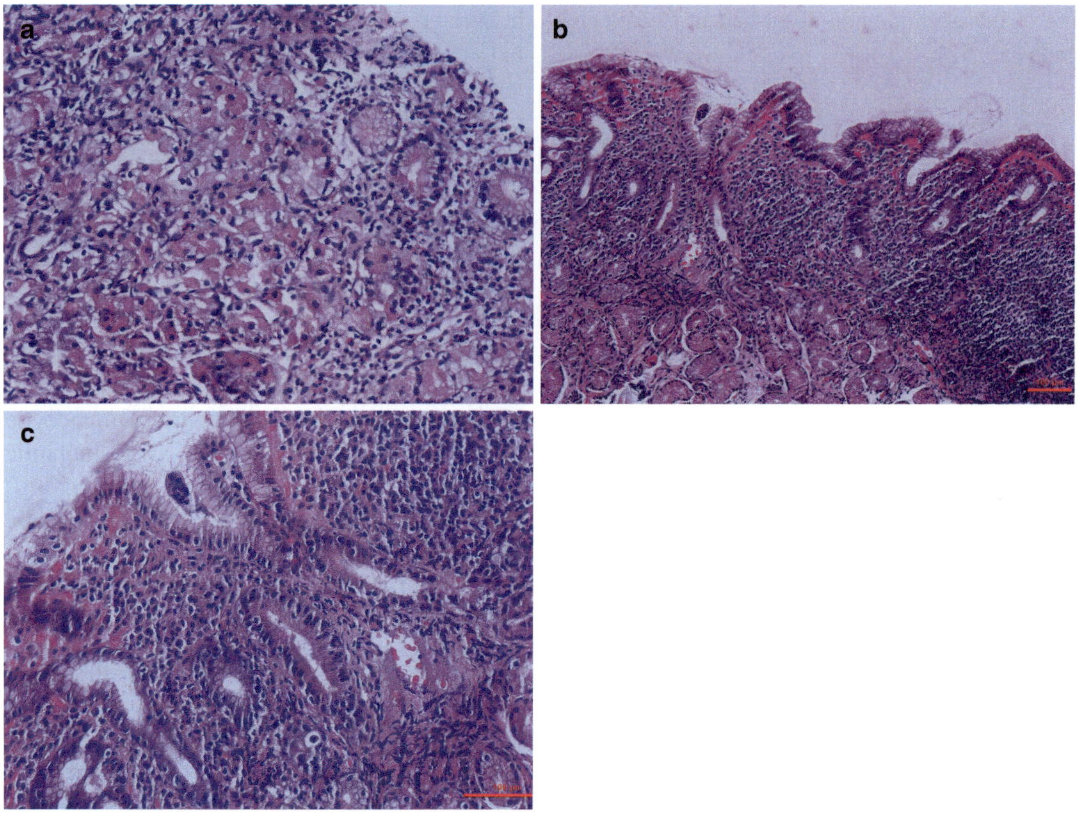

Fig. 8.6 A—photomicrograph of gastric fundus biopsy showing active destruction of parietal cells by lymphocytes with moderately heavy lamina propria lymphocytic infiltration (HE, x300). B and C—photomicrographs of antrum and body biopsies, respectively, showing heavy mucosal inflammation mainly comprising of lymphocytes with plasma cells and lymphoid follicles. There is gross increase in intra-epithelial lymphocytes of foveolae and glands, relatively sparing the surface lining epithelial cells. No infective agent identified (HE, x300)

Chemical gastritis can be diagnosed quite accurately as it has classic morphological features of cock screw like appearances of the gastric foveolae due to increased cell regenerative activity in response to destruction and degeneration taking place, with variable degree of associated changes and inflammation (Fig. 8.7 A to C). All these changes may also be associated with streaks of lamina propria fibrosis with reduction in the specialized gastric glands. When one sees presence of epithelioid cell granuloma in a given endoscopic gastric biopsy, the above-mentioned conditions will definitely be considered in the differential diagnosis by taking the clinical history and other investigative parameters. Foreign body granuloma, the histological appearance of the granuloma will show foreign type of multinucleated giant cells with bubbly or foamy cytoplasm, tend to be more superficially located. Certain granulomas may be correlated with the other infiltrating cells, blood vessel involvement and presence of necrosis. In our setting until and unless there is specific reason irrespective of the type of the granuloma, every granulomatous inflammatory condition to be subjected to Z N stain to look for acid fast bacilli. A diagnosis of idiopathic granulomatous gastritis may be entertained when all the investigative parameters are non-contributory for any condition that may be related to the gastric granulomas. Granuloma with heavy eosinophilic infiltration will definitely point towards a diagnosis of eosinophilic granuloma. Eosinophilia with vasculitis will help to make a diagnosis of Churg–Strauss vasculitis.

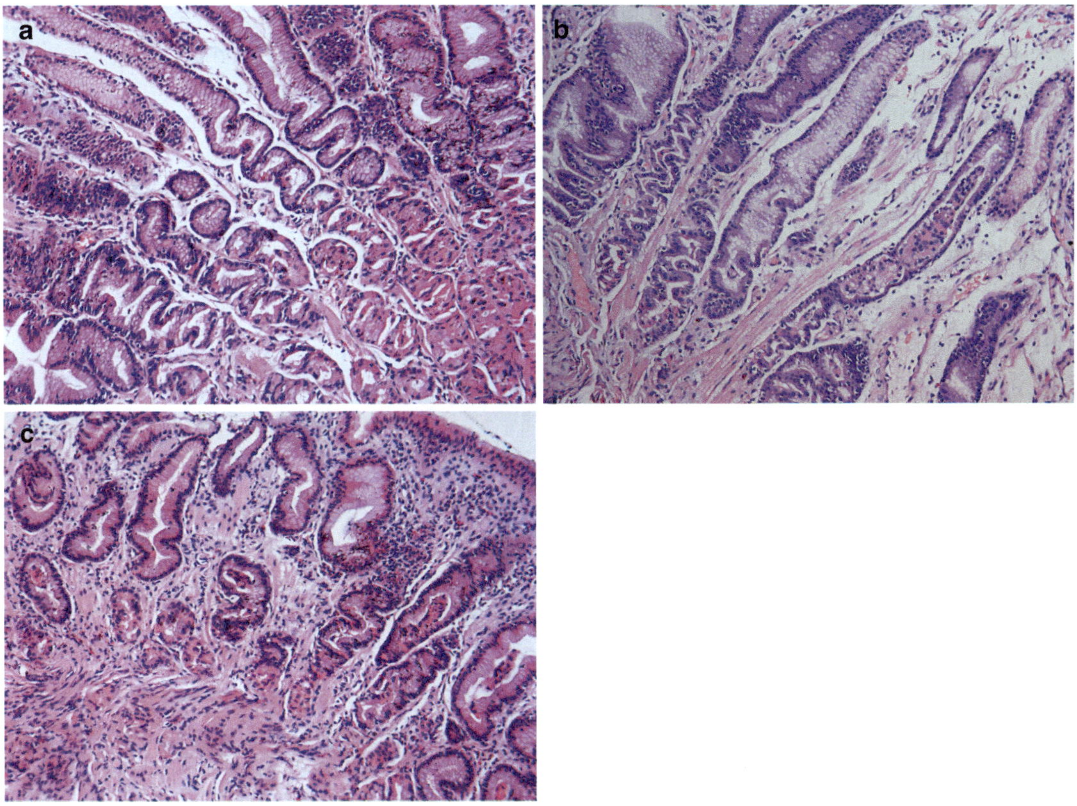

Fig. 8.7 A—Low-power photomicrograph of an endoscopic biopsy sampled from thicken gastric body mucosal folds showing grossly elongated and coiled cock screw like gastric foveolae, few intact parietal cells are identified on the deeper portion of the picture. Lamina propria inflammatory cells are distinctly minimal; B—Photomicrograph of another biopsy showing similar features as in A but with fine fibrosis in between the coiled foveolae containing clusters of apoptotic bodies; C—Another photomicrograph to show lesser degree of foveolar changes however, associated with heavier mononuclear cell infiltration of the lamina propria along with fibrosis and active glandular destruction. Fibrosis is also seen involving the muscularis mucosae. (HE, x250)

In fungal or any other infective associated granuloma, the causative organism should be demonstrable in the granulomas. Similarly for amyloid granuloma, the amyloid material should be demonstrable. Epithelioid cell granulomas in response to malignancy will also show areas of the tumour in the biopsy tissue pieces.

Eosinophilic gastritis, formerly was known as allergic gastritis, as an isolated condition is rare and usually is a part of the condition of eosinophilic gastroenteritis. Usually, it is seen in children or young adults presenting with vomiting, diarrhoea, protein losing enteropathy, food sensitivity, growth failure with history of some known allergic. The affected individual may have anaemia, blood eosinophilia, increased serum IgE level. Stomach is the most common site of involvement but primary eosinophilic gastritis without involvement of oesophagus or duodenum is uncommon. Presenting symptoms will be related to involved segment and extent or depth of involvement of gut wall that can be limited mucosa or may be transmural or serosal dominant. Mucosal biopsy may be normal when the disease is deep seated. In serosal disease, the patient may present with ascites and eosinophilia. These patients may have a + ive skin test, no anaphylaxis, suggestive of type IV hypersensitivity reaction. In histology, the endoscopic mucosal biopsy will show features of florid inflammation, which dominantly be comprising of eosinophils in the lamina propria intermixed with variable number of lymphoplasmacytic cells. Usually, the involvement in eosinophilic gastritis is pyloric antrum dominant, focally also the other parts of the stomach [57] (Fig. 8.8). Occasionally there could be some biopsies dominantly comprising of plasma cell infiltrate, sometimes may be with Russel body, which may be superficial and full thickness with glandular destruction qualifying for the diagnosis of plasma cell gastritis or Russel body gastritis (Fig. 8.8 B and C).

Classification of chronic gastritis is complex and none of the classification is satisfactory. Firstly, irrespective of the underlying aetiology, chronic gastritis may be morphologically classified into under two main headings, i.e. non-atrophic and atrophic gastritis depending upon

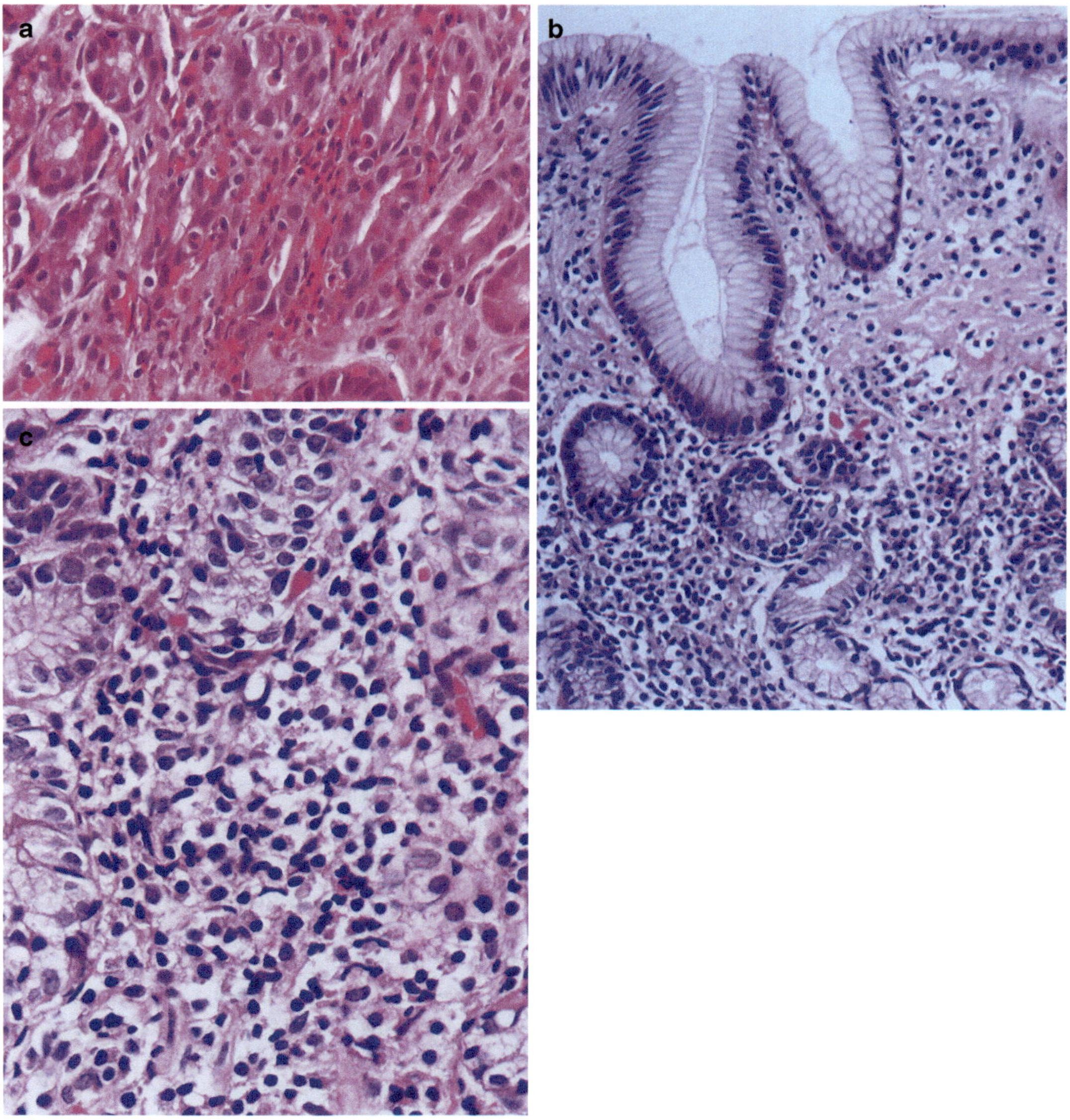

Fig. 8.8 A—medium-power photomicrograph of gastric body biopsy to show predominant eosinophil infiltration accompanied by active glandular destruction (HE, x500). B and C—medium- and high-power views to highlight the lamina propria infiltrate to be of plasma cells only. In Fig. 8.8 B—there is also deposition of pinkish amorphous material (para-amyloid) along with plasma cells and 8.8 C in addition also shows plasma cells infiltrating the glandular epithelial cells (HE, x300 and x500, respectively)

the distribution of maintenance of the gastric glandular components both in antrum and body mucosae. Depending upon the distribution pattern it may be grouped into three types, i.e. i) pangastritis where both antrum and body may be patchily involved, ii) antrum predominant where antral mucosa is almost totally or diffusely showing features of chronic gastritis and is also known as diffuse antral gastritis and iii) corpus predominant or autoimmune gastritis or Type A gastritis. Alternatively, non-atrophic gastritis may be subgrouped into three, first two are *H. pylori* associated, i.e. chronic superficial gastritis and diffuse antral gastritis where both are associated with hypersecretion; the third subgroup is the one associated with irritants like bile or chemicals and is named as reflux or reactive gastritis. The first two conditions show normal or mild increase in serum gastrin level with little or no gastric glandular loss and duodenal ulcer. Long-standing gastric mucosal inflammation results in mucosal atrophy and hypo or achlorhydria [58, 59]. In such situation, HP tends to migrate towards proximal stomach resulting in different forms of gastritis, i.e. either a diffuse corporal or patchy and multifocal. Regenerating epithelial cells tend to undergo metaplasia of either pyloric and/or intestinal type. These metaplastic epithelia may be the leading point in the development of gastric carcinomas [3, 14, 51, 60–64]. Under the atrophic group, it can be either diffuse corporal or autoimmune gastritis (also known as Type A atrophic gastritis) and multifocal or environmental and *H. pylori* associated gastritis where both antral and body can be patchily involved (also known as Type B atrophic gastritis). Type A gastritis is the one where the patients usually present with refractile megaloblastic anaemia and hypochlorhydria [20, 22–24, 30, 57, 58].

It has been postulated that sequence of mucosal changes takes place in *H. pylori* infection which will lead ultimately in the development of gastric cancer (GC). The first foremost mucosal change is that of chronic inflammation followed by atrophy, metaplasia, dysplasia and GC, which may continue over decades and this sequence has been described in Correa's hypothesis [65]. A meta-analysis of many studies has documented a strong relationship between HP eradication and GC [66]. Contrary to this meta-analysis, a study in Japanese population showed that persistence of mucosal changes related to chronic HP infection might still be important factors in the development of GC in spite of HP eradication [65]. Development of GC involves both genetic and epigenetic changes, and majority of these are supposedly related to long-standing HP infection [67–71].

Sydney Systems have given uniform criteria including the visual analogue system in the diagnosis of gastritis worldwide, though these systems do not talk about component of prognostication [39, 41]. These systems have their own limitations due to the manyfold parameters that have been incorporated in the systems and make the systems to be cumbersome for routine diagnostic activities [66, 67]. A group of gastroenterologists and pathologists proposed a reporting system, i.e. Operative Link for Gastritis Assessment [OLGA] for gastritis known as OLGA staging system by arranging histological features along a scale of increasing risk for GC ranging from stage 0 to stage IV [66]. Histological features used are gastritis grade, atrophy and metaplastic epithelium. The system refers to issue of making physician to be aware of the significance of the clinical, serological or endoscopic management for each patient. It has also been observed in many developing countries that in spite of a high incidence of *H. pylori* infection and its associated gastric mucosal atrophy, incidence of GC has not shown any significant increase in the last few decades [66–69]. Though OLGA staging system is simple for routine use, it requires validation in context to different epidemiology [68, 70, 71]. OLGA system has been found to be helpful as a positive correlation between mild chronic inflammation and total OLGA score was observed; however, its failure in applicability has been found between presence of features of chronicity with dysplasia or cancer ($P > 0.05$) [69]. However, contradictory to this study, there are many other studies which had observed OLGA staging system to be useful in predicting development of gastric cancer specially OLGA stage III and IV [68, 70, 71].

The extent of inflammation in gastritis may be graded into mild, moderate and severe depending upon the extent of inflammatory cell infiltration in the lamina propria. Inflammatory cell infiltrate may be graded as mild if the infiltrating cells are sparse, lying in between the glands and foveolae where the distance between the glands and gastric pits is normal or near normal and no undue increased in thickness of the mucosa; The inflammation may be graded as moderate when there is a significant increase in inflammatory cells in between the glandular structures and gastric pits, where the spaces occupy by the inflammatory cells in between are almost or double and also associated with increase in mucosal thickness. And the infiltrate may be graded as severe or extensive when the inflammatory cells are present in large number exhibiting gross broadening of the spaces between the gastric glands and foveolae, due to which the widely spaced gastric glands give an appearance of glandular, but it is associated with increase in mucosal thickness. There is no true loss or reduction of the epithelial components or no replacement fibrosis in lamina propria. In all the three grades specially in moderate and severe grades, there will be relatively loss of mucous and the glands or the epithelial cells will look dysplastic specially cells in the neck region of the foveolae but no dysplasia in the true sense. These gradings may be applicable both for superficial and full-thickness gastritis with or without activity and atrophy. There may be lymphoid follicles; however, the areas where lymphoid follicles are present should be avoided in consideration for the gradings of inflammation [16].

8.2 Chronic Superficial Gastritis

This is one of the most frequently encountered morphological features amongst the gastric biopsies in routine practice and can be seen in biopsies from any portion of the stomach. There is a band like infiltration of the superficial half of the lamina propria by lymphocytes and plasma cells occasionally intermixed with scattered eosinophils and believed to be preceded by *H. pylori* associated acute gastritis. Most of the acute gastritis progresses to develop chronic superficial gastritis. The intensity of the inflammatory cell infiltrate is variable, most frequently it is heavy and dense expanding the lamina propria resulting in wide spacing of the gastric foveolae and epithelial structures. The glandular component is relatively spared though there may be extension of the inflammatory cells patchily to the deeper mucosa in between the gastric glands but with no obvious glandular loss of replacement fibrosis. There may be focal neutrophilic infiltration in close proximity or infiltrating the epithelial cells specially in the foveolae neck region which may exudate out into the lumen forming microabscesses or it may remain in between the epithelial cells qualifying for the diagnosis of recent onset activity. This feature of recent onset activity is most likely due to *H. pylori* infection. Due to the ongoing inflammation the epithelial cells will look mucodepleted, regenerative activity simulating dysplasia accompanied by distortion of the glandular architecture. Chronic superficial gastritis may be observed in biopsies from any portion of the stomach, however it is most frequently in antral biopsy with sparing of the body mucosa or involving the body mucosa with sparing of the antral mucosa, sometimes it may multifocal and patchy in distribution.

No clear clinical syndrome has been defined with respect to chronic superficial gastritis and lack of co-relationship between the clinical symptom and histological features [72]. According to Lambert the term gastritis is very frequently been used incorrectly as clinical term to account for the non-ulcer dyspeptic symptoms [73]. However, the sensation of bloating, epigastric pain, heartburn, nausea and vomiting have been more frequently associated with chronic gastritis [14]. It is a frequently observed feature in gastric biopsies unrelated to stomach problem or in routine investigations for chronic anaemia. Thus, it may represent an early stage of developing atrophic gastritis or it may be just a nonspecific finding which undergoes healing of itself with no specific treatment being given to the patient. Gastric mucosal inflammation confining to the upper half of the lamina propria is most likely to be related to injurious or irritants present within the gastric lumen. In human it has been associated with intake of spicy and salty food, alcohol and NSAIDs [74–76].

Chronic superficial gastritis is one condition where there may be no good co-relationship between endoscopic findings and histological features. Endoscopic examination may show no obvious finding or a normal appearing mucosa. *H. pylori* may be frequently found both in the antral and body biopsies showing chronic superficial gastritis. Though the inflammation is superficial, there may be associated features of chronic gastritis in the form of crypt hyperplasia and regenerative and metaplastic epithelium, along with elongation of the foveolae and distortion with coiling, which are classically indicative of a long-standing exposure to irritants or infection. These changes are more frequently seen in antral biopsies with normal body biopsies. These foveolar changes in reactive gastropathy may be accompanied by hyperplasia of the specialized glands like parietal cells which possibly will be indicative long-standing NSAIDs intake. Features of atrophy, dysplasia and malignancy are seldom observed in such biopsy [48, 49, 66, 67].

Functional disturbance observed in superficial gastritis is little known as there may be wide variation amongst the population. It has been shown that serum gastrin level is reported to be slightly higher in chronic superficial gastritis compared to normal population [77]. It is a frequent finding in patients who presents with unrelated disease conditions and during routine screening process for gastric cancer. Thus, it may be initial stage of developing atrophic gastritis or a condition which may undergo self-healing process and it has been associated with ingestion of alcohol, spicy and salty foods and analgesic intake [78].

8.3 Diffuse Antral Gastritis

It is a term introduced by Correa in *H. pylori* related gastritis [51]. Antral gastritis type is unique in that it selectively involves the antrum, sparing the rest of the stomach and shows heavy lymphoid cell infiltration with many lymphoid follicles with germinal centres in the deeper portion of the mucosa and the superficial mucosa infiltrated by lymphocytes intermixed with plasma cells. These infiltrates result in wide separation of the epithelial components, giving a look of atrophy; however, due to the heavy infiltrate, the mucosa is thicker than thinning. The epithelial cells will show variable degree of evidence of inflammation visible as mucodepleted, foveolar hyperplasia and disorganization of the glands due to regenerative activities, with or without intestinal metaplasia (Fig. 8.9 A and B). Diffuse antral gastritis is a part of the nosological entity of peptic ulcer disease of duodenum and pyloric ring [73, 79]. This condition is characterized by excessive acid and pepsin secretion,

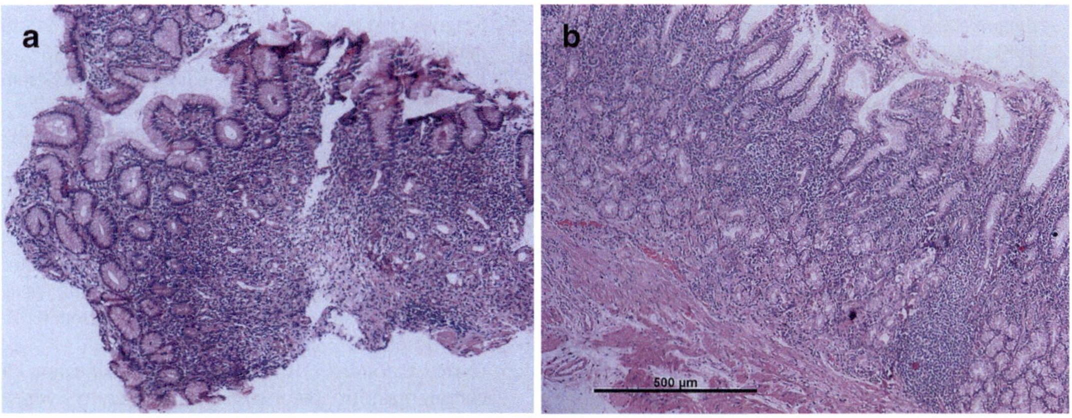

Fig. 8.9 A—low-power view of a pyloric antral biopsy to show full-thickness diffuse dense inflammatory cell infiltration of lamina propria with loss of antral glands. Inflammatory cells are mainly comprising of lymphomononuclear cells along with hyperplastic foveolae; B—another picture to show similar features with lymphoid follicles. (HE, x250)

possibly with gastrin hypersecretion, though all patients of duodenal and pyloric sphincter ulcers will not present with hyperacidity. Hence, the ulcers may be induced by some other aetiological factor like drugs or other irritant food particles. Clinically this group of patients will come with classic duodenal peptic ulcer disease. More recently majority of this condition has been associated with *H. pylori* infection documented in antral biopsy; however, different morphological spectrum produced by *H. pylori* is not very clear. Possibly one explanation is that heavy lymphoid aggregates are partly inhibited by parietal cells, hence sparing the gastric body and fundus [80]. This type more frequently involves elderly. This may be associated with various infective agents like viruses, bacteria, exposure to factors that may produce injury to mucosa and may be following administration of certain medication. This condition is less frequent compared to *H. pylori* associated chronic gastritis. These patients usually present clinically with problems of long-standing indigestion and duodenal peptic ulcer disease. Though relatively rarer, these patients also may present with the typical gastritis associated problems of epigastric discomfort, nausea, bloating, flatulence and changes in stool colour [80].

References

1. Siurala M, Sipponen P, Kekki M. Chronic gastritis: dynamic and clinical aspects. Scand J Gastroenterol. 1985;20(sup109):69–76.
2. Sipponen P, Maaroos HI. Chronic gastritis. Scandinavian Journal of Gastroenterol. 2015;50:657–67.
3. IARC. Schistosomes, liver flukes and helicobacter pylori. IARC working group on the evaluation of carcinogenic risks to humans. Lyon, 7-14 June 1994. IARC Monogr Eval Carcinog Risks Hum. 1994;61:1–241.
4. Schindler R. Chronic gastritis. Klin Wochenschr. 1966;44:601–12.
5. Siurala M. The story of gastritis. Scand J Gastroenterol Suppl. 1991;186:1–3.
6. Telaranta-Keerie A, Kara R, Paloheimo L, et al. Prevalence of undiagnosed advanced atrophic corpus gastritis in Finland: an observational study among 4,256 volunteers without specific complaints. Scand J Gastroenterol. 2010;45:1036–41.
7. Szabo IL, Cseko K, Czimmer J et al (2012) Diagnosis of gastritis – Review from early pathological evaluation to present day management. Mozsik G, ed. Current Topics in Gastritis. Rijeka, Croatia: In Tech; 2012. Chap 1.
8. Warren JR, Marshall B. Unidentified curved bacilli on gastric epithelium in active chronic gastritis. Lancet. 1983;1(8336):1273–5.
9. Cruveilhier J. Traite d'anatomie pathologique generale. Paris: Balliere; 1862. p. p484.
10. Fenwick S. On atrophy of stomach. Lancet. 1870;2:78.
11. Szabo IL, Cseko K, Czimmer J, Mozsik G (2012) Diagnosis of gastritis – Review from early pathological evaluation to present day management. Mozsik G, ed. Current Topics in Gastritis. Rijeka, Croatia: In Tech; 2012. Chap 1.
12. Schmidt A. Untersuchugen ulcer des menschliche Magenepitel unter normalen und pathologischen Verhaltnissen. Virchows Arch (A). 1896;143: 477–508.
13. Bonne L, Harzt P, Clerks JV. Morphology of the stomach and gastric secretions in Malays and Chinese and the different incidence of gastric ulcer and gastric cancer in those races. Am J Cancer. 1938;3:265–79.
14. Correa P, Haenszel W, Cuello C, et al. A model for gastric cancer epidemiology. Lancet. 1975;2:58–60.
15. Motteram RA. A biopsy study of chronic gastritis and gastric atrophy. J Path Bact. 1951;63:389–94.
16. Rao SS, Krasner N, Thomson TJ. Chronic gastritis—a simple classification. J Pathol. 1975;117:93–6.
17. Joske RA, Finkh ES, Wood IJ. Gastric biopsy: a study of 1000 consecutive successful gastric biopsies. Quart J Med. 1955;2:269.
18. Brus I, Siegel H, Yamaguchi N, et al. Immunoglobulins IgA and IgG in gastric mucosa of patients with atrophic gastritis and pernicious anemia. Scand J Gastroenterol. 1968;3:43–57.
19. Faber K, Bloch CE. Uber die pathologischen Verenderungen am digestion tractus bei die perniciosen anemia and ulcer die Sogennante. Dermat Z Klin Med. 1900;40:98.
20. Magnus HA. A re-assessment of the gastric lesion in pernicious anaemia. J Clin Path. 1958;11:289–95.
21. Lambert R. Chronic gastritis. Digestion. 1972;7:83–126.
22. Strickland RG, Mackay IR. A reappraisal of the nature and significance of chronic atrophic gastritis. Am J Dig Dis. 1973;18:426–40.
23. Price AB. The Sydney system: histological division. J Gastroenterol Hepatol. 1991;6:209–22.
24. Stolte M, Meining A. The updated Sydney system: classification and grading of gastritis as the basis of diagnosis and treatment. Can J Gastroenterol. 2001;15:591–8.
25. Correa P, Yardley JH. Grading and classification of chronic gastritis: one American response to Sydney system. Gastroenterol. 1992;102:355–9.
26. Correa P. The epidemiology and pathogenesis of chronic gastritis. Three aetiologic entities. Front Gastroenterol Res. 1980;6:98–108.

27. Marshall BJ, Warren JR. Unidentified curved bacilli in the stomach of patients with gastritis and peptic ulceration. Lancet. 1984;323:1311–5.
28. Valle J, Seppälä K, Sipponen P, et al. Disappearance of gastritis after eradication of helicobacter pylori. A morphometric study. Scand J Gastroenterol. 1991;26:1057–65.
29. Hojo M, Miwa H, Ohkusa T, et al. Alteration of histological gastritis after cure of helicobacter pylori infection. Aliment Pharmacol Ther. 2002;16:1923–32.
30. Annibale B, Di Giulio E, Caruana P, et al. The long-term effects of cure of helicobacter pylori infection on patients with atrophic body gastritis. Aliment Pharmacol Ther. 2002;16:1723–31.
31. Mehrabani S. Helicobacter pylori infection in children: a comprehensive review. Maedica (Bucur). 2019;14:292–7.
32. Rajindrajith S, Devanarayana NM, De Silva HJ. Helicobacter pylori infection in children. Saudi J Gastroenterology (official journal of the Saudi Gastroenterology Association). 2009;2:86.
33. Suerbaum S, Michetti P. Helicobacter pylori infection. N Engl J Med. 2002;15:1175–86.
34. Mourad-Baars PE, Verspaget HW, Mertens BJ, et al. Low prevalence of helicobacter pylori infection in young children in the Netherlands. Eur J Gastroenterol; Hepatol. 2007;3:213–6.
35. Opekun AR, Gilger MA, Denyes SM, et al. Helicobacter pylori infection in children of Texas. J Ped Gastroenterol Nutr. 2000;4:405–10.
36. Rothenbacher D, Bode G, Berg G, et al. Prevalence and determinants of helicobacter pylori infection in preschool children: a population-based study from Germany. Inter J Epidem. 1998;1:135–41.
37. Maaroos HI, Kekki M, Villako K, et al. The occurrence and extent of helicobacter pyloric colonization and antral and body gastritis profiles in an Estonian population sample. Scand J Gastroenterol. 1990;25:1010–7.
38. Kekki M, Siurala M, Varis K, et al. Classification principles and genetics of chronic gastritis. Scand J Gastroenterol Suppl. 1987;141:1–28.
39. Dixon MF, Genta RM, Yardley JH, et al. Classification and grading of gastritis. The updated Sydney system. International workshop on the histopathology of gastritis, Houston 1994. Am J Surg Pathol. 1996;20:1161–81.
40. Correa P. Chronic gastritis: a clinico-pathological classification. Am J Gastroenterol. 1988;83:504–9.
41. Sipponen P, Kekki M, Siurala M. The Sydney system: epidemiology and natural history of chronic gastritis. J Gastroenterol Hepatol. 1991;6:244–51.
42. Lhamäki T, Sipponen P, Varis K, et al. Characteristics of gastric mucosa which precede occurrence of gastric malignancy: results of long-term follow-up of three family samples. Scand J Gastroenterol Suppl. 1991;186:16–23.
43. Maaroos HI, Rägo T, Sipponen P, et al. Helicobacter pylori and gastritis in children with abdominal complaints. Scand J Gastroenterol. 1991;26:95–9.
44. Rautelin H, Sipponen P, Seppälä K, et al. Gastric inflammation and neutrophil activating and cytotoxin-producing helicobacter pylori strains. Scand J Gastroenterol. 1996;31:639–42.
45. Maaroos HI, Vorobjova T, Sipponen P, et al. An 18-year follow-up study of chronic gastritis and helicobacter pylori association of CagA positivity with development of atrophy and activity of gastritis. Scand J Gastroenterol. 1999;34:864–9.
46. Lhamäki T, Kekki M, Sipponen P, et al. The sequelae and course of chronic gastritis during a 30- to 34-year bioptic follow-up study. Scand J Gastroenterol. 1985;20:485–91.
47. Valle J, Kekki M, Sipponen P, et al. Long term course and consequences of helicobacter pylori gastritis. Results of a 32-year follow-up study. Scand J Gastroenterol. 1996;31:546–50.
48. Siurala M, Sipponen P, Kekki M. Chronic gastritis: dynamic and clinical aspects. Scand J Gastroenterol Suppl. 1985;109:69–76.
49. Correa P, Villako K, Kekki M, et al. Chronic gastritis: progression of inflammation and atrophy in a six-year endoscopic follow-up of a random sample of 142 Estonian urban subjects. Scand J Gastroenterol Suppl. 1991;186:135–41.
50. Villako K, Kekki M, Maaroos HI, et al. A 12-year follow-up study of chronic gastritis and helicobacter pylori in a population-based random sample. Scand J Gastroenterol. 1995;30:964–7.
51. Correa P, Haenszel W, Cuello C, et al. Gastric precancerous process in a high-risk population: cohort follow-up. Cancer Res. 1990;50:4737–40.
52. Correa P, Piazuelo MB. The gastric precancerous cascade. J Dig Dis. 2012;13:2–9.
53. Lehours P. Actual diagnosis of helicobacter pylori infection. Minerva Gastroenterol Dietol. 2018;64:267–79.
54. Xiong X, Liu F, Zhao W, et al. Cytomegalovirus infective gastritis in an immunocompetent host misdiagnosed as malignancy on upper gastrointestinal endoscopy: a case report and review of literature. Hum Pathol. 2019;92:107–12.
55. Kasper DL, Braunwald E, Fauci A et al (2006) Gastritis. Harrison's Principles of Internal Medicine: Companion Handbook. 16th ed. McGraw-Hill: Part 12, Chapter 274.
56. Srivastava A, Lauwers GY. Pathology of non-infective gastritis. Histopathol. 2007;50:15–29.
57. Goldman H, Proujansky R. Allergic proctitis and gastroenteritis in children. Clinical and mucosal biopsy features in 53 cases. Am J Surg Pathol. 1986;10:75–86.
58. Sipponen P, Ranta P, Helske T, et al. Serum levels of amidated gastrin-17 and pepsinogen I in atrophic gastritis: an observational case-control study. Scand J Gastroenterol. 2002;37:785–91.
59. Väänänen H, Vauhkonen M, Helske T, et al. (2—3) non-endoscopic diagnosis of atrophic gastritis with a blood test. Correlation between gastric histology and serum levels of gastrin-17 and pepsinogen I: a multicentre study. Eur J Gastroenterol Hepatol. 15:885–91.

60. Correa P. Helicobacter pylori and gastric carcinogenesis. Am J Surg Pathol. 1995;19(Suppl 1):S37–43.
61. Take S, Mizuno M, Ishiki K, et al. The long-term risk of gastric cancer after the successful eradication of helicobacter pylori. J Gastroenterol. 2011;46:318–24.
62. Sipponen P, Hyvärinen H. Role of helicobacter pylori in the pathogenesis of gastritis, peptic ulcer and gastric cancer. Scand J Gastroenterol Suppl. 1993;196:3–6.
63. Kikuchi S, Wada O, Nakajima T, et al. Serum anti-helicobacter pylori antibody and gastric carcinoma among young adults. Research group on prevention of gastric carcinoma among young adults. Cancer. 1995;75:2789–93.
64. Kokkola A, Valle J, Haapiainen R, et al. Helicobacter pylori infection in young patients with gastric carcinoma. Scand J Gastroenterol. 1996;31:643–7.
65. Tanaka A, Watari J, Tanabe H, et al. Effect of eradication of helicobacter pylori on genetic instabilities in gastric intestinal metaplasia. Aliment Pharmacol Ther. 2006;24(Suppl 4):194–202.
66. Rugge M, Genta RM. Staging gastritis: an international proposal. Gastroenterol. 2005;129:1807–8.
67. Rugge M, Genta RM. Staging and grading of chronic gastritis. Hum Pathol. 2005;36:228–33.
68. Rugge M, Meggio A, Pennelli G, et al. Gastritis staging in clinical practice: the OLGA staging system. Gut. 2007;56:631–6.
69. Molaei M, Ehtiati A, Mashayekhi R, et al. Gastric atrophy: use of OLGA staging system in practice. Gastroenterol Hepatol Bed Bench. 2016;9:25–9.
70. Rugge M, de Boni M, Pennelli G, et al. Gastritis OLGA-staging and gastric cancer risk: a twelve-year clinico-pathological follow-up study. Aliment Pharmacol Ther. 2010;31:1104–11.
71. Satoh K, Osawa H, Yoshizawa M, et al. Assessment of atrophic gastritis using the OLGA system. Helicobacter. 2008;13:225–9.
72. Siurala M, Isokoski M, Varis K, et al. Prevalence of gastritis in a rural population. Bioptic study of subjects selected at random. Scand J Gastroenterol. 1968;3:211–23.
73. Lambert R. Chronic gastritis. A critical study of the progressive atrophy of the gastric mucosa. Digestion. 1972;7:83–126.
74. MacDonald WC, Anderson FH, Hashimoto S. Histological effect of certain pickles on the human gastric mucosa. A preliminary report. Can Med Assoc J. 1967;96:1521–5.
75. Palmer ED. Gastritis, a re-evaluation. Medicine. 1954;33:199–290.
76. Edwards FC, Coghill NF. Aetiological factors in chronic atrophic gastritis. Br Med J. 1966;2:1409–15.
77. Creutzfeldt W, Lamberts R. Inter-relationship between serum gastrin levels. Gastric Mucosal Histology and Gastric Endocrine Cell Growth Digestion. 1992;51(Suppl 1):76–81.
78. Sipponen P, Maaroos HI. Chronic gastritis. Scand J Gastroenterol. 2015;50:657–67.
79. Gear MW, Truelove SC, Whitehead R. Gastric ulcer and gastritis. Gut. 1971;12:639–45.
80. Chen XY, Liu WZ, Shi Y, et al. Helicobacter pylori associated gastric diseases and lymphoid tissue hyperplasia in gastric antral mucosa. J Clin Pathol. 2002;55:133–7.

9 Precancerous Lesions: Atrophic Gastritis, Intestinal Metaplasia, Natural Course of Chronic Gastritis and Associated Risk Factors

9.1 Atrophic Gastritis

Atrophic gastritis (AG) refers to a condition where there is loss of gastric glands associated with mucosal thinning and a variable amount of inflammatory cell infiltration in lamina propria [1]. It is usually the effect of a long-standing mucosa inflammation and is accompanied by reduction in gastric secretory function giving rise to a state of achlorhydria or hypochlorhydria and has a significant risk of development of gastric cancer (GC) [2, 3]. There are studies that had shown presence of AG and intestinal metaplasia (IM) in the setting of chronic gastritis predisposes to a higher risk of cancer development compared to individual who has only features of chronic gastritis without AG or IM. And AG is relatively high in countries having high prevalence of *H. pylori* infection [4, 5]. The converse is also true in certain countries with low incidence of GC and precancerous lesions with high incidence of HP infection. This has been described as the phenomenon of geographical enigmas and the countries with such enigma are Africa, Asia including India and Costa Rica [6–8]. Duodenal ulcer is known to be associated with antral dominant non-atrophic gastritis, reportedly is low risk for GC [9, 10]. GC and peptic ulcer occupy opposite ends in the spectrum of *H. pylori*-related gastritis. Individuals with AG have been documented to exhibit a stepwise reduction in serum pepsinogen I and I/II ratio, thereby is a good modality in clinical evaluation of AG in patients who are documented with chronic gastritis in biopsy samples [11, 12].

9.2 Endoscopic Features of Atrophic Gastritis

Endoscopic features described for AG and IM are non-specific and variable with a wide inter-observer variation, and AG is considered when gastric mucosa shows prominent mucosal vascular pattern along with loss of gastric mucosal folds [13]. HP-related AG progresses from antrum to corpus along lesser curvature [14]. Kimura-Takemoto classifies gastric mucosa atrophy appearances in endoscopy as—i) closed-type where atrophic border remains on lesser curvature; ii) open type when atrophic border is not limited to lesser curvature but extends much beyond on anterior as well as posterior walls [15]. Endoscopic diagnosis of atrophy mucosal changes was found to be non-specific, especially in individuals less than 50 years of age and was inaccurate, majority of the mild changes appeared normal [16]. Equally, sensitivity and specificity for IM were also observed to be low [17]. Specialized techniques like chromoendoscopy and narrow band imaging (NBI) enhances identification of the abnormal mucosa bearing IM and dysplasia [18]. Other high resolution magnifying endoscopies have also been found to be superior

K. Vaiphei, *Interpretation of Endoscopic Biopsy - Gastritis, Gastropathies and Beyond*,
https://doi.org/10.1007/978-981-16-6026-9_9

to conventional endoscopes in identifying the abnormal mucosa associated with HP infection, IM and dysplasia [19, 20]. NBI has been found to have good sensitivity and specificity in identifying gastric precancerous lesions [21, 22].

In routine practice to assess histological grades and changes of gastritis, adequate number of samples (at least 5 to 6 pieces) should be taken from different segments and identifiable lesions of the stomach, orienting them on filter papers and putting them into separately labelled vials. The reason for taking multiple biopsy specimens from different areas of the gastric mucosa is due to the patchy and focal nature of environmental gastritis; hence most of the pathologies occur in a haphazard manner with irregular distribution [1, 5]. Hence, biopsy samples covering different areas of the mucosa are necessary to determine the type of the gastritis and its associated mucosal pathology. Multiple specimens from: a) antral biopsies—along lesser and greater curvatures of antrum within 2 to 3 cm from pylorus; b) transition zone between antrum and body at incisura angularis; c) corpus biopsies—from the lesser curvature of the corpus about 4 cm proximal to incisura angularis and from the mid-portion of greater curvature of the corpus approximately 8 cm from cardia [23]. Additional biopsy is indicated from an endoscopically visible abnormal area(s), i.e. ulcer, erosion or any depressed or nodular area. This pattern of sampling helps to detect any unsuspected premalignant focus and its distribution [24]. Biopsy of gastric body and fundic mucosa are valuable to assess effects of proton pump inhibitor and demonstration of HP that tends to colonize in this region. Characterization of gastritis is all the time better if each biopsy includes the muscularis mucosae representing a full-thickness mucosa. Assessment of atrophy is reliable if the sample includes at least 15–20 gastric pit areas [23]. In the Sidney system, presence of *H. pylori*, neutrophils, mononuclear cells, loss of specialized glands and intestinal metaplasia are given descriptive graded values ranging from 0 for absent, 1 for mild, 2 for moderate and 3 for marked (or severe) changes [1]. Other nongraded variables include changes in surface lining cells, status of the mucin content, surface epithelial cell denudation or erosion, presence of lymphoid cell in aggregates, foveolae epithelial cell status, pyloric gland and pancreatic or acinar metaplasia, and neuroendocrine cell hyperplasia. Some of these factors do help in identifying HP-related mucosal inflammation from other subtypes of gastritis.

Histology of normal gastric mucosa is site specific and identifiable from the different population of glands, i.e. mucous and oxyntic types are normal components of antrum and corpus respectively and these normal glands are equipped with appropriate function for the site [25–27] Fig. 9.1 A and B). Recommended number of biopsy samples are from five locations, i.e. two from antrum, one from incisura and two from corpus [1]. When sampling from incisura is difficult, it may be avoided. As individual ages, the atrophy changes progress from incisura along lesser curvature reaching almost to GEJ in elderly individuals. Hence, examination of specimens from antrum and corpus along lesser as well as greater curvatures are essential to evaluate AG and IM [28–30]. Histological interpretation may face difficulties when sampling is inadequate. In biopsies bearing heavy inflammation obscures the glands and epithelial cells, which may result in overestimation of atrophy. In such situation, the biopsy may be labelled as "indefinite for atrophy" and a repeat biopsy may be advised after controlling active inflammation [26].

Occasionally in routine reporting, there may be a small focus of metaplastic/goblet cells along the foveolar epithelium which may be termed as foveolar restricted intestinal metaplasia with normal and appropriate glands for the biopsy site. Histological feature to label a gastric biopsy showing atrophy is reduced or near-total loss of appropriate glands for the site of biopsy. It is important to remember the type of the glands as mucus glands replacing the corpus glands will qualify for a diagnosis of atrophy (Fig. 9.2 A to E). Ruggae et al (2011) formulated a simplified way to classify the histological spectrum of atrophy [31]. Loss of the specialized glands may take place in different forms: i) complete absence of the glands associated with replacement fibrosis and expansion of the lamina propria and ii) the

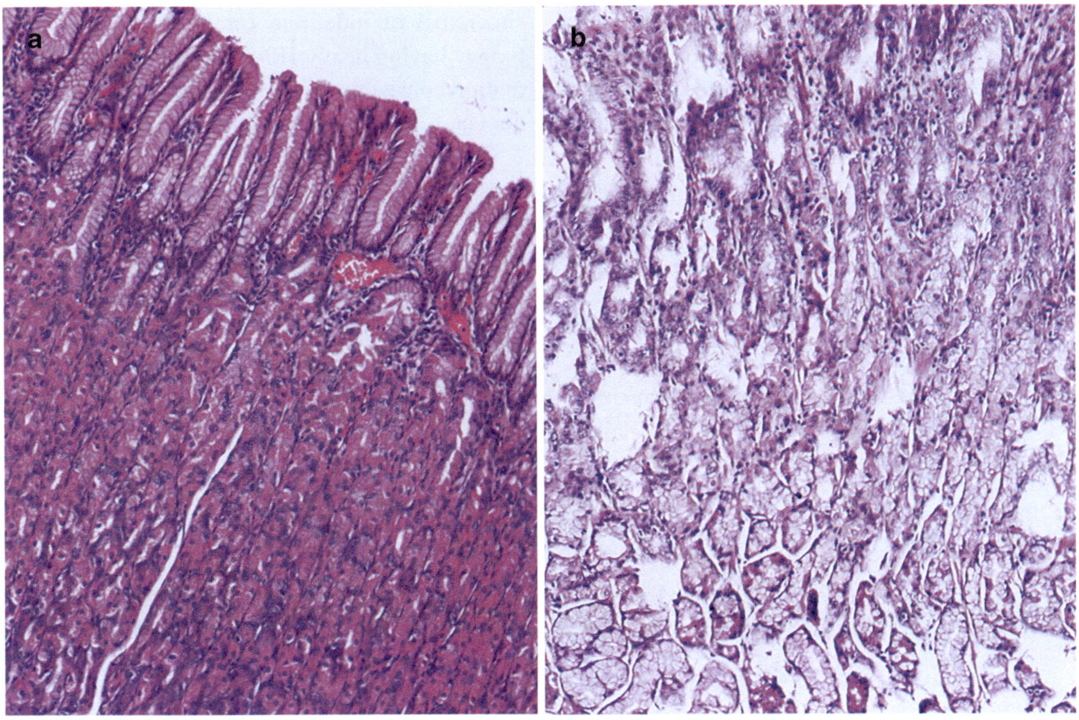

Fig. 9.1 A and B—Photomicrographs showing normal body and pyloric antral mucosa (HE, x250)

native glands may be replaced by metaplastic gland like the pyloric gland in corpus biopsy associated with intestinal metaplasia. The second type may not have true reduction of glands. Metaplasia is a process of transformation of native committed cell to another type that will not be associated with dedifferentiation. Two main types of gastric gland metaplasia have been recognized. The first one being pseudopyloric metaplasia or spasmolytic polypeptide-expressing metaplasia [SPEM]) of oxyntic mucosa and is identified by antral-like mucosa in biopsies obtained from corpus/fundus [32–34]. It re-iterates the importance of submitting appropriately labelled biopsy for histopathology analysis. Character of the native oxyntic mucosa in cases of pseudo-pyloric metaplasia may be confirmed by demonstrating the presence of pepsinogen I positive cells [35, 36]. Second type is intestinal metaplasia (IM) may arise in any type of mucosa, that may be complete or small intestinal mucosal type or incomplete where it resembling colonic mucosa [35, 36]. Loss of normal gland is the first specific recognizable step in atrophy, metaplastic and precancerous cascade indicating long-standing inflammatory process giving rise to multifocal atrophic gastritis (MAG). These histological changes are progressive with time and glandular loss possibly is followed by fibrosis. Serology indicator for oxyntic mucosal atrophy is pepsinogen I (PGI) where the level progressively reduces. Pepsinogen II (PGII) is secreted by foveolar glands in antrum and body mucosa and an increased serum value is related to mucosal and foveolar epithelial cell proliferation both in benign hyperplasia and neoplasia. Hence, the ratio of PGI/PGII may be used as an indicator of corporal atrophy [36, 37].

A good biopsy should include the whole thickness of mucosa, fixed in fixative adequately, orientated and the glass slide having adequate number of ribbon sections [38]. For routine H&E staining, sections should be obtained at least at three levels from paraffin block. In addition to the H&E staining, special stains like alcian blue–periodic acid–Schiff staining detects metaplastic epithelial cell [1, 38–41] (Fig. 9.3 A and B). A biopsy may be labelled negative for atrophy if glands are identified in appropriate number and there may be minimal isolated intestinal metaplasia. Label of indefinite for atrophy refers to a biopsy having heavy HP-related mucosal inflammation consisting of dense lamina propria mononuclear cells, frequently with lymphoid

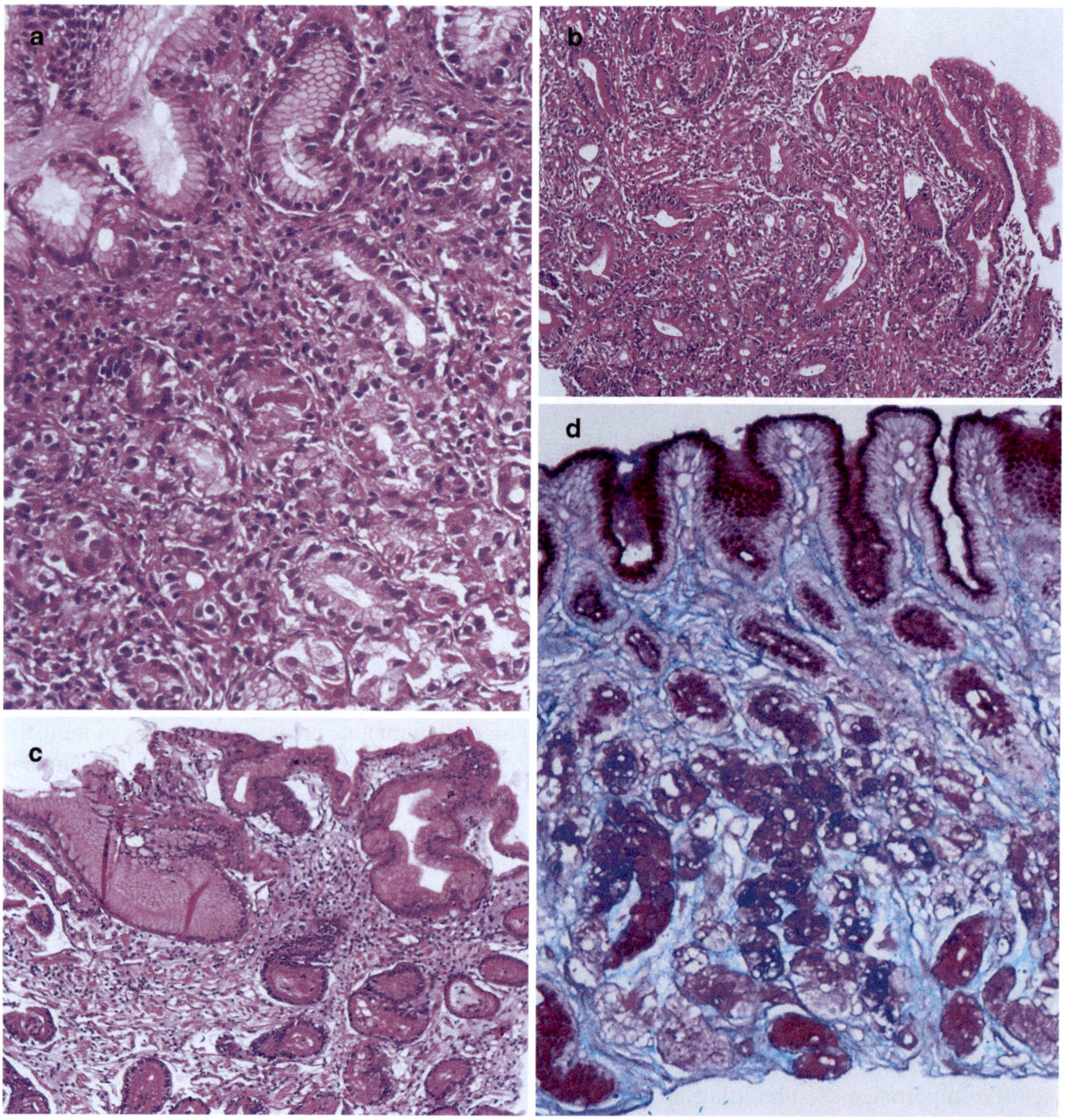

Fig. 9.2 A, B and C—Photomicrographs showing different grades of atrophy changes in a body mucosa; A—no significant reduction in the number of glandular components, to be noted is the antral type of glands present amongst the fundic glands; B—reduction in the number of glandular components along with patchy fibrosis and moderately heavy chronic inflammatory cell infiltration, to be noted is the presence of goblet cells amongst the glandular lining epithelium; C—significant loss of the specialized glands and replacement fibrosis with mucinous degeneration, minimal inflammatory cell infiltration and a few goblet cell metaplasia. (HE, x250); D—the picture highlights the different mucin characters ranging from the normal magenta colour gastric foveolar mucin to blue colour intestinal mucin to intermediate colour of bluish purplish colour mucin (AB-PAS, x250) and E—picture shows a mild increase in enterochromaffin-like cells indicated in immunohistochemistry using chromogranin A primary antibody (PAP, x300)

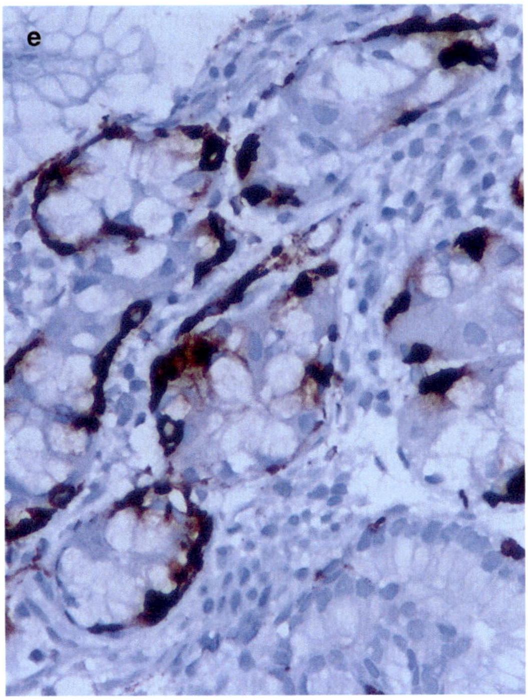

Fig. 9.2 (continued)

aggregates or follicles, obscuring antral or oxyntic glands; this term should be avoided in the presence of metaplasia involving one entire gland, which is an objective evidence of atrophy. Atrophy refers to gastric mucosa having loss of native glands; metaplastic atrophy there is replacement of the native glands by metaplastic epithelium and in non-metaplastic group there is decreased density of native glands with increase inter-glandular extracellular matrix. Metaplastic and non-metaplastic patterns may coexist in the same atrophy mucosal biopsy [42–45].

Atrophy associated with metaplasia: Defining atrophy includes intestinalized glands representing mucosal atrophy that involves a complete native glandular unit. Metaplasia may be restricted only to foveolar cells with no glandular loss. Such metaplasia should be labelled as foveolar restricted metaplasia. Sometimes, when metaplasia is more extensive, the glandular unit may have an irregular outline. Such kind of metaplasia frequently associates with increased loose matrix in lamina propria, but the metaplastic glands maintain normal configuration with a minimal amount of stromal component. In grading metaplastic atrophy, three levels have been identified following the scheme suggested by visual analogue scales of the updated Sydney system [1, 46]. Mild atrophic associated with sporadic glands with intestinal type of metaplastic epithelium; when the biopsy shows extensive metaplasia, it equalizes with severe atrophy, and intermediate grade of atrophy with metaplasia refers to a biopsy exhibiting moderate degree of morphological changes (See Figs. 4.14, 4.15, 4.16, 4.18, 8.2 and 8.3), where the native fundic and body glands are replaced by foveolar cells or mucus glands called as pseudo-pyloric metaplasia [45, 47]. This type of morphological change may be observed in any form of chronic gastritis including autoimmune gastritis. Frequently there is associated enterochromaffin-like (ECL) cell hyperplasia [1, 48–51] (see Figs. 5.1, 5.7, and 5.10). Lamina propria stromal component may not be increased with an apparent look of normal glands. However obviously oxyntic glands are replaced. Problem may arise while dealing with a biopsy sampled from incisura and transition zone in distinguishing between an inflamed antral mucosa and body mucosa with pseudo-pyloric metaplasia [41, 52]. A helpful tip in such a situation will be the presence of IM as a reliable feature for atrophy.

Gastric intestinal metaplasia or GIM is defined as intestinal epithelium replacing gastric epithelium identifiable in HE staining and is believed to be the result of long-standing inflammation [53, 54]. The process of metaplasia taking place in inflamed gastric mucosa possibly is to adapt the inciting agent producing gastritis, destruction of the glands, and replacement fibrosis of the gastric mucosa. A good exemplification will be HP-associated gastritis [53]. Jason Mills stated that it was Rudolph Virchow who had coined metaplasia at VIII International Medical Congress in Copenhagen in 1884 [54]. George Adami illustrated that stem cell generates normal cells and tissue; and under unfavourable situation a differentiated cell is capable of proliferation and differentiating into some other cell type [55]. This view was not accepted by many developmental biologists, rather embraced Conrad Waddington's proposal that stem cell differentiates in one particular direction [56].

More recently, the concept of intestinal metaplasia being congenital has become obsolete and since the late 1930s, IM has been accepted as a metaplasia caused by gastritis [57]. In 1970, Japanese pathologists described IM to be of two types having malignant potential [58]. About a decade later, Jass and Filipe categorize 2 types of gastric IM based on their mucin histochemistry [59] (Fig. 9.3 A and B). Type I refers to complete metaplasia having both absorptive and goblet cells containing sialomucin. Type II or incomplete metaplasia refers to the presence of goblet cells with foveolar cells and this may be further subcategorized into IIB expressing hindgut type sulfomucin and IIA expressing with no sulfomucin. In the 1990s, Correa followed by Megan et al. proposed that HP gastritis with IM is a precancerous condition [60, 61]. Hayakawa et al. observed that Mist1 messenger RNA expressing cells include chief cells and quiescent stem cells in the isthmus of body mucosa [62]. Chief cell ablation experiments suggested that Mist1+ isthmus stem cells could be used for lineage tracing of body mucosa. Inducing K-ras mutation, Mist1+ stem cells were found to be the cells of origin for IM and thereby in cancer development [62].

Atrophy without metaplasia. The term gastric antral atrophy without intestinal metaplasia has been questioned by many gastroenterologists and pathologists. The epidemiology and clinical aspect of this condition have been documented [44, 51, 52, 63–66]. More recently Ruiz et al. have validated the existence of antral mucosal atrophic changes even in the absence of metaplastic changes [67]. Landis and Koch had documented antral mucosal atrophy changes many years ago and the best way to identify is by studying number of glands in cross-sections observed at intermediate magnification [68]. The three-tiered visual analogue scales proposed in the updated Sydney System may be utilized to grade non-metaplastic atrophy into mild, moderate and severe [1, 46]. In this condition, there is expan-

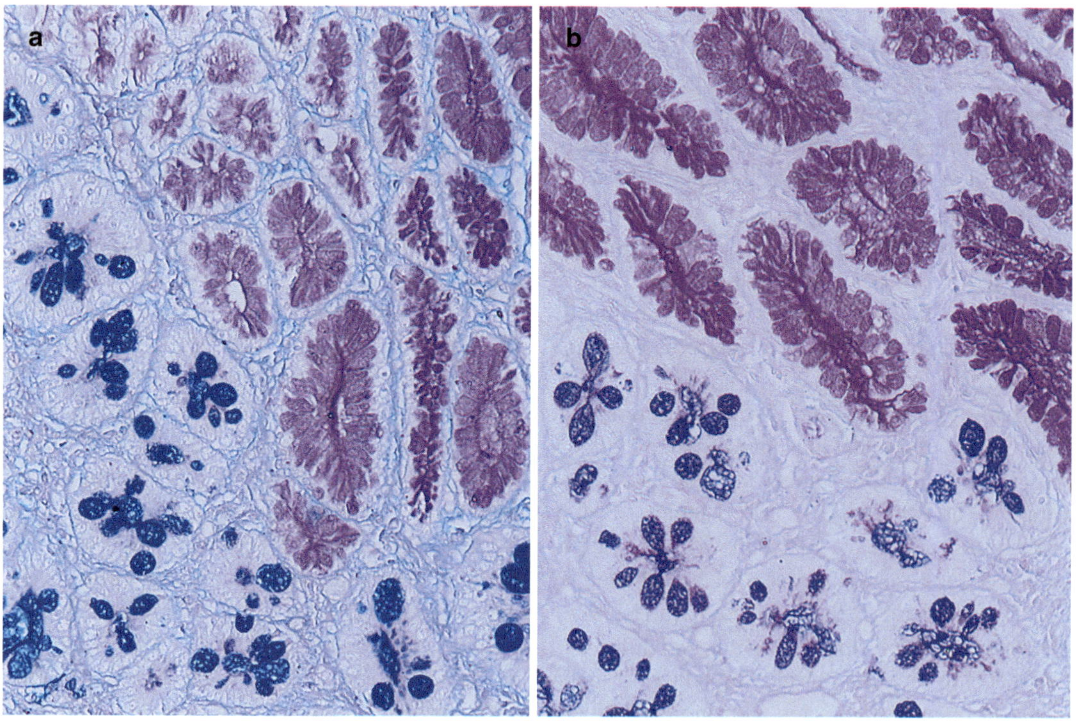

Fig. 9.3 A and B—the two photomicrographs look almost similar, however, both the staining were carried out using alcian blue at pH 2.5 and 1, respectively, to identify the sialomucin and sulfomucin components in the intestinal metaplastic epithelium in a gastric biopsy (AB-PAS at pH 2.5 and 1, x250)

sion of the lamina propria with collagenization and reduction in the number of branching foveolae. And in body and fundic mucosa, the native oxyntic tubules become shortened with increased expansion of the inter-glandular lamina propria by collagenization. In a patient with severe atrophic changes, mucosa appears distinctly different, losing its normal shining mucosal fold pattern and becomes granular and white [26].

Gastric atrophy with limited involvement of oxyntic mucosa is a manifestation of pernicious anaemia syndrome, frequently observed in Scandinavian and northern European countries. Gastric mucosal changes observed in this condition is called autoimmune gastritis or type A gastritis showing features of severe and diffuse loss of oxyntic glands and normal antral mucosa [68, 69]. This condition is not known to be associated with the development of peptic ulcer disease. The other type of gastric mucosal atrophy is antral dominant gastritis and this group of patients are prone to develop duodenal ulcer [65–67]. The third type refers to multifocal type or type B atrophic gastritis and is usually associated with environmental factors, most frequently *H. pylori*-related gastritis. This group of patients is prone to have gastric peptic ulcer disease [68, 69]. In mild form of atrophic gastritis, the lesions are patchy and may be present in some of the biopsy samples. In *H. pylori*-associated gastritis, biopsy from angularis incisura shows the histological changes most frequently. Presence of HP is to be mentioned in the report, though a semi-quantitative assessment of HP has little or no clinical implication. Patients receiving proton pump inhibitors, antral biopsy may be negative for HP but the presence of inflammatory cells (polymorphs and lymphoid infiltrate) may suggest the presence of the organism.

9.3 Documentation of Histopathology Report

1. Biopsy sample(s) submitted needs to be identified by matching with the requisition form. 2. Clinical history, endoscopic findings and site of biopsies are essential components for interpretation of gastric biopsies. 3. Number of tissue fragments present on the filter papers at the time of grossing requires to be matched with the number of tissue pieces observed in the ribbon sections present on glass slides and it is imperative to examine every fragment. I like to scan them under low power and start with the least involved fragment on medium or higher power lenses according to the need. 4. Biopsies were taken from different areas of the stomach to be read, interpreted and described separately. 5. While mentioning the findings like inflammation and metaplasia, to be graded and the pattern of distribution should be mentioned in the report clearly. 6. Presence of history of intake of certain chemicals or drugs should be taken into consideration while interpreting the biopsy with the effort of making a relevant histological diagnosis. Presence of such histories will not exclude the possibility of being infective aetiology or coexistence of both conditions. Semi-quantitative scoring to be done for some of the elementary lesions, such as (a) lymphomononuclear inflammation, (b) polymorphs and eosinophils, (c) atrophic changes to be distinguished as metaplastic and non-metaplastic type, and also the extend, (d) metaplasia—type and extend to be mentioned, (e) *H. pylori* status, (f) foveolar hyperplasia, (g) regenerative epithelium, (h) any atypia or dysplasia and (i) any other significant findings including mucosal and submucosal vascular changes. According to OLGA staging system, the final assessment should be based on the overall extent and severity of gastritis which may be mentioned as grade and possible underlying aetiology.

9.4 Gastric Intestinal Metaplasia

The two types of Gastric Intestinal Metaplasia (GIM) may be observed—i) absorptive type enterocytes having brush border and goblet cells and ii) columnar cells with no brush border [42] (see Figs. 4.14 to 4.19). GIM may be further divided into 3 phenotypes depending on mucin character on histochemistry using alcian blue and high iron diamine [70]. Type I refers to a complete or small intestinal type. Type II GIM is positively stained for sialomucin in goblet and columnar cells, whereas type III shows positivity for sulfomucin. Type I may also have Paneth cell. These changes are progressive. Normal gastric mucosa is MUC5AC positive along the surface and MUC6 in the deeper glands; and is of neutral pH, take-up magenta colour in periodic acid Schiff staining. In IM, cytoplasmic mucin is mostly stained with alcian blue at pH 2.5 indicating it to be mostly sialic acid and shows MUC2 positivity in IHC (Fig. 9.4 A to C). Sialomucin may be seen in combination with neutral mucin [72]. Over the years, metaplastic focus expands spreading over large areas acquiring new phenotypes. Type II IM tends to show a mixture of goblet and mucous cells showing positive staining for both sialo and neutral mucin. Type III has tortuous and branched crypts lined by columnar and goblet cells positive for sulfo- and sialomucin [1]. IM exhibiting the colonic type of metaplasia, i.e. both type II and III are classified as incomplete as it has phenotype of large bowel in morphology and mucin character but lacking digestive enzymes partially or completely. These cells also have the potential to re-express neutral mucin and lack brush border, their mucin droplets are of variable sizes and shapes. A gastric biopsy showing features of atrophic gastritis with IM frequently contains foci of both complete and incomplete IM and may be classified according to the dominant type. Incomplete or type III GIM is considered to have a higher cancer risk than other types [70, 72–74]. The significance of type III GIM as a precursor lesion in the development of gastric cancer remains controversial as some consider it to be of limited value as an indicator of risk of gastric cancer [74–78]. Hence, in addition to the type of IM, extent and

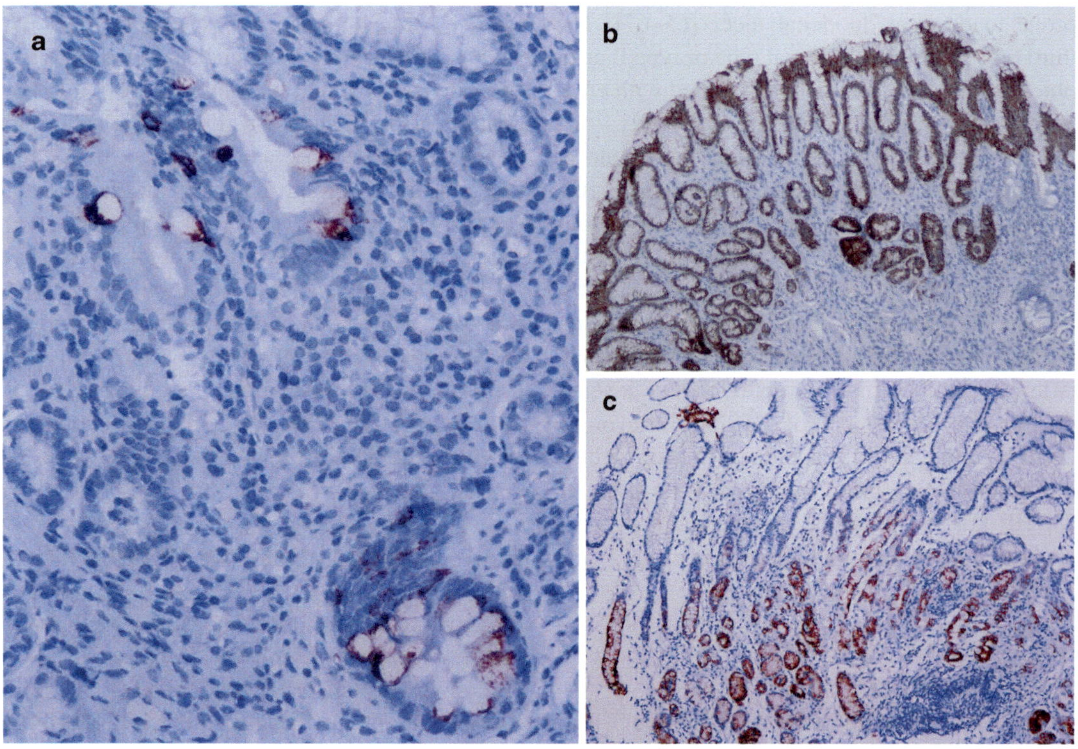

Fig. 9.4 A to C—panels of the photomicrographs of immunohistochemistry stain sections showing MUC6, MUC5Ac and MUC 2 positivity in an antral mucosal biopsy (PAP, x250). A—medium-power view showing MUC positively stained goblet cells in gastric biopsy to indicate complete metaplasia (PAP, x250); B—another picture where MUC5a had been used to stain the normal gastric foveolar cells (PAP, x250) and C—another picture of gastric biopsy where MUC6 had been used to stain the antral glands positively (PAP, x250)

severity of atrophy changes are considered as the most significant predictor for cancer risk [79–81]. There are some studies which had reported that intestinal-type gastric cancers do not necessarily arise from a precursor lesion of GIM, raising the question of the significance of GIM [81, 82]. There has been a study in which IM was not always demonstrable surrounding intestinal-type GC, questioning the significance of IM in cancer development [83].

In conjunction with histochemistry, IM may be typed using IHC and more than 20 mucin (MUC) associated proteins have been identified. Of which most commonly used proteins are MUC1, MUC2, MUC5AC and MUC6. Incomplete type IM, similar to large intestine in pathologic features, is positive for MUC5AC, MUC6 and MUC2 [84, 85] (Fig. 9.1 A to C). High iron diamine-alcian blue staining is helpful in classifying IM, type I expresses the only sialomucin seen as bright blue and, type II and III express both sialomucin and sulfomucin seen as black colour [84]. Because *H. pylori* are not demonstrable in the gastric mucosa with IM due to changing pH milieu in the background of gastric mucosa with IM and atrophy, which have been interpreted by some as protection against *H. pylori* infection or physiologic adaptation to altered bacterial flora [23]. It is a matter of debate on the clonality of gastric gland with IM and suggestion has been made that IM is a result of mutation and normal glands are replaced by metaplastic glands by crypt fission [71]. IM is the result of alteration in gastric epithelial stem and progenitor cells [83]. A study in experimental animals demonstrated conversion of gastric epithelium into intestinal type on transgenic expression of CDX2 suggesting role of stem cells in initiating IM [71, 86].

9.5 Natural Course of Chronic Gastritis

Chronic gastritis, if left unattended, is progressive lifelong inflammatory condition. The process of superficial chronic gastritis usually starts in childhood as mononuclear inflammation coexisting with acute inflammation. The inflammation progresses to atrophic gastritis characterized by loss of normal specialized gastric glands that may affect glands in antrum or corpus and fundus or all different sites [36, 87–89]. Age-specific prevalence of gastritis tends to increase with age and is more frequently occurred in developing countries than in the developed country. It has been reported to involve more than 50% of young children in developing countries and a lesser percentage has been reported in developed countries [87, 88]. Loss of native mucosal glands in atrophic gastritis is replaced by new immature glandular and epithelial elements, i.e. glands of intestinal type resembling colonic or small intestinal epithelium and/or with pyloric type resembling pyloric glands and epithelium with no G cell [1, 43, 44, 86–88]. The first morphological change observed in *H. pylori* infection was antral dominant inflammation. Inflammation confining to superficial half of gastric mucosa comprising lymphoplasmacytic cells has been referred to as superficial gastritis. Intensity of acute or active components of chronic gastritis is likely to depend on the cytotoxicity of *H. pylori* strain [89, 90]. It has been estimated that about 50% of HP-infected patients in their lifetime will develop atrophic gastritis. A pure antral phenotype of HP gastritis may extend to remaining gastric mucosa giving the morphology of multifocal or corpus dominant gastritis. Proximal extension of the pathology associates with functional abnormality of gastric mucosa resulting in hypochlorhydria, reduction or absence of intrinsic factor and affects the synthesis and secretion of gastrin by antral G cells. Antral limited severe atrophic changes are extremely rare condition. An advanced atrophy involving body mucosa alone or with involvement of the antral mucosa simultaneously is relatively common. Long-term follow-up studies revealed that as the HP infection progresses towards the corpus, antral gastritis may get resolved. Along the process of development of atrophic phenotypes, perhaps there is coincidental triggering of carcinogenic pathway, as has been suggested by Correa's cascade [1, 36, 43, 86, 87, 89, 91, 92].

9.6 Risk Factors for Atrophic Gastritis and Intestinal Metaplasia

Diets that have been associated with e development of atrophic gastritis (AG), intestinal metaplasia (IM) and cancer are HP infection, excess amount of salt intake, deficient in vitamin C and insufficient carotenoid [60, 91, 93–96]. *Helicobacter pylori*-related bacterial virulence genes such as cagA and VacA have been found to be risk factors for AG, IM and GC [91–95]. A follow-up study to evaluate the role of HP-associated antigens, cagA was found to be more virulent than any other antigens and risk for gastric cancer was increased by 1.64 in meta-analysis [95–99]. cagA protein produces its cytotoxic effect by getting translocated into the cytoplasm via its type IV secretion system. cagA interrupts signalling pathways by phosphorylation resulting in modification of cytoskeletal, motility and cellular activities [100–102]. Other well well-known vacA associated virulence factors are s1 and m1, which are related to gastric epithelial damage, AG and gastric cancer [100]. A high association between the presence of AG or IM and prevalence of VacA s1, m1 and cagA strains of *H. pylori* genotypes. IM was associated with VacA s1, VacA m1 and cagA [101, 102]. In another study, the outer membrane protein of *H. pylori* SabA positive individuals were found to have association with the presence of AG, IM and GC [103]. In a multicentric prospective study, risk factors were found to be influenced by the age of the patients. In those who are older than 60 years of age, risk factors were cagA and VacA m1 positivity for the development of atrophic gastritis. And the risk factors for IM in a similar age group were more than 61 years of age, HP infection per se, spicy food, smoking and production of IL10 [104]. Many of the studies that have referred have shown that VacA and cagA genotypes of HP were not distributed uniformly in different parts of the world and a significant difference in HP genotypes was documented between Asian and European and American countries, which possibly is the reason for the differences in incidences of gastric cancer.

References

1. Dixon MF, Genta RM, Yardley JH, et al. Classification and grading of gastritis. The updated Sydney system. International workshop on the histopathology of gastritis, Houston 1994. Am J Surg Pathol. 1996;20:1161–81.
2. Lechago J, Correa P. Prolonged achlorhydria and gastric neoplasia: is there a causal relationship? Gastroenterol. 1993;104:1554–7.
3. de Vries AC, Haringsma J, Kuipers EJ. The detection, surveillance and treatment of premalignant gastric lesions related to helicobacter pylori infection. Helicobacter. 2007;12:1–15.
4. Kim N, Park YS, Cho SI, et al. Prevalence and risk factors of atrophic gastritis and intestinal metaplasia in a Korean population without significant gastroduodenal disease. Helicobacter. 2008;13:245–55.
5. Sipponen P, Kekki M, Haapakoski J, et al. Gastric cancer risk in chronic atrophic gastritis: statistical calculations of cross-sectional data. Int J Cancer. 1985;35:173–7.
6. Graham DY, Lu H, Yamaoka Y. African, Asian or Indian enigma, the east Asian helicobacter pylori: facts or medical myths. J Dig Dis. 2009;10:77–84.
7. Miwa H, Go MF, Sato N. H. Pylori and gastric cancer: the Asian enigma. Am J Gastroenterol. 2002;97:1106–12.
8. Goh KL. Epidemiology of helicobacter pylori infection in Malaysia--observations in a multiracial Asian population. Med J Malaysia. 2009;64:187–92.
9. Uemura N, Okamoto S, Yamamoto S, et al. Helicobacter pylori infection and the development of gastric cancer. N Engl J Med. 2001;345:784–9.
10. Mera R, Fontham ET, Bravo LE, et al. Long term follow up of patients treated for helicobacter pylori infection. Gut. 2005;54:1536–40.
11. Miki K, Ichinose M, Shimizu A, et al. Serum pepsinogens as a screening test of extensive chronic gastritis. Gastroenterol Jpn. 1987;22:133–41.
12. Ichinose M, Yahagi N, Oka M, et al. Screening for gastric cancer in Japan. In: Wu GY, Aziz K, editors. Cancer screening for common malignancies. Totowa, New Jersey: Humana Press 2001; 2001. p. 87–102.
13. Lee JY, Kim N, Lee HS, et al. Correlations among endoscopic, histologic and serologic diagnoses for the assessment of atrophic gastritis. J Cancer Prev. 2014;19:47–55.
14. Kimura K, Satoh K, Ido K, et al. Gastritis in the Japanese stomach. Scand J Gastroenterol Suppl. 1996;214:17–20. discussion 21-3
15. Kono S, Gotoda T, Yoshida S, et al. Can endoscopic atrophy predict histological atrophy? Historical study in United Kingdom and Japan. World J Gastroenterol. 2015;21:13113–23.
16. Eshmuratov A, Nah JC, Kim N, et al. The correlation of endoscopic and histological diagnosis of gastric atrophy. Dig Dis Sci. 2010;55:1364–75.

17. Lim JH, Kim N, Lee HS, et al. Correlation between endoscopic and histological diagnoses of gastric intestinal metaplasia. Gut Liver. 2013;7:41–50.
18. Dinis-Ribeiro M, da Costa-Pereira A, Lopes C, et al. Magnification chromoendoscopy for the diagnosis of gastric intestinal metaplasia and dysplasia. Gastrointest Endosc. 2003;57:498–504.
19. Anagnostopoulos GK, Yao K, Kaye P, et al. High-resolution magnification endoscopy can reliably identify normal gastric mucosa, helicobacter pylori-associated gastritis, and gastric atrophy. Endoscopy. 2007;39:202–7.
20. Gonen C, Simsek I, Sarioglu S, et al. Comparison of high-resolution magnifying endoscopy and standard videoendoscopy for the diagnosis of helicobacter pylori gastritis in routine clinical practice: a prospective study. Helicobacter. 2009;14:12–21.
21. Kadowaki S, Tanaka K, Toyoda H, et al. Ease of early gastric cancer demarcation recognition: a comparison of four magnifying endoscopy methods. J Gastroenterol Hepatol. 2009;24:1625–30.
22. Capelle LG, Haringsma J, de Vries AC, et al. Narrow band imaging for the detection of gastric intestinal metaplasia and dysplasia during surveillance endoscopy. Dig Dis Sci. 2010;55:3442–8.
23. Crafa P, Russo M, Miraglia C, et al. From Sidney to OLGA: an overview of atrophic gastritis. Acta Biomed. 2018;89(Supplement 8):93–9.
24. Sugano K, Tack J, Kuipers EJ, et al. Kyoto global consensus report on helicobacter pylori gastritis. Gut. 2015;64:1–15.
25. Ruiz B, Garay J, Correa P, et al. Morphometric evaluation of gastric antral atrophy: improvement after cure of helicobacter pylori infection. Am J Gastroenterol. 2001;96:3281–7.
26. Rugge M, Correa P, Dixon MF, et al. Gastric mucosal atrophy: interobserver consistency using new criteria for classification and grading. Aliment Pharmacol Ther. 2002;16:1249–59.
27. Rugge M, Meggio A, Pennelli G, et al. Gastritis staging in clinical practice: the OLGA staging system. Gut. 2007;56:631–6.
28. Jönsson KA, Gotthard R, Bodemar G, et al. The clinical relevance of endoscopic and histologic inflammation of gastroduodenal mucosa in dyspepsia of unknown origin. Scand J Gastroenterol. 1989;24:385–95.
29. Lim JH, Kim N, Lee HS, et al. Correlation between endoscopic and histological diagnoses of gastric intestinal metaplasia. Gut Liver. 2013;7:41–50.
30. Lee JY, Kim N, Lee HS, et al. Correlations among endoscopic, histologic and serologic diagnoses for the assessment of atrophic gastritis. J Cancer Prev. 2014;19:47–55.
31. Ruggea M, Pennellia G, Pilozzic E, et al. Gastritis: the histology report. Dig Liv Dis. 2011;2011: S373–84.
32. Gutiérrez-Gonzalez L, Wright NA. Biology of intestinal metaplasia in 2008: more than a simple phenotypic alteration. Dig Liver Dis. 2008;40:510–22.
33. Weis VG, Goldenring JR. Current understanding of SPEM and its standing in the preneoplastic process. Gastric Cancer. 2009;12:189–97.
34. Nam KT, Lee HJ, Sousa JF, et al. Mature chief cells are cryptic progenitors for metaplasia in the stomach. Gastroenterol. 2010;139:2028–37.
35. Niwa T, Tsukamoto T, Toyoda T, et al. Inflammatory processes triggered by helicobacter pylori infection cause aberrant DNA methylation in gastric epithelial cells. Cancer Res. 2010;70:1430–40.
36. Correa P. Chronic gastritis: a clinico-pathological classification. Am J Gastroenterol. 1988;83:504–9.
37. Vannella L, Lahner E, Osborn J, et al. Risk factors for progression to gastric neoplastic lesions in patients with atrophic gastritis. Aliment Pharmacol Ther. 2010;31:1042–50.
38. Cassaro M, Di Mario F, Leandro G, et al. The dark side of the gastric biopsy. Hum Pathol. 1999;30:741–4.
39. Owen DA. Normal histology of the stomach. Am J Surg Pathol. 1986;10:48–61.
40. Satoh K, Kimura K, Taniguchi Y, et al. Biopsy sites suitable for the diagnosis of helicobacter pylori infection and the assessment of the extent of atrophic gastritis. Am J Gastroenterol. 1998;93:569–73.
41. Van Zanten SJ, Dixon MF, Lee A. The gastric transitional zones: neglected links between gastroduodenal pathology and helicobacter ecology. Gastroenterol. 1999;116:1217–29.
42. Filipe MI, Munoz N, Matko I, et al. Intestinal metaplasia types and the risk of gastric cancer: a cohort study in Slovenia. Int J Cancer. 1994;57:324–9.
43. Sipponen P, Stolte M. Clinical impact of routine biopsies of the gastric antrum and body. Endoscopy. 1997;29:671–8.
44. Correa P, Haenszel W, Cuello C, et al. Gastric precancerous process in a high risk population: cross-sectional studies. Cancer Res. 1990;50:4731–6.
45. Hattori T. Development of adenocarcinomas in the stomach. Cancer. 1986;57:1528–34.
46. Genta RM. Recognizing atrophy: another step toward a classification of gastritis. Am J Surg Pathol. 1996;20(Suppl.1):S23–30.
47. Wright NA. Migration of the ductular elements of gut-associated glands gives clues to the histogenesis of structures associated with responses to acid hypersecretory state: the origins of gastric metaplasia in the duodenum of the specialized mucosa of Barrett's esophagus and of pseudopyloric metaplasia. Yale J Biol Med. 1996;69:147–53.
48. Solcia E, Fiocca R, Villani L, et al. Morphology and pathogenesis of endocrine hyperplasia, precarcinoid lesions, and carcinoids arising in chronic atrophic gastritis. Scand J Gastroenterol. 1991;26(Suppl. 180):146–59.
49. Strickland RG, Mackay IR. A reappraisal of the nature and significance of chronic atrophic gastritis. Am J Dig Dis. 1973;18:426–40.
50. Lechago J. Gastrointestinal neuroendocrine cell proliferations. Hum Pathol. 1994;25:1114–22.

51. Dixon MF. Autoimmune reactions in type a and H. pylori gastritis. Helicobacter. 1998;3:222.
52. Kimura K. Chronological transition of the fundic–pyloric border determined by stepwise biopsy of the lesser and greater curvatures of the stomach. Gastroenterol. 1972;63:584–92.
53. Corbett JL, Tosh D. Conversion of one cell type into another: implications for understanding organ development, pathogenesis of cancer and generating cells for therapy. Biochem Soc Trans. 2014;42:609–16.
54. Spechler SJ, Merchant JL, Wang TC, et al. A summary of the 2016 James W. Freston conference of the American Gastroenterological Association: intestinal metaplasia in the Esophagus and stomach: origins, differences, similarities and significance. Gastroenterol. 2017;153:e6–e13.
55. Adami JG. On growth and overgrowth and on the relationship between cell differentiation and proliferative capacity; its bearing upon the regeneration of tissues and the development of tumors. In: Huber F, Sondern FE, editors. Festschrift in honor of Abraham Jacobi. New York: The Knickerbocker Press; 1900. p. 422–32.
56. Waddington CH. How do cells differentiate? Scientific Am. 1953;189:108–16.
57. Spechler SJ. Editorial. Of mice and men and metaplasia. Cell Mol Gastroenterol Hepatol. 2017;4:183–4.
58. Kawachi T, Kurisu M, Numanyu N, et al. Precancerous changes in the stomach. Cancer Res. 1976;36:2673–7.
59. Jass JR, Filipe MI. The mucin profiles of normal gastric mucosa, intestinal metaplasia and its variants and gastric carcinoma. Histochem J. 1981;13:931–9.
60. Correa P. Human gastric carcinogenesis: a multistep and multifactorial process—first American Cancer Society award lecture on cancer epidemiology and prevention. Cancer Res. 1992;52:6735–40.
61. Megan D, Burclaff RJ, Willet SG, et al. Metaplastic cells in the stomach Arise, independently of stem cells, via dedifferentiation or trans differentiation of chief cells. Gastroenterol. 2018;154:839–43.
62. Hayakawa Y, Ariyama H, Stancikova J, et al. Mist1 expressing gastric stem cells maintain the normal and neoplastic gastric epithelium and are supported by a perivascular stem cell niche. Cancer Cell. 2015;28:800–14.
63. Correa P, Haenszel W, Cuello C, et al. Gastric precancerous process in a high-risk population: cohort follow-up. Cancer Res. 1990;50:4737–40.
64. Correa P, Fontham ET, Bravo JC, et al. Chemoprevention of gastric dysplasia: randomized trial of antioxidant supplements and anti-helicobacter pylori therapy. J Natl Cancer Inst. 2000;6:1881–8.
65. Bertges LC, Dibai FN, Bezerra G, et al. Comparison between endoscopic findings and histological diagnosis of antral gastritis. Arq Gastroenterol. 2018;55:212–5.
66. Dhakhwa R, Acharya IL, Shrestha HG, et al. Histopathologic study of chronic antral gastritis. J Nepal Health Res Counc. 2012;10:57–60.
67. Ruiz B, Garay J, Johnson W, et al. Morphometric assessment of gastric antral atrophy: comparison with visual evaluation. Histopathol. 2001;39:235–42.
68. Landis JR, Koch GG. The measurement of observer agreement for categorical data. Biometrics. 1977;33:159–74.
69. Correa P. The epidemiology and pathogenesis of chronic gastritis: three etiologic entites. Front Gastrointest Res. 1980;6:98–108.
70. Filipe MI, Jass J. Intestinal metaplasia subtypes and cancer risk. In: Filipe MI, Jass JR, editors. Gastric carcinoma. Churchill Livingston: Edinburgh; 1986. p. 212–36.
71. Correa P, Blanca M, Piazuelo MB. The gastric precancerous cascade. J Dig Dis. 2012;13:2–9.
72. Filipe MI, Muñoz N, Matko I, et al. Intestinal metaplasia types and the risk of gastric cancer: a cohort study in Slovenia. Int J Cancer. 1994;57:324–9.
73. González CA, Pardo ML, Liso JM, et al. Gastric cancer occurrence in preneoplastic lesions: a long-term follow-up in a high-risk area in Spain. Int J Cancer. 2010;127:2654–60.
74. Rokkas T, Filipe MI, Sladen GE. Detection of an increased incidence of early gastric cancer in patients with intestinal metaplasia type III who are closely followed up. Gut. 1991;32:1110–3.
75. Kumamoto M, Nakae Y, Ishiguro S, et al. Histological risk markers for non-cardia early gastric cancer. Pattern of mucin expression and gastric cancer. Virchows Arch. 2006;449:652–9.
76. Ectors N, Dixon MF. The prognostic value of sulphomucin positive intestinal metaplasia in the development of gastric cancer. Histopathol. 1986;10:1271–7.
77. Ramesar KC, Sanders DS, Hopwood D. Limited value of type III intestinal metaplasia in predicting risk of gastric carcinoma. J Clin Pathol. 1987;40:1287–90.
78. El-Zimaity HM, Ramchatesingh J, Saeed MA, et al. Gastric intestinal metaplasia: subtypes and natural history. J Clin Pathol. 2001;54:679–83.
79. Tosi P, Filipe MI, Luzi P, et al. Gastric intestinal metaplasia type III cases are classified as low-grade dysplasia on the basis of morphometry. J Pathol. 1993;169:73–8.
80. Matsukuma A, Mori M, Enjoji M. Sulphomucin-secreting intestinal metaplasia in the human gastric mucosa. An association with intestinal-type gastric carcinoma. Cancer. 1990;66:689–94.
81. Antonioli DA. Precursors of gastric carcinoma: a critical review with a brief description of early (curable) gastric cancer. Hum Pathol. 1994;25:994–1005.
82. Sasaki I, Yao T, Nawata H, et al. Minute gastric carcinoma of differentiated type with special reference to the significance of intestinal metaplasia, proliferative zone, and p53 protein during tumor development. Cancer. 1999;85:1719–29.
83. Mills JC, Ramesh AS. Gastric epithelial stem cells. Gastroenterol. 2011;140:412–24.
84. Reis CA, David L, Correa P, et al. Intestinal metaplasia of human stomach displays distinct patterns

of mucin (MUC1, MUC2, MUC5AC, and MUC6) expression. Cancer Res. 1999;59:1003–7.
85. Babu SD, Jayanthi V, Devaraj N, et al. Expression profile of mucins (MUC2, MUC5AC and MUC6) in helicobacter pylori infected pre-neoplastic and neoplastic human gastric epithelium. Mol Cancer. 2006;5:10.
86. Price AB. The Sydney system: histological division. J Gastroenterol Hepatol. 1991;6:209–22.
87. Siurala M. The story of gastritis. Scand J Gastroenterol Suppl. 1991;186:1–3.
88. Valle J, Kekki M, Sipponen P, et al. Longterm course and consequences of helicobacter pylori gastritis. Results of a 32-year follow-up study. Scand J Gastroenterol. 1996;31:546–50.
89. Maaroos HI, Vorobjova T, Sipponen P, et al. An 18-year follow-up study of chronic gastritis and helicobacter pylori association of CagA positivity with development of atrophy and activity of gastritis. Scand J Gastroenterol. 1999;34:864–9.
90. Rautelin H, Sipponen P, Seppälä K, et al. Gastric inflammation and neutrophil activating and cytotoxin-producing helicobacter pylori strains. Scand J Gastroenterol. 1996;31:639–42.
91. IARC. Schistosomes, liver flukes and helicobacter pylori. IARC working group on the evaluation of carcinogenic risks to humans. Lyon,7-14 June 1994. IARC Monogr Eval Carcinog Risks Hum. 1994;61:1–241.
92. You WC, Li JY, Blot WJ, et al. Evolution of precancerous lesions in a rural Chinese population at high risk of gastric cancer. Int J Cancer. 1999;83:615–9.
93. Stemmermann GN, Mower H. Gastritis, nitrosamines, and gastric cancer. J Clin Gastroenterol. 1981;3:23–7.
94. Uemura N, Okamoto S, Yamamoto S, et al. Helicobacter pylori infection and the development of gastric cancer. N Engl J Med. 2001;345:784–9.
95. Ohata H, Kitauchi S, Yoshimura N, et al. Progression of chronic atrophic gastritis associated with helicobacter pylori infection increases risk of gastric cancer. Int J Cancer. 2004;109:138–43.
96. Kim N, Park RY, Cho SI, et al. Helicobacter pylori infection and development of gastric cancer in Korea: long-term follow-up. J Clin Gastroenterol. 2008;42:448–54.
97. Atherton JC. The clinical relevance of strain types of helicobacter pylori. Gut. 1997;40:701–3.
98. Kuipers EJ, Pérez-Pérez GI, Meuwissen SG, et al. Helicobacter pylori and atrophic gastritis: importance of the cagA status. J Natl Cancer Inst. 1995;87:1777–80.
99. Huang JQ, Zheng GF, Sumanac K, et al. Meta-analysis of the relationship between cagA seropositivity and gastric cancer. Gastroenterol. 2003;125:1636–44.
100. Basso D, Zambon CF, Letley DP, et al. Clinical relevance of helicobacter pylori cagA and VacA gene polymorphisms. Gastroenterol. 2008;135:91–9.
101. Nogueira C, Figueiredo C, Carneiro F, et al. Helicobacter pylori genotypes may determine gastric histopathology. Am J Pathol. 2001;158:647–54.
102. Wroblewski LE, Peek RM Jr, Wilson KT. Helicobacter pylori and gastric cancer: factors that modulate disease risk. Clin Microbiol Rev. 2010;23:713–39.
103. Yamaoka Y. Increasing evidence of the role of helicobacter pylori SabA in the pathogenesis of gastroduodenal disease. J Infect Dev Ctries. 2008;2:174–81.
104. Kim N, Park YS, Cho SI, et al. Prevalence and risk factors of atrophic gastritis and intestinal metaplasia in a Korean population without significant gastroduodenal disease. Helicobacter. 2008;13:245–55.

10 Gastric Epithelial Dysplasia: Grading, Significance in Endoscopic Biopsy, Genetic and Epigenetic Alterations

Dysplasia grading was a three-tiered system—mild, moderate and severe, in the early 1980s [1–6]. World Health Organization (WHO) defines gastric dysplasia (also called intra-epithelial neoplasia) as an unequivocal neoplastic lesion (depressed, flat or elevated) without evidence of stromal invasion. And it has been graded dichotomously into low or high grade, and the degree of differentiation has been consistently shown to be directly correlate with the development of gastric cancer risk [7]. WHO has further subclassify dysplasia into the following subtypes, i.e. serrated dysplasia, intestinal type of dysplasia, foveolar type of dysplasia, gastric pit/crypt dysplasia, all subtypes may be either low- or high-grade dysplasia. Gastric dysplasia is frequently observed in antral biopsy, though it may be seen in biopsies from any compartment of the stomach and distributions of gastric mucosal dysplasia show similar incidence to early differentiated type of adenocarcinoma in similar incidences of occurrences in gastric antrum, body and fundus [8, 9]. Clinically dysplasia per se does not add any clinical problem to the patient, the patient will be presenting with underlying dyspeptic features or if associated with ulcer, may present with upper gastrointestinal bleeding or anaemia. Endoscopically, gastric dysplasia may present as flat, depressed or elevated polypoidal lesion, along with erosion or ulcer and colour tone change. Gastric dysplasia has a prevalence that mirrors gastric cancer (GC) with male predominance and higher incidence in Asian countries compared to North American countries [10, 11]. Average age of the patients ranges from fifth to seventh decade of life (range 28 to 86 years) [12–16]. A dysplastic gastric mucosa shows certain histological changes, i.e. reduction in the cytoplasmic mucin content, nuclear crowding, increased N:C, nuclear pleomorphism, hyperchromatism and stratification and increased mitosis. The glandular component tends to show disarray and budding with irregular branching along with irregularity and dilatation of gastric pits. These cellular and nuclear changes are present in a dysplastic mucosa along the full length of the pit and surface epithelium [17]. Changes along the surface epithelium has significant role in the diagnosis of dysplasia as a preneoplastic GIT mucosa is believed to lose differentiation capacity; hence presence of maturation along the surface epithelium with atypical changes in deeper area in a mucosal biopsy is considered to be a feature regeneration [18–20]. However, a term referred as gastric pit dysplasia has been used by Nari et to refer to dysplasia involving pit epithelial cells without involving surface lining [17]. Gastric pit dysplasia has been observed frequently in association with certain features of gastric cancer like significantly higher age of presentation, carcinoma with intestinal type, low-grade and stage 1 tumours, higher rate of co-existence with chronic gastritis, atrophy

K. Vaiphei, *Interpretation of Endoscopic Biopsy - Gastritis, Gastropathies and Beyond*,
https://doi.org/10.1007/978-981-16-6026-9_10

and intestinal metaplasia [17, 18, 21]. These dysplastic mucosae have high Ki-67 index and positive for MUC6 [22, 23]. Long-term follow-up studies have observed that these surface lesions get converted into full-thickness dysplasia in quarter of individuals who have features of chronic gastritis [9, 24, 25]. Hence, gastric pit dysplasia has been identified as precursor mucosa in carcinogenetic pathway. Histomorphologically, dysplasia may have intestinal and foveolar or gastric type morphology [26, 27] and there could be cases having hybrid morphology comprising of both intestinal and gastric type of dysplastic epithelium and the hybrid type has shown significantly higher grades of dysplasia [8]. The dysplastic cells in intestinal type may have tubular, villous or tubule-villous pattern of arrangement. The cells are columnar, nuclei are enlarged, elongated, hyperchromatic and stratified with variably eosinophilic cytoplasm. They may also show differentiation towards absorptive cells, goblet cells, endocrine and even Paneth cell differentiation. Foveolar type dysplasia is characterized by tubulovillous epithelial fonds, it may also show serrated configuration. The cells are cuboidal to low columnar resembling foveolar cells. The cells have round to oval nuclei with visible or prominent nucleoli. These cells usually have pale eosinophilic cytoplasm with apical mucous globules of neutral mucin character [28]. The two types may be distinguished by immunoexpression of the mucin in immunohistochemistry profiles, i.e. intestinal type—MUC2, CD10 and CDX2, and gastric/foveolar type—MUC5AC and/or MUC6, and absence of CD10 and low or absent expression of CDX2 [8, 20, 22, 28, 29]. Biopsies with hybrid differentiation may not have any specific expression and also there may be cases which fail to express any of the aforementioned markers.

Grading of gastric dysplasia is based on both nuclear, cytoplasmic and architectural changes; extend of nuclear atypia is indicated by nuclear crowding, hyperchromasia, stratification and mitosis; cytoplasmic differentiation and architectural disorganization or distortion [19, 20, 28–30]. A low-grade dysplasia is indicated by minimal architectural disorganization along with mild to moderate nuclear and cytological atypia [9, 22, 24]. The nuclei are hyperchromatic, mildly enlarged and elongated in intestinal type of dysplasia, whereas in foveolar type, the nuclei are round to oval. In both types, the nuclei maintain polarity and are basally located. Mitosis may be mildly increased and are basally located. The glandular architecture observed in low-grade dysplasia is similar to the native glands and exhibits minimal disorganization. In high-grade dysplasia, the cuboidal to columnar epithelial cells exhibit prominent cytological atypia, enlarged nuclei with increased nucleocytoplasmic ratio with prominent nucleoli. Nuclear stratification is a prominent feature where the nuclei will be located towards the lumen of the glands, mitosis including atypical form is a prominent feature with luminal location. The glandular architecture is usually distorted and is complex with infoldings and serrations; closely pack glands may be prominent mimicking lamina propria infiltration. However the glands with high-grade cytological features intact basement membrane along with myoepithelial cell layer and loss of these two structures will indicate lamina propria infiltration and is the feature for an intramucosal carcinoma. In doubtful cases, examination of the step serial sections is rewarding. Contrast to the intestinal type, foveolar type dysplasia may not exhibit marked cytological atypia, however, if it is associated with grossly disorganized glandular architecture, a diagnosis of high-grade dysplasia should be entertained [31]. In this category, carcinoma in situ is frequently observed and p53 overexpression is also another characteristic [24].

10.1 Significance of Diagnosing Dysplasia in Endoscopic Gastric Biopsy

Gastric adenomas are precursor lesion of gastric cancer [32]. Dysplastic mucosal focus is composed of either a flat, a plaque, a raised, depressed or ulcerated area. Adenoma refers to raised mucosal lesion composed of dysplastic epithelium [33, 34]. Gastric dysplasia may be co-existing with gastric cancer [35]. Hence, an adenoma diagnosed by endoscopic biopsy may have invasive component in resected specimens including endoscopic resection (ER) (range, 4–30%) [31, 36, 37]. One-piece complete and en-bloc resected specimen from cases diagnosed to harbour adenoma is to be analysed for completeness of the resection margins. This may be accomplished by carrying out endoscopic mucosal resection (EMR) or endoscopic submucosal dissection (ESD) as the choice of treatment for polyps irrespective of the grades of dysplasia [38]. Many endoscopists prefer ESD as it can be used to resect large and depressed lesions [39–41]. An adenoma with HGD may be treated by ESD according to the revised Vienna classification recommendation, whereas adenoma with LGD, it may be treated either by ESD or by follow-up simply [42]. European guidelines recommneds ESD for all adenomas irrespective of the grade of dysplasia for a better assessment of dysplasia in the resected one-piece specimen [32, 43]. The recommendation by the European group has been criticized by Park et al. (2020) in their long-term follow-up of patients with adenomas showing low-grade dysplasia [44]. There is a lack of documentation on exact time line on follow-up endoscopic biopsy and also the incidence of metachronous cancer in adenoma cases [36, 38, 41, 44, 45]. Relationship between adenoma size and tumour recurrence had been analysed and a direct relationship was observed between large adenoma i.e. larger than 2 cms to be associated with high recurrence rate [43, 46, 47].

10.2 Molecular Alterations in Gastric Mucosal Precancerous Lesions

Exact pathways through which gastric cancer (GC) develops is not very clearly understood, though several pathways have been proposed. Some of the hypothetical pathways have been studied and documented the abnormalities. One of the extensively studied mechanisms is DNA methylation in which cytosines acquire methyl group in 5'position, only if it is followed by a guanine site resulting in silencing of the gene [48, 49]. There are two published studies that have reported higher methylation index in IM gastric mucosa than AG mucosa and no difference between IM and dysplasia [48–51]. Specific genes such as p16 shows four-fold increase methylation while progressing from dysplasia to cancer [52] and DNA methylation of CDH-1 gene had also been associated with H. pylori infection where H. pylori eradication resulted in reversal of aberrant DNA methylation [53, 54]. Twenty differentially expressed miRNAs had been identified from H. pylori related AG and IM gastric mucosa by Wang et al. An *in-silico* approach from Gene Expression Omnibus datasets [55] and these miRNAs played key roles in signal transduction, cell proliferation and death and also regulated RAB22A, SOX4, IKZF2, PLAG1 and BTBD7 genes. Another study documented knockdown of miR-204 in HP related AG promoted uncontrolled cell growth and invasion in vitro, downregulation of miR204 enhances epithelial mesenchymal transition by up-regulating SOX4 [56, 57]. There are many studies that had reported varied incidences of GC in the background of atrophic gastritis and IM; reported incidence for AG ranges from 0 to 2%; for IM and dysplasia it ranges from 0 to 10% and 0–73% per year, respectively [58, 59]. And these wide variations have been attributed to difference in pattern of design and different population, also to certain extend depend upon sex of the individual and in defining IM and dysplasia [58, 59].

Besides the histological morphology to document presence of IM in a given biopsy, it also has been found to express gut-specific transcription factors like CDX-1 and CDX-2 [60–62]. Another study had documented downregulation of both transcription factors GC and in metaplastic epithelium, CDX2 expression preceded CDX1 [63–65]. Many other oncoproteins are also expressed by these lesions, e.g. associated with IM are COX-2, TP53, TGF alpha and EGFR, and cyclins E, D2 and p16 in adenoma/dysplasia [4, 66–71]. Both types of mucosal lesions express C-MET protein [70], Dysplastic epithelium was found to exhibit decreased expressions for hMLH1, FHIT and E-cadherin (CDH1) proteins [70–72]. Large number of cases with IM (47–79%) and chronic gastritis (23%) express human telomerase reverse transcriptase (hTERT) gene, and about 30% of IM also expresses CD44 [73–75]. Padova international classification has been based on both molecular and cellular profiles [4, 76].

10.3 Epigenetic Alterations

Normal ageing process is known to produce methylation of CpG focus, which may result in epigenetic mutations. CpG island methylation is an important pathway underlying malignancy. In a study conducted in autopsy samples of benign gastric mucosa, adenomatous polyposis coli (APC) gene undergoes methylation in almost 50% of individuals less than 32 years of age who were subjected to routine autopsy in subjects who died due to non-GI conditions. And in individuals who were older than 40 years, many genes like CDH1 (70%), p16 (20%), RASSF1A (7%) and RUNX3 (8%) showed methylation, however hMLH1 gene rarely showed methylation [77, 78]. In the process of chronic gastritis to adenoma to dysplasia to carcinoma is associated with increased promoter methylation of multiple genes, and RUNX3 and hMLH1 methylation have been reported in 45 and 32%, respectively [79, 80]. Another study had reported p16 methylation 7% in IM, 18% in adenomas, 29% in adenomas associated with adenocarcinoma and 44% in adenocarcinomas [81]. Some other groups have also documented similar molecular changes in the process of development of gastric cancer [72, 82]. Cumulative methylation of p16, hMLH1, COX2 and RUNX3 in a precancerous lesion might serve as a biomarker for an increased risk of malignant transformation [4].

References

1. Morson BC, Sobin LH, Grundmann E, et al. Precancerous conditions and epithelial dysplasia in the stomach. J Clin Pathol. 1980;33:711–21.
2. Riddell RH, Goldman H, Ransohoff DF, et al. Dysplasia in inflammatory bowel disease: standardized classification with provisional clinical applications. Hum Pathol. 1983;14:931–68.
3. Ming SC, Bajtai A, Correa P, et al. Gastric dysplasia significance and pathologic criteria. Cancer. 1984;54:1794–801.
4. Yashima K, Sasaki S, Koda M, et al. Premalignant lesions in gastric cancer. Clin J Gastroenterol. 2010;3:6–12.
5. Chung GE, Chung SJ, Yang JI, et al. Development of metachronous tumors after endoscopic resection for gastric neoplasm according to the baseline tumor grade at a health checkup center. Korean J Gastroenterol. 2017;70:223–31.
6. Kang GH, Lee S, Kim JS, et al. Profile of aberrant CpG island methylation along the multistep pathway of gastric carcinogenesis. Lab Investig. 2003;83:635–41.
7. WHO classification of tumours. Digestive system tumours. 5th ed. France, Lyon: WHO; 2019. p. 66.
8. Park DY, Srivastava A, Kim GH, et al. Adenomatous and foveolar gastric dysplasia, distinct patterns of mucin expression and background intestinal metaplasia. Am J Surg Pathol. 2008;32:524–33.
9. Valente P, Garrido M, Gullo I, et al. Epithelial dysplasia of the stomach with gastric immunophenotype shows features of biological aggressiveness. Gastric Cancer. 2015;18:720–8.
10. Hamashima C, Okamoto M, Shabana M, et al. Sensitivity of endoscopic screening for gastric cancer by the incidence method. Int J Cancer. 2013;133:653–9.
11. Kang JH, Lim YJ, Yang JN, et al. Prevalence of precancerous conditions and gastric cancer based upon the National Cancer Screening Program in Korea for 7 years, single center experience. Gastroenterol Res Pract. 2015;15:571965.
12. Arnold M, Ferlay J, van Berge Henegouwen MI, et al. Global burden of oesophageal and gastric cancer by histology and subsite in 2018. Gut. 2020;69:1564–71.
13. Rugge M, Farinati F, Baffa R, et al. Gastric epithelial dysplasia in the natural history of gastric cancer: a multicenter prospective follow-up study. Interdiscip Grp Gastric Epithelial Dysplasia Gastroenterol. 1994;107:1288–96.
14. Rugge M, Farinati F, Di Mario F, et al. Gastric epithelial dysplasia: a prospective multicenter follow-up study from the interdisciplinary group on gastric epithelial dysplasia. Hum Pathol. 1991;22:1002–8.
15. Ming SC, Camilleri JP, Potet F, et al. Gastric mucosal dysplasia: preliminary results of a prospective study of patients followed for periods of up to six years. In: Ming S-C, editor. Precursors of gastric cancer, vol. 18984. New York: Praeger. p. 83–92.

16. Farinati F, Rugge M, Di Mario F, et al. Early and advanced gastric cancer in the follow-up of moderate and severe gastric dysplasia patients. A prospective study. Endoscopy. 1993;25:261–4.
17. Nari S, Hong-Jae J, Woo-Kyung K, et al. Gastric pit dysplasia in adjacent gastric mucosa in 414 gastric cancers: prevalence and characteristics. Am J Surg Path. 2011;35:1021–9.
18. Agoston AT, Odze RD. Evidence that gastric pit dysplasia-like atypia is a neoplastic precursor lesion. Hum Pathol. 2014;45:446–55.
19. Rugge M, Correa P, Dixon MF, et al. Gastric dysplasia: the Padova international classification. Am J Surg Pathol. 2000;24:167–76.
20. Schlemper RJ, Riddell RH, Kato Y, et al. The Vienna classification of gastrointestinal epithelial neoplasia. Gut. 2000;47:251–5.
21. Jhi JH, Kim GH, Kim A, et al. Negative pathology after endoscopic resection of gastric epithelial neoplasms: importance of pit dysplasia. Korean J Intern Med. 2017;32:647–55.
22. Gullo I, Carneiro F, Oliveira C, et al. Heterogeneity in gastric cancer: from pure morphology to molecular classifications. Pathobiology. 2018;85:50–63.
23. Abraham SC, Montgomery EA, Singh VK, et al. Gastric adenomas: intestinal-type and gastric-type adenomas differ in the risk of adenocarcinoma and presence of background mucosal pathology. Am J Surg Pathol. 1996;26:1276–85.
24. Kushima R, Müller W, Borchard F, et al. Differential p53 protein expression in stomach adenomas of gastric and intestinal phenotypes: possible sequences of p53 alteration in stomach carcinogenesis. Virchows Arch. 1996;428:223–7.
25. Abraham SC, Park SJ, Lee JH, et al. Genetic alterations in gastric adenomas of intestinal and foveolar phenotypes. Mod Pathol. 2003;18:786–95.
26. Nogueira AM, Machado JC, Carneiro F, et al. Patterns of expression of trefoil peptides and mucins in gastric polyps with and without malignant transformation. J Pathol. 1999;187:541–8.
27. Park DY, Srivastava A, Kim GH, et al. CDX2 expression in the intestinal type gastric epithelial neoplasia: frequency and significance. Mod Pathol. 2010;23:54–61.
28. Rugge M, Capelle LG, Cappellesso R, et al. Precancerous lesions in the stomach: from biology to clinical patient management. Best Pract Res Clin Gastroenterol. 2013;27:205–23.
29. Rugge M, Genta RM, Di Mario F, et al. Gastric cancer as preventable disease. Clin Gastrol Hepatol. 2017;15:1833–43.
30. Day DW, Jass JR, Price AB, et al. Morson and Dawson's gastrointestinal pathology. 4th ed. Wiley: Blackwell Science Ltd; 2003.
31. Sakurai U, Lauwers GY, Vieth M, et al. Gastric high-grade dysplasia can be associated with submucosal invasion: evaluation of its prevalence in a series of 121 endoscopically resected specimens. Am J Surg Pathol. 2014;38:1545–50.
32. Robinson JC, Hoffman B, Sun S. Gastric Adenomas. Pathol Case Rev. 2013;18:70–4.
33. Fujiwara Y, Arakawa T, Fukuda T, et al. Diagnosis of borderline adenomas of the stomach by endoscopic mucosal resection. Endoscopy. 1996;28:425–30.
34. Orlowska J, Jarosz D, Pachlewski J, et al. Malignant transformation of benign epithelial gastric polyps. Am J Gastroenterol. 1995;90:2152–9.
35. Cho SJ, Choi IJ, Kim CG, et al. Risk of high-grade dysplasia or carcinoma in gastric biopsy-proven low-grade dysplasia: an analysis using the Vienna classification. Endoscopy. 2011;43:465–71.
36. Choi CW, Kang DH, Kim HW, et al. Endoscopic submucosal dissection as a treatment for gastric adenomatous polyps: predictive factors for early gastric cancer. Scand J Gastroenterol. 2012;47:1218–25.
37. Kim YJ, Park JC, Kim JH, et al. Histologic diagnosis based on forceps biopsy is not adequate for determining endoscopic treatment of gastric adenomatous lesions. Endoscopy. 2010;42:620–6.
38. Moon HS, Yun GY, Kim JS, et al. Risk factors for metachronous gastric carcinoma development after endoscopic resection of gastric dysplasia: retrospective, single-center study. World J Gastroenterol. 2017;23:4407–15.
39. Ohkuwa M, Hosokawa K, Boku N, et al. New endoscopic treatment for intramucosal gastric tumors using an insulated-tip diathermic knife. Endoscopy. 2001;33:221–6.
40. Ono H, Kondo H, Gotoda T, et al. Endoscopic mucosal resection for treatment of early gastric cancer. Gut. 2001;48:225–9.
41. Choi CW, Kim HW, Shin DH, et al. The risk factors for discrepancy after endoscopic submucosal dissection of gastric category 3 lesion (low grade dysplasia). Dig Dis Sci. 2014;59:421–7.
42. Dixon MF. Gastrointestinal epithelial neoplasia: Vienna revisited. Gut. 2002;51:130–1.
43. Banks M, Graham D, Jansen M, et al. British Society of Gastroenterology guidelines on the diagnosis and management of patients at risk of gastric adenocarcinoma. Gut. 2019;68:1545–75.
44. Park TY, Jeong SJ, Kim TH, et al. Long-term outcomes of patients with gastric adenoma in Korea: a retrospective observational study. Medicine. 2020;99:12(e19553).
45. Lee HJ, Lee YJ, Lee JY, et al. Characteristics of synchronous and metachronous multiple gastric tumors after endoscopic submucosal dissection of early gastric neoplasm. Clin Endosc. 2018;51:266–73.
46. Bae SE, Jung HY, Kang J, et al. Effect of helicobacter pylori eradication on metachronous recurrence after endoscopic resection of gastric neoplasm. Am J Gastroenterol. 2014;109:60–7.
47. Nam HS, Choi CW. Endoscopic predictive factors associated with local recurrence after gastric endo-

scopic submucosal dissection. Scand J Gastroenterol. 2018;53:1000–7.
48. Chenand ZX, Riggs AD. DNA methylation and demethylation in mammal. J Biol Chem. 2011;286:18347–53.
49. Nishizawa T, Suzuki H. Gastric carcinogenesis and underlying molecular mechanisms: helicobacter pylori and novel targeted therapy. Biomed Res Int. 2015;2015. Article ID 794378, 7 pages. https://doi.org/10.1155/2015/794378
50. Kang GH, Shim YH, Jung HY, et al. CpG island methylation in premalignant stages of gastric carcinoma. Cancer Res. 2001;61:2847–51.
51. Park SY, Yoo EJ, Cho NY, et al. Comparison of CpG island hypermethylation and repetitive DNA hypomethylation in premalignant stages of gastric cancer, stratified for helicobacter pylori infection. J Pathol. 2009;219:410–6.
52. Goto T, Mizukami H, Shirahata A, et al. Methylation of the p16 gene is frequently detected in lymphatic-invasive gastric cancer. Anticancer Res. 2010;30: 2701–3.
53. Chan AOO, Lam SK, Wong BCY, et al. Promoter methylation of E-cadherin gene in gastric mucosa associated with helicobacter pylori infection and in gastric cancer. Gut. 2003;52:502–6.
54. Leung WK, Man EPS, Yu J, et al. Effects of helicobacter pylori eradication on methylation status of E-cadherin gene in non cancerous stomach. Clin Cancer Res. 2006;12:3216–21.
55. Wang XW, Wu Y, Wang D, et al. Micro RNA network analysis identifies key micro rnas and genes associated with precancerous lesions of gastric cancer. Gen Mol Res. 2014;13:8695–703.
56. Zhou X, Li L, Su J, et al. Decreased miR-204 in H. pylori-associated gastric cancer promotes cancer cell proliferation and invasion by targeting SOX4. PLoS One. 2014;9:101457.
57. de Vries AC, Haringsma J, Kuipers EJ. The detection, surveillance and treatment of premalignant gastric lesions related to helicobacter pylori infection. Helicobacter. 2007;12:1–15.
58. de Vries AC, van Grieken NCT, Looman CWN, et al. Gastric cancer risk in patients with premalignant gastric lesions: a nationwide cohort study in the Netherlands. Gastroenterology. 2008;134:945–52.
59. Dinis-Ribeiro M, Areia M, de Vries AC, et al. Management of precancerous conditions and lesions in the stomach (MAPS): guideline from the European Society of Gastrointestinal Endoscopy (ESGE), European helicobacter study group (EHSG), European Society of Pathology (ESP), and the Sociedade Portuguesa de Endoscopia Digestiva (SPED). Endoscopy. 2012;44:74–94.
60. Beck F. The role of cdx genes in the mammalian gut. Gut. 2004;53:1394–6.
61. Silberg DG, Furth EE, Taylor JK, et al. CDX1 protein expression in normal, metaplastic, and neoplastic human alimentary tract epithelium. Gastroenterology. 1997;113:478–86.
62. Yuasa Y. Control of gut differentiation and intestinal-type gastric carcinogenesis. Nat Rev Cancer. 2003;3:592–600.
63. Busuttil RA, Boussioutas A. Intestinal metaplasia: a premalignant lesion involved in gastric carcinogenesis. J Gastroenterol Hepatol. 2009;24:193–201.
64. Boussioutas A, Li H, Liu J, et al. Distinctive patterns of gene expression in premalignant gastric mucosa and gastric cancer. Cancer Res. 2003;63:2569–77.
65. Eda A, Osawa H, Yanaka I, et al. Expression of homeobox gene CDX2 precedes that of CDX1 during the progression of intestinal metaplasia. J Gastroenterol. 2002;37:94–100.
66. Sung JJ, Leung WK, Go MY, et al. Cyclooxygenase-2 expression in helicobacter pylori-associated premalignant and malignant gastric lesions. Am J Pathol. 2000;157:729–35.
67. Fenoglio-Preiser CM, Wang J, Stemmermann GN, et al. TP53 and gastric carcinoma: a review. Hum Mutat. 2003;21:258–70.
68. Filipe MI, Osborn M, Linehan J, et al. Expression of transforming growth factor alpha, epidermal growth factor receptor and epidermal growth factor in precursor lesions to gastric carcinoma. Br J Cancer. 1995;71:30–6.
69. Oshimo Y, Nakayama H, Ito R, et al. Promoter methylation of cyclin D2 gene in gastric carcinoma. Int J Oncol. 2003;23:1663–70.
70. Sun Y, Li JY, He JS, et al. Tissue microarray analysis of multiple gene expression in intestinal metaplasia, dysplasia and carcinoma of the stomach. Histopathology. 2005;46:505–14.
71. Hara A, Yashima K, Yasugi A, et al. Expression of Fhit, Mlh1, p16INK4A and E-cadherin in early gastric neoplasia: correlation with histological grade and gastric phenotype. Oncol Rep. 2007;18:553–9.
72. Kawaguchi K, Yashima K, Koda M, et al. Fhit expression in human gastric adenomas and intramucosal carcinomas: correlation with Mlh1 expression and gastric phenotype. Br J Cancer. 2004;90:672–7.
73. Suzuki K, Kashimura H, Ohkawa J, et al. Expression of human telomerase catalytic subunit gene in cancerous and precancerous gastric conditions. J Gastroenterol Hepatol. 2000;15:744–51.
74. Jong HS, Park YI, Kim S, et al. Up-regulation of human telomerase catalytic subunit during gastric carcinogenesis. Cancer. 1999;86:559–65.
75. Yao XX, Yin L, Sun ZC. The expression of hTERT mRNA and cellular immunity in gastric cancer and precancerosis. World J Gastroenterol. 2002;8:586–90.
76. Jin Z, Tamura G, Honda T, et al. Molecular and cellular phenotypic profiles of gastric noninvasive neoplasia. Lab Investig. 2002;82:1637–45.
77. Waki T, Tamura G, Sato M, et al. Age-related methylation of tumor suppressor and tumor-related genes: an analysis of autopsy samples. Oncogene. 2003;22:4128–33.
78. Waki T, Tamura G, Tsuchiya T, et al. Promoter methylation status of E-cadherin, hMLH1, and p16 genes

in nonneoplastic gastric epithelia. Am J Pathol. 2002;161:399–403.
79. Waki T, Tamura G, Sato M, et al. Promoter methylation status of DAP-kinase and RUNX3 genes in neoplastic and non-neoplastic gastric epithelia. Cancer Sci. 2003;94:360–4.
80. Lee JH, Park SJ, Abraham SC, et al. Frequent CpG island methylation in precursor lesions and early gastric adenocarcinomas. Oncogene. 2004;23:4646–54.
81. Kang GH, Shim YH, Jung HY, et al. CpG island methylation in premalignant stages of gastric carcinoma. Cancer Res. 2001;61:2847–51.
82. Sun Y, Deng D, You WC, et al. Methylation of p16 CpG islands associated with malignant transformation of gastric dysplasia in a population-based study. Clin Cancer Res. 2004;10:5087–93.

11 Controversies in the Diagnosis of Early Gastric Cancer

It is interesting to go through the evolvement of the term "early gastric cancer (EGC)". The term was coined by Murakami in 1979 and referred to mucosal and submucosal carcinomas without taking into account lymph node involvement [1, 2]. The term EGC had been used unanimously and has been used by different groups as there was a consensus meeting held by the Japanese Endoscopic Society in 1962 in context to minute early gastric mucosal tumour regardless of depth of invasion [3]. Saeki in 1938 evaluated histological depth of invasion with 5-year survival in 202 gastrectomized patients and observed 91% survival in tumours limited to submucosa [4]. The term carcinoma in situ had been used for epithelial malignant lesion with no lamina propria invasion and is believed to be with no metastatic potential [5]. Over the years these groups of tumours have also been found to have metastasized to regional lymph nodes in 4.0 to 11.8% of cases [6–9]. EGC has three gross types, i.e. protruded/type I, superficial/type II which can be flat, elevated or depressed lesion and excavated/type III. The mucosal lesions observed in subgroups of type II are less than that of type I and III [3, 10]. The gross appearance of a particular tumour may not fit into the above five types that have been mentioned but it may have combinations of two or more types by writing the prominent type first and it may be written as IIa+IIc or IIc+III. Other types of mucosal lesions like a polypoid growth or deep ulcerating lesions are not used in this classification [11].

Initially, EGCs had been frequently reported from Japan [12, 13], however, increasing number of cases are recorded from other parts of the world [14–18]. In most of the advanced centres worldwide, EGCs are managed by a minimally invasive surgical technique like therapeutic endoscopic submucosal dissection (ESD) [19, 20]. In spite of the fact that ESD has been found to be an excellent technique, lately there have been concerns with increased number of cases having a local recurrence and early cancer-related deaths [21, 22]. Outcome of ESD depends upon the criteria for case selection, preferably with no regional lymph node involvement and free resection margins [23, 24], though diagnostic criteria for EGC do not consider lymph node status [1, 25, 26]. Many of the studies had analyzed for the plausible key parameters for treatment failure [27–30]. There is a lack of agreement in microscopic features and staging with and without lymph not metastasis. A drastic survival benefit of 98–100% has been observed in patients without lymph node involvement compared to the ones with lymph node metastasis of 15–20% where the survival rate drops down to 70% and the most important factor that has been observed is depth of tumour invasion [27, 28, 30]. Some studies also had observed similar outcomes in 5-year survival rates which were 100% only with mucosal lesions and 90% with submucosal

K. Vaiphei, *Interpretation of Endoscopic Biopsy - Gastritis, Gastropathies and Beyond*,
https://doi.org/10.1007/978-981-16-6026-9_11

invasion [14, 31] and a number of lymph node metastases also had a role in patient outcome, i.e. N0 overall survival rate of 99% and for N1 it was 73%. Many other groups also documented an increased number of lymph node involvement with submucosal extension [20, 32–35]. Kodama et al. [36] divided EGC into superficial spreading and deep penetrating types; superficially spreading type refers to mucosal indurated growth measuring over 4 cm in diameter that may be confined to mucosa or partly submucosal involvement; and a lesion <4.0 cm in diameter which has penetrated into submucosa, that may invade through muscularis mucosae, maybe with destruction of muscularis mucosae, or the tumour may have expansile and fenestrated pattern of infiltration into muscularis mucosae. There may be mixed types and larger lesions, i.e. >4 cm usually invades into submucosa. A tumour <4.0 cm in diameter with or without submucosal invasion is designated as a small mucosal type. EGCs having 3 or more lymph nodes metastasis are associated with poor prognosis [37–40]. Lymph node metastases have been associated with lymphovascular emboli and tumour with features of poor differentiation [34, 39, 41–46] and tumour having a diffuse pattern and >2 cm [47–51]. Based on these publications, incidences of lymph node metastases were—9% with no lymphovascular emboli, 13% in well-differentiated and 34% in poorly differentiated tumours. According to the Paris classification, the probability of lymph node metastases is 2.3 times higher for depressed lesions compared to elevated ones [52]. Some other studies quoted risk of lymph node metastases to be 15–24% [53–55]. Saragoni had referred to the significance of lymph node involvement in prognostication of EGCs, which is particularly true with respect to case selection for ESD [56].

Endoscopic mucosal resection (EMR) was introduced for the first time in 1987 by the National Cancer Centre Hospital Tokyo had used the technology lesion smaller than 15 mm [57]. Criteria by the Japanese Gastric Cancer Association (JGCA) for endoscopic submucosal dissection (ESD) are—non-ulcerated <2 cm size mucosal tumour with glandular differentiation with no ulcer and negative margins [58]. JGCA has recently redefined criteria for ESD which include non-ulcerated T1a tumour having either a well differentiated which may be >3 cm in diameter or a tumour with diffuse morphology not larger than 2 cm [3, 20]. The standard criteria between Western and Eastern pathologists differ to a certain extent. EGC diagnosis is based on cytomorphological atypia and disorganization of the architecture in the East whereas tumour invasion into proper lamina has been acknowledge in the West [59, 60]. Vienna classification has addressed these issues of differences by clubbing all non-invasive neoplastic lesions into category 4 amenable by local resection [61, 62].

WHO 2019 writes a note saying that there is limited consensus regarding the diagnostic criteria of gastric dysplasia and adenocarcinoma, especially between pathologists in Japan and those in North America, Europe and the Republic of Korea [63]. Japanese pathologists give importance to the cytoarchitectural pattern whereas pathologists in North America, Europe and the Republic of Korea based their diagnosis of adenocarcinoma presence of disruption of basement membrane with infiltration into lamina propria [63]. In Japan, a diagnosis of non-invasive carcinoma is established based on a non-invasive neoplastic lesion with high-grade cellular and/or architectural atypia, whereas the same lesion will be diagnosed as high-grade dysplasia by many pathologists in other countries [64]. Seventh edition of GI tumour classification by WHO defined only invasive tumours as EGCs and, low and high-grade intraepithelial lesions were classified on the presence of cytological atypia [65] (Fig. 11.1a–d). Criteria for invasiveness may be subjective not easily definable and reproducible depending upon subjective evaluation. In an endoscopic biopsy, invasion into the lamina propria may be commented upon. There had been incidences where biopsy had been labelled as high-grade dysplasia according to the Western criteria showed features of EGC in ESD specimen [66]. Saragoni et al. in their case series made efforts looking for new features to provide an updated definition of EGC [18, 56]. Proposals were made to label EGC in those limited to mucosa

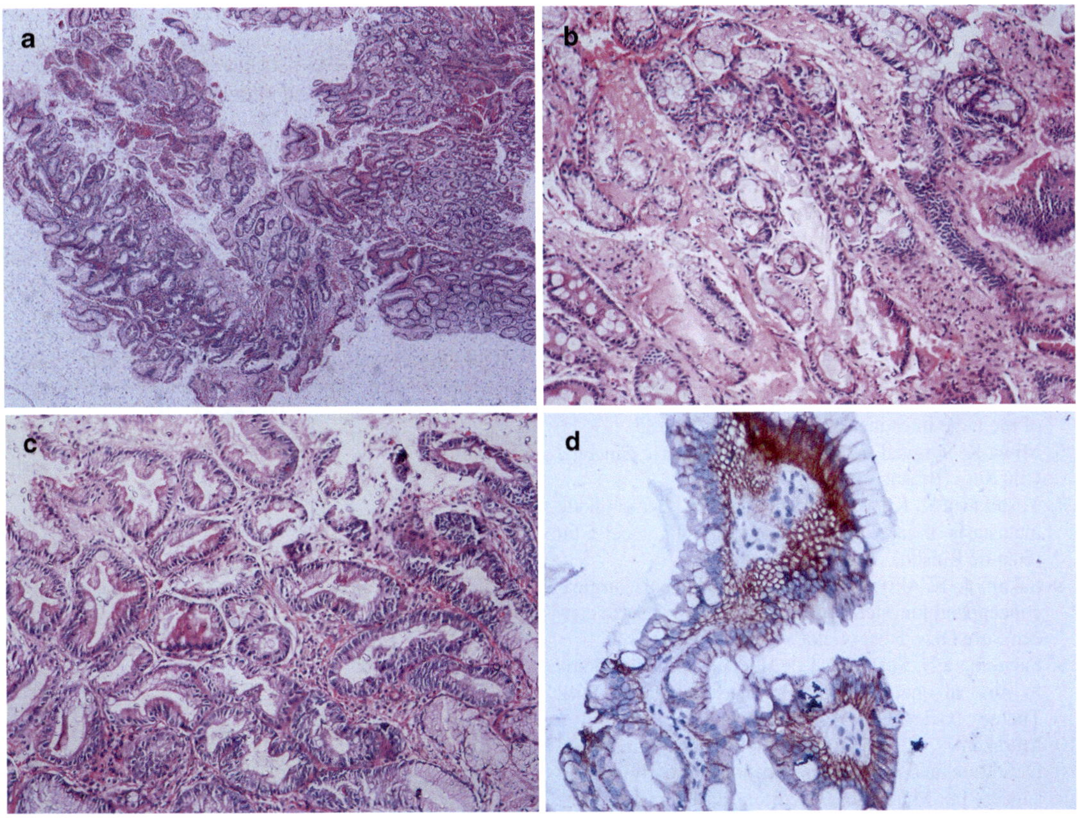

Fig. 11.1 (**a**) Low power photomicrograph of an endoscopic biopsy from suspicious mucosal lesion in gastric body and pyloric junction, showing two mucosal pieces. The one on the right side shows foveolar hyperplasia, loss of the native glands and extensive intestinal metaplasia. The second piece on the left hand shows many atypical glands arranged haphazardly (HE, x150). (**b**) Higher power view of the atypical glands showing focal back-to-back arrangement and micropapillary fronds of the abnormal glands having many goblet cells along with focal collection of extracellular mucin and acquisition of abnormal stroma (HE, x250). (**c**) The same tissue piece is another area on a higher power to show the atypical glands with atypical lining epithelial cells including many goblet cells. Majority of these atypical glands contain many micropapillary fronds (HE, x250). (**d**) A high-power photomicrograph of an immunostained section using E-cadherin primary antibody to show the loss of E-cadherin by the proliferating multilayered cells along the papillary fronds, though many of the cells maintained positive staining along the intercellular junctions. Loss of E-cadherin in IHC indicates mutation in CDH1 gene associated with familial gastric cancer (PAP, x500)

or minimal submucosal invasion with no potential risk for lymph node metastases, and followed-up revealed the risk factors were tumour >2 cm, submucosal infiltration, diffuse morphology and Kodama's PEN A type [56]. Submucosal depth invasion according to Parish endoscopic classification is a maximum of 500 microns [52].

In brief, important points to remember with EGCs are—(i) it has been most frequently observed along lesser curvature at cardia in elderly and angularis in mid and elderly individuals; (ii) hereditary carcinomas involves corpus and fundus in young women; (iii) tubular adenocarcinoma is most common starting in the neck region of gastric pits; (iv) papillary type is associated with worse prognosis related to deeper penetration, frequent lymphovascular emboli, liver and nodal metastases, and v) intramucosal signet ring cell carcinoma tends to have low nodal metastasis compared to intestinal type [67].

References

1. Murakami T. Early cancer of the stomach. World J Surg. 1979;3:685–92.
2. Kitamura K, Yamaguchi T, Okamoto K, et al. Early gastric lymphoma: a clinicopathologic study of ten patients, literature review, and comparison with early gastric adenocarcinoma. Cancer. 1996;77:850–7.
3. Murakami T. Early cancer of the stomach. World J Surg. 1979;3:685–91.
4. Saeki J. Iber die histologische Prognostik des Magenkarzinoms. Mitteilungen der Medizinischen Gesellschaft zu Tokyo (Tokyo Igakukai Zasshi). 1938;52:191.
5. Morson BC. Precancerous and early malignant lesions of the large intestine. Br J Surg. 1968;55:725.
6. Miwa K. Surgical treatment of early gastric cancer. J Clin Surg (Rinsho Geka). 1972;27:45.
7. Yoshikawa K, Kitaoka H, Sano R, et al. Lymph node metastasis of early gastric cancer. Jpn J Cancer Clin (Gan no Rinsho). 1969;15:699.
8. Sakamoto K, Akiyama H, Sakakibara Y, et al. Surgical concept and long-term prognosis of early gastric cancer. Surg Diag Treat (Geka Shinryo). 1971;13:37.
9. Sakakibara N, Suzuki H, Lde H, et al. Some problems in surgical operation for early gastric cancer. Surg Therapy (Geka Chiryo). 1975;33:113.
10. Murakami T. Pathomorphological diagnosis. Definition and gross classification of early gastric cancer. In: Murakami T, editor. Early gastric cancer, Gann Monograph on Cancer Research, vol. 11. Tokyo: University of Tokyo Press; 1971. p. 53–66.
11. Japanese Research Society for Gastric Cancer and National Cancer Center. Annual Report of National Registration of Gastric Cancer, Vol 2, Miwa K, editor. Tokyo; 1969, p 40
12. Japanese Research Society for Gastric Cancer. Japanese classification of gastric carcinoma. Tokyo: Kanehara & Co., Ltd.; 1995.
13. Sano T, Sasako M, Kinoshita T, et al. Maruyama K. Recurrence of early gastric cancer. Follow-up of 1475 patients and review of the Japanese literature. Cancer. 1993;72:3174–8.
14. Yuan Y. A survey and evaluation of population-based screening for gastric cancer. Cancer Biol Med. 2013;10:72–80.
15. Green PH, O'Toole KM, Slonim D, et al. Increasing incidence and excellent survival of patients with early gastric cancer: experience in a United States medical center. Am J Med. 1988;85:658–61.
16. Rokkas T, Filipe MI, Sladen GE. Detection of an increased incidence of early gastric cancer in patients with intestinal metaplasia type III who are closely followed up. Gut. 1991;32:1110–3.
17. Shoropad V, Berdov B, Zagrebin V. Clinicopathological features and outcome of surgical treatment of 149 patients with early (pT1) gastric cancer. Onkologie. 2005;28:247–52.
18. Saragoni L, Morgagni P, Gardini A, et al. Early gastric cancer: diagnosis, staging, and clinical impact. Evaluation of 530 patients. New elements for an updated definition and classification. Gastric Cancer. 2013;16:549–54.
19. Yada T, Yokoi C, Uemura N. The current state of diagnosis and treatment for early gastric cancer. Diagn Ther Endosc. 2013;2013:241320.
20. Gotoda T, Ho KY, Soetikno R, et al. Gastric ESD: current status and future directions of devices and training. Gastrointest Endosc Clin N Am. 2014;24:213–33.
21. Takenaka R, Kawahara Y, Okada H, et al. Risk factors associated with local recurrence of early gastric cancers after endoscopic submucosal dissection. Gastrointest Endosc. 2008;68:887–94.
22. Lian J, Chen S, Zhang Y, et al. A meta-analysis of endoscopic submucosal dissection and EMR for early gastric cancer. Gastrointest Endosc. 2012;76:763–70.
23. Japanese Gastric Cancer Association. Japanese classification of gastric carcinoma: 3rd English edition. Gastric Cancer. 2011;14:101–12.
24. Soetikno R, Kaltenbach T, Yeh R, et al. Endoscopic mucosal resection for early cancers of the upper gastrointestinal tract. J Clin Oncol. 2005;23:4490–8.
25. Gotoda T. Endoscopic resection of early gastric cancer: the Japanese perspective. Curr Opin Gastroenterol. 2006;22:561–9.
26. Kitaoka H, Yoshikawa K, Hirota T, et al. Surgical treatment of early gastric cancer. Jpn J Clin Oncol. 1984;14:283–93.
27. Abe S, Yoshimura H, Nagaoka S, et al. Long-term results of operation for carcinoma of the stomach in T1/T2 stages: critical evaluation of the concept of early carcinoma of the stomach. J Am Coll Surg. 1995;181:389–96.
28. Folli S, Dente M, Dell'Amore D, et al. Early gastric cancer: prognostic factors in 223 patients. Br J Surg. 1995;82:952–6.
29. Saragoni L, Gaudio M, Vio A, et al. Early gastric cancer in the province of Forlì: follow-up of 337 patients in a high risk region for gastric cancer. Oncol Rep. 1998;5:945–8.
30. Saragoni L, Gaudio M, Morgagni P, et al. The role of growth patterns, according to Kodama's classification, and lymph node status, as important prognostic factors in early gastric cancer: analysis of 412 cases. Gastric Cancer. 2000;3:134–40.
31. Inoue K, Tobe T, Kan N, et al. Problems in the definition and treatment of early gastric cancer. Br J Surg. 1991;78:818–21.
32. Sano T, Kobori O, Muto T. Lymph node metastasis from early gastric cancer: endoscopic resection of tumour. Br J Surg. 1992;79:241–4.
33. Folli S, Morgagni P, Roviello F, et al. Risk factors for lymph node metastases and their prognostic significance in early gastric cancer (EGC) for the Italian Research Group for Gastric Cancer (IRGGC). Jpn J Clin Oncol. 2001;31:495–9.

34. Tachibana M, Takemoto Y, Monden N, et al. Clinicopathological features of early gastric cancer: results of 100 cases from a rural general hospital. Eur J Surg. 1999;165:319–25.
35. Shimada S, Yagi Y, Honmyo U, et al. Involvement of three or more lymph nodes predicts poor prognosis in submucosal gastric carcinoma. Gastric Cancer. 2001;4:54–9.
36. Kodama Y, Inokuchi K, Soejima K, et al. Growth patterns and prognosis in early gastric carcinoma. Superficially spreading and penetrating growth types. Cancer. 1983;51:320–6.
37. Degiuli M, Calvo F. Survival of early gastric cancer in a specialized European center. Which lymphadenectomy is necessary? World J Surg. 2006;30:2193–203.
38. Gertler R, Stein HJ, Schuster T, et al. Prevalence and topography of lymph node metastases in early esophageal and gastric cancer. Ann Surg. 2014;259:96–101.
39. An JY, Baik YH, Choi MG, et al. Predictive factors for early gastric cancer with submucosal invasion: analysis of a single institutional experience. Ann Surg. 2007;246:749–53.
40. Waddell T, Verheij M, Allum W, et al. Gastric cancer: ESMO-ESSO-ESTRO Clinical Practice Guidelines for diagnosis, treatment and follow-up. Ann Oncol. 2013;24(Suppl 6):57–63.
41. Hayes N, Karat D, Scott DJ, et al. Radical lymphadenectomy in the management of early gastric cancer. Br J Surg. 1996;83:1421–3.
42. Gotoda T, Yanagisawa A, Sasako M, et al. Incidence of lymph node metastasis from early gastric cancer: estimation with a large number of cases at two large centers. Gastric Cancer. 2000;3:219–25.
43. Hyung WJ, Cheong JH, Kim J, et al. Application of minimally invasive treatment for early gastric cancer. J Surg Oncol. 2004;85:181–5.
44. Nasu J, Nishina T, Hirasaki S, et al. Predictive factors of lymph node metastasis in patients with undifferentiated early gastric cancers. J Clin Gastroenterol. 2006;40:412–5.
45. Ishikawa S, Togashi A, Inoue M, et al. Indications for EMR/ESD in cases of early gastric cancer: relationship between histological type, depth of wall invasion, and lymph node metastasis. Gastric Cancer. 2007;10:35–8.
46. Hirasawa T, Gotoda T, Miyata S, et al. Incidence of lymph node metastasis and the feasibility of endoscopic resection for undifferentiated-type early gastric cancer. Gastric Cancer. 2009;12:148–52.
47. Ha TK, An JY, Youn HK, et al. Indication for endoscopic mucosal resection in early signet ring cell gastric cancer. Ann Surg Oncol. 2008;15:508–13.
48. Ye BD, Kim SG, et al. Predictive factors for lymph node metastasis and endoscopic treatment strategies for undifferentiated early gastric cancer. J Gastroenterol Hepatol. 2008;23:46–50.
49. Li H, Lu P, Lu Y, et al. Predictive factors of lymph node metastasis in undifferentiated early gastric cancers and application of endoscopic mucosal resection. Surg Oncol. 2010;19:221–6.
50. Wang Z, Zhang X, Hu J, et al. Predictive factors for lymph node metastasis in early gastric cancer with signet ring cell histology and their impact on the surgical strategy: analysis of single institutional experience. J Surg Res. 2014;191:130–3.
51. Nesi G, Basili G, Girardi LR, et al. Pathological predictors of lymph node involvement in submucosal gastric carcinoma: a retrospective analysis of long-term outcome. In Vivo. 2009;23:337–41.
52. The Paris endoscopic classification of superficial neoplastic lesions. Esophagus, stomach, and colon: November 30 to December 1, 2002. Gastrointest Endosc. 2003;58:S3–S43.
53. Sano T, Sasako M, Kinoshita T, et al. Recurrence of early gastric cancer. Follow-up of 1475 patients and review of the Japanese literature. Cancer. 1993;72:3174–8.
54. Park DJ, Lee HK, Lee HJ, et al. Lymph node metastasis in early gastric cancer with submucosal invasion: feasibility of minimally invasive surgery. World J Gastroenterol. 2004;10:3549–52.
55. Maruyama K, Gunvén P, Okabayashi K, et al. Lymph node metastases of gastric cancer. General pattern in 1931 patients. Ann Surg. 1989;210:596–602.
56. Saragoni L. Upgrading the definition of early gastric cancer: better staging means more appropriate treatment. Cancer Biol Med. 2015;12:355–61.
57. Ono H, Kondo H, Gotoda T, et al. Endoscopic mucosal resection for treatment of early gastric cancer. Gut. 2001;48:225–9.
58. Tanabe S, Ishido K, Higuchi K, et al. Long-term outcomes of endoscopic submucosal dissection for early gastric cancer: a retrospective comparison with conventional endoscopic resection in a single center. Gastric Cancer. 2014;17:130–6.
59. Jung HY. Endoscopic resection for early gastric cancer: current status in Korea. Dig Endosc. 2012;24:159–65.
60. Probst A, Schneider A, Schaller T, et al. Endoscopic submucosal dissection for early gastric cancer: are expanded resection criteria safe for Western patients? Endoscopy. 2017;49:855–65.
61. Schlemper RJ, Riddell RH, Kato Y, et al. The Vienna classification of gastrointestinal epithelial neoplasia. Gut. 2000;47:251–5.
62. Stolte M. The new Vienna classification of epithelial neoplasia of the gastrointestinal tract: advantages and disadvantages. Virchows Arch. 2003;442:99–106.
63. Nagtegaal ID, Odze RD, Klimstra D, et al. A Cree for the WHO Classification of Tumours Editorial Board. The 2019 WHO classification of tumours of the digestive system. Histopathology. 2020;76:182–8.
64. Sekine S, Yoshida H, Jansen M, et al. The Japanese Viewpoint on the Histopathology of Early Gastric Cancer. Adv Exp Med Biol. 2016;908:331–46.

65. World Health Organization. Pathology and Genetics of tumours of the digestive system. 4th ed. Lyon: IARC press; 2010.
66. Sakurai U, Lauwers GY, Vieth M, et al. Gastric high-grade dysplasia can be associated with submucosal invasion: evaluation of its prevalence in a series of 121 endoscopically resected specimens. Am J Surg Pathol. 2014;38:1545–50.
67. Huang Q, Zou X. Clinicopathology of early gastric carcinoma: an update for pathologists and gastroenterologists. Gastrointest Tumors. 2016;3:115–24.

Handling of Endoscopic Resected Specimen: Indication for ESD and Grossing of ESD Specimen

12

Endoscopically resected specimen may be either endoscopic mucosal resection (EMR) or endoscopic submucosal dissection (ESD). These are carried out for a high-grade premalignant and superficial malignant lesions of the gastrointestinal tract (GIT). However, the drawback associated with EMR is that ablation therapies increase risk stricture at the site of resection. The main disadvantages of ablative therapies are the lack of tissue for histopathological examination [1]. The role of pathologists in reporting endoscopic resection samples is to confirm the endoscopic diagnosis and to provide information that may be of importance in determining further management, staging and follow-up of the patient [2].

EMR is a safe technology in the management of well-to-moderately differentiated GI carcinomas that are confined to mucosa with no lymph node involvement or any metastatic disease (T1m N0 M0). It is also very helpful for staging early GI cancers because it can provide a larger specimen than conventional biopsies [3–5]. There are several techniques to perform EMR that include injection-, cap- and ligation-assisted techniques [6]. The basic principle in all the methods is to identify and demarcate the lesions clearly and to inject along the submucosa of solutions such as saline, methylene blue and epinephrine to lift the lesion. The resection may be carried out either by ligation, cap-assisted suction technique or using the rubber band. In the cap-assisted technique, the resected piece of the mucosal lesion is sucked into the cap after grasping it a snare for resection. In the rubber band technique, the affected site to be resected is tied with a rubber band producing a raised polypoidal structure, the base of which is cut with a snare. In all the methods, a bit of the surrounding uninvolved mucosa and/or submucosa is usually included in the resected specimen [7, 8].

The resected EMR specimen should be submitted immediately to the pathology lab in the fresh state so that the specimen can be oriented with respect to the resection margins on a flat wax surface and leave it for fixation in 10% buffered formalin overnight [9]. Labelling the one particular position of the specimen, like 12 o'clock position, is enough for complete orientation. Alternately, the better can be by labelling the specimen as proximal and distal margins. EMR/ESD specimens are usually round to oval in shape [10]. Stepwise approach of handling the specimen by a pathologist: (i) Base and lateral mucosal margins should be inked with different colours. (ii) The resected specimen should be stretched and fixed mucosal side up onto a rigid support such as a block of wax or a corkboard. The fresh resected specimen is best to handle by fixing it immediately in order to preserve near to the in vivo shape and size. One should try to avoid pinning or poking the suspicious-looking area(s) and the obvious lesion. The specimen should be optimally stretched as overstretching may alter the shape, the size and also the thickness of the specimen and the lesional area [11, 12]. Once the speci-

K. Vaiphei, *Interpretation of Endoscopic Biopsy - Gastritis, Gastropathies and Beyond*,
https://doi.org/10.1007/978-981-16-6026-9_12

men has been appropriately displayed and placed, a representative gross photograph with a scale may be taken to document the lesion for future reference, or if photography is not feasible, a representative picture may be obtained with the help of a hand-drawn diagram. These documentations may be used to compare the findings observed in the resected specimen with the endoscopic features that have been recorded by the endoscopist. In some cases, the specimens need to be evaluated using a dissecting microscope to confirm the orientation and assess the margins [12]. Once the specimen is fixed, after removal from the board, it should be sliced serially at an interval of 2 to 3 mm thickness parallel along the long axis [13]. Ideally, the specimen may be embedded in toto, taking care to embed the sections sequentially, processed and stained with Haematoxylin and Eosin [7].

In larger and wider samples, appropriate sectioning that may be radial to be sampled for a microscopic study of the resection limits. In situations where the gross lesion is located just about 1 or more mm from the resection margin, it is essential to include both the narrow margins while sampling for proper comments with regards to involvement by the tumour. For small EMR specimens, perpendicular sections are to be sampled to include both the lesion and the resection margins. EMR specimens may be received in piecemeal and fragmented and are difficult to take appropriate sections to comment for the deep and lateral resection margins and to carry out accurate staging. Resection of the early lesions that are larger than 2 cms requires more than en-bloc resection by EMR, as it is observed that en bloc resection by EMR alone resulted in frequent local recurrence [9]. In order to solve these problems, deeper resection of the mucosa lesions by a technique called endoscopic submucosal dissection (ESD) in 1990 was developed enabling the lesion to be excised en bloc [14, 15]. As the resection is more complete by this new technology, more accurate examination of the resected specimen could be carried out. Ultimately this technology has been implicated as an established modality of treatment based on data compiled over 50 years of practice by Japanese physicians, surgeons, radiologists and pathologists [9]. ESD was used selectively only for EGC, now it has been used for many other lesions at different locations. Eligibility criteria for ESD therapy guidelines were described by the Japanese Gastric Cancer Association [16, 17] and the described selection criteria are tumour size and location appropriate for en bloc resection extremely low probability of lymph node involvement. And the absolute criteria are a differentiated adenocarcinoma cT1a of 2 cm or less size with no ulcer or scar [18–21]. More recently ESD has been performed for tumours which are—(i) >2 cm with no ulceration, (ii) differentiated type adenocarcinoma of 3 cm or less with ulcer and (iii) undifferentiated adenocarcinoma of 2 cm or less without ulceration [22–25]. And all these lesions should not ideally be with no lymphatic or vascular emboli (Table 12.1).

Table 12.1 Indications for endoscopic resection of early gastric cancer [22, 23]

Absolute indications: Histology with differentiated type, mucosal lesion of <2 cm with no ulcer, lymphatic or vascular invasion.
Expanded indications:
– Differentiated histology type, no ulcer, lymphatic or vascular invasion irrespective of tumour size.
– Differentiated histology, ulcerated, <3 cm size with no lymphatic vascular invasion.
– Differentiated minute lesion, size 500 μm or less.
– Submucosal invasive lesion <3 cm in size with vascular emboli.
– Undifferentiated type, <2 cm, no ulcer, lymphatic or vascular invasion.

12.1 Handling of ESD Sample

Evaluation of resection margins is undoubtably essential to determine completeness of the procedure. The specimens and also the lesions are smaller than what is observed in a standard surgical operation material, a careful and meticulous handling and examination are desired. Endoscopically resected specimens are to be placed on a tray containing a board on which the specimen can be pin-up using rust-proof pins under formalin solution taking care to spread out the specimen optimally near to its vivo size and shape, to be left overnight. Proper care is to be taken while spreading out the specimen so that resection margins can be sampled properly. Ideally, filter paper can be placed between the specimen and the board to enhanced fixation.

Macroscopic examination: The endoscopist while submitting the specimen to the pathology lab should be labelled by identifying the proximal and distal margins including the location of the tumour and also by mentioning important clues for specimen orientation in the requisition form. Specimens bearing small ulcer or ulcer scar with suspicion for submucosal invasion, the exact suspicious site to be identified do that representative block may be sampled from this site. A video recording or multiple photographs of the fresh and or the fixed specimens should be taken having labelled appropriately with markers. While taking photography putting labels to identify the lesion and the resection margins along with a scale should not be forgotten. A gross photograph with cutting lines through the main lesion is recommended a correlative study of naked appearances and the microscopy of the lesion and this may be supplemented with a hand-drawn diagram. The mucosal lesion appearance may be enhanced while taking a gross photograph by painting it with haematoxylin and immersing it underwater [9]. While serially slicing, the cut should be along the closest or closure resection margin(s), also traversing through the main lesion. While describing the closest margin distance from the main lesion should be mention, also describing the wider resection margins as well. The main lesion should also be described appropriately mentioning the shape, the size and also the thickness through the wall of the resected specimen, presence of ulcer, appearances of the mucosal lesion, and the resection margins; All the important landmarks of the specimen may be represented by making diagrams along with the descriptions. The width of the serial cuts or sections may be placed at a distance of 2 to 3 mm apart using a sharp knife [16]. ESD treatment outcome is assessed according to its relationship to extend of regional lymph node involvement. While taking blocks for microscopic examination of the mucosal lesion, there should not be any cut through the main mucosal lesion, it should be sampled in toto so that proper assessment of the extend of the lesion may be determined and the block should be placed edgewise within the cassettes. While reporting, in addition to the morphology of the mucosal lesion, its extent and involvement of submucosa, presence of lymphovascular emboli, adjoining mucosal histological status, resection margins play important role in commenting on the completeness of the resection. Major histological type of the tumour is usually taken as the final pathological diagnosis [15, 16]. Histological types may be differentiated and undifferentiated or diffuse type in Laurén's classification [26]. A differentiated cell type has lesser chances of vascular invasion and nodal metastasis. If a tumour exhibits a mixed morphology of differentiated and undifferentiated types may be labelled as high-risk type. In cases where there is submucosal invasion, histological type of the invasive front is to be mentioned as it will determine requirement for any additional treatment [9]. pT1b tumour may be grouped into two according to the depth of invasion, i.e. pT1b1 if <0.5 mm from the lower limit of muscularis mucosae and pT1b2 if invasion is 0.5 mm or more from lower edge of muscularis mucosae, and the second group has a higher risk of lymph node metastases [9]. In a situation where muscularis mucosae is difficult to distinguish from proliferating myofibroblasts, it will be wise to utilize the help of immunohistochemistry for desmin. There are a few available methods used to measure the depth of infiltration of 0.5 mm by placing a transparent scale on the desired area of the glass slide or a microscopic digital camera or using the micrometer attached to the eyepiece or a scale loupe [9]. Measurement of depth of invasion is of value only in those cases where the deep resection plane is free of tumour and if the deep plane is involved, the histological features should be described appropriately; Example pT1b2/SM2 and mentioning the distance of invasion from muscularis mucosae. Presence of any lymphatic permeation and vascular invasion are important factors for additional therapy. If need be additional immunohistochemistry staining like D2-40, CD31 or CD34 may be carried out for lymphatics and or vascular invasion. Sometimes even elastic Van Gieson stain may be of help [27–29]. If presence of invasion is clear in HE stained sections, special stains may not be necessary. Presence of an ulcer scar requires histological confirmation, not endoscopically. A biopsy scar is not a real ulcer scar, confirmation with the previous history of biopsy with respect to exact site of biopsy is essential and this can be clarified by the endoscopist who had carried out the previous biopsy before the procedure of ESD.

While evaluating horizontal surgical margins, the first and last sections of the whole length of the sections sampled from the resected specimen and both sides of all other sections are to be examined. In cases with negative horizontal margins, ideally, the distances to the margin from the lesion should be recorded. In a biopsy having positive margins, number of sections with positive margins may be mentioned. Presence of crushed or cautery artefacts along resection margins may be the reason for difficulty in clearly documenting involvement. In such situation, clear description may be given in the report of the difficulties resulting in inability to interpret. Crush artefacts may sometimes be the result of rough handling during the process of sampling in the pathology laboratory and also may be the result of utilization of blunt instruments, which are easily avoidable. A careful microscopic examination evaluating the cytomorphology of the suspicious cells present along the margins along with analysis of the associated structural changes in other tissues may help. In such a difficult situation, immunohistochemistry staining for p53 and Ki-67 may be of help sometimes to label the suspicious cells along the edges [30]. The deep resection plane through which the submucosa dissection has been carried out, is free of invasion by the cancer cell, then a diagnosis of negative vertical or deep margin can be documented and at the same time, the depth of invasion may also be documented. A positive vertical/deep margin, i.e. submucosa and the distance from the lower edge of muscularis mucosae to the positive margin site is the one to be recorded and may be useful information at the time of follow-up. Sometimes isolated tumour cells or there is extensive cautery of crushed artefacts are present resulting in difficulty to be able to identify the cancer cell(s), help of certain ancillary technique like immunohistochemistry stain may be of help using p53, Ki67 or a keratin primary antibody to highlight the cancer cell(s) better [31]. Sometimes a false cut through the specimen resulting in a falsely positive margin may be concerned. A cut made during the time of grossing usually gives a clean and straight cut, compared to the cuts made at the time of endoscopic dissection as the resected tissue undergoes retraction by the inherent presence of smooth muscles, nerves and blood vessels and also shrinkage due to fixation. Multiple deep cuts or step serial sections may be of help occasionally in a controversial situation. Since examination by re-embedding often does not work well as a part of the tissue has already been lost at the time of rough trimming of the paraffin blocks and fine microtomy sectioning, it is better to avoid such an approach.

ESD has its applicability besides the routine utilization for EGC, it has been used for high-risk patients with intractable diseases who are not fit for surgery [32]. Early detection of the precancerous and the early cancerous lesion is the deciding factor for a curative application of ESD [33, 34]. The more advanced endoscopy like narrow-band imaging and magnifying endoscopy have helped in tissue characterization by outlining the microvascular patterns and mucosal glandular architecture [32–34]. For a complete en-block dissection of the mucosal lesion, having a clear-cut resection margins is indispensable. This step is usually executed with completeness with the help of chromoendoscopy using indigo carmine and acetic acid to outline the desired land markings [32–34]. The changes and the gross improvement in these techniques had taken place over the last few years [9, 15, 16].

The unmistakable benefits of ESD over the years has been indicated by its successful expanded indications compared to surgical procedure for high-risk patients. ESD patients have exhibited limited complications, lesser days of hospital stay, limited but preservation of the stomach with lesser post-operative gastric-related complications enabling the patients' to have a better quality of life [34–39]. However, there are certain disadvantages that are involved with ESD, post-operative patients reported a larger number of second tumour in the stomach, which may be manageable with another session of ESD if detected early. These unwanted post-operative complications in the local site warrant a need for endoscopy surveillance [40].

12.2 Molecular Factors Influencing Outcome of Intramucosal Gastric Carcinomas

There has been a gross increase in the number of early gastric carcinomas (EGC) because of advancements in technics in radiographic and endoscopic examinations. EGC are subjected to minimal surgery like EMR and ESD for the small and differentiated types as these techniques offer a better quality of life. In previous chapters, it has been mentioned about the tumour criteria for application of these special techniques and their associated prognosis. However, certain groups of differentiated type carcinomas occasionally have been observed to have a more aggressive outcome, similar to poorly differentiated tumours by exhibiting a tendency for invasion and metastasis [41]. Conventionally gastric carcinomas are classified into intestinal and diffuse types [26] or differentiated and undifferentiated types [41]. Gastric carcinomas may have gastric or intestinal phenotype by immunohistochemical or mucin-histochemistry [42–44]. GC can be grouped into 3 phenotypes, i.e. intestinal type—complete or incomplete, and gastric type by its expression pattern for CD10 (CALLA), expressed by intestinal brush border [45], and MUC2 indicative of goblet cell differentiation [46] and human gastric mucin (HGM) indicating foveolar epithelial mucin [47]. GC exhibiting predominant gastric phenotypic have been found to be aggressive than those with intestinal phenotypic [47–50]. Hence, a phenotypic subclassification may require a better analysis and understanding of these tumours so that appropriate therapeutic measures can be taken. Gastric phenotype carcinomas associate with overexpression of MMPs, which possibly has the potential to degrade the extracellular matrix, compared to intestinal phenotype gastric carcinomas [40].

References

1. Vieth M, Langner C, Neumann H, et al. Barrett's esophagus. Practical issues for daily routine diagnosis. Pathol Res Pract. 2012;208:261–8.
2. Bejarano PA, Berho M. Examination of surgical specimens of the esophagus. Arch Pathol Lab Med. 2015;139:1446–54.
3. Participants in Paris Workshop. The Paris endoscopic classification of superficial neoplastic lesions: esophagus, stomach, and colon. Gastrointest Endosc. 2003;58:S3–S43.
4. Brahmania M, Lam E, Telford J, et al. Endoscopic mucosal resection: early experience in British Columbia. Can J Gastroenterol. 2010;24:239–44.
5. Scudiere JR, Montgomery EA. New treatments, new challenges: Pathology's perspective on esophageal carcinoma. Gastroenterol Clin N Am. 2009;38:121–33.
6. Geramizadeh B, Owen D. Handling and pathology reporting of gastrointestinal endoscopic mucosal resection. Middle East J Dig Dis. 2017;9:5–11.
7. Inoue H, Minami H, Kaga M, et al. Endoscopic mucosal resection and endoscopic submucosal dissection for esophageal dysplasia and carcinoma. Gastrointest Endosc Clin N Am. 2010;20:25–34.
8. Zhou PH, Schumacher B, Yao LQ, et al. Conventional vs. waterjet-assisted endoscopic submucosal dissection in early gastric cancer: a randomized controlled trial. Authors Endoscopy. 2014;46:836–42.
9. Nagata K, Shimizu M. Pathological evaluation of gastrointestinal endoscopic submucosal dissection materials based on Japanese guidelines. World J Gastrointest Endosc. 2012;4:489–99.
10. Höbel S, Dautel P, Baumbach R, et al. Single center experience of endoscopic submucosal dissection (ESD) in early Barrett's adenocarcinoma. Surg Endosc. 2015;29:1591–7.
11. Chevaux JB, Piessevaux H, Jouret-Mourin A, et al. Clinical outcome in patients treated with endoscopic submucosal dissection for superficial Barrett's neoplasia. Endoscopy. 2015;47:103–12.
12. Mino-Kenudson M, Brugge WR, Puricelli WP, et al. Management of superficial Barrett's epithelium-related neoplasms by endoscopic mucosal resection: clinicopathologic analysis of 27 cases. Am J Surg Pathol. 2005;29:680–6.
13. Oyama T, Tomori A, Hotta K, et al. Endoscopic submucosal dissection of early esophageal cancer. Clin Gastroenterol Hepatol. 2005;3:S67–70.
14. Ono H. Early gastric cancer: diagnosis, pathology, treatment techniques and treatment outcomes. Eur J Gastroenterol Hepatol. 2006;18:863–6.

15. Japanese gastric cancer association. Gastric cancer treatment guidelines. 3rd ed. Tokyo: Kanehara; 2010.
16. Japanese Gastric Cancer Association. Japanese gastric cancer treatment guidelines 2010 (ver. 3). Gastric Cancer. 2011;14:113–23.
17. Abe N, Watanabe T, Suzuki K, et al. Risk factors predictive of lymph node metastasis in depressed early gastric cancer. Am J Surg. 2002;183:168–72.
18. Kunisaki C, Takahashi M, Nagahori Y, et al. Risk factors for lymph node metastasis in histologically poorly differentiated type early gastric cancer. Endoscopy. 2009;41:498–503.
19. Yamao T, Shirao K, Ono H, et al. Risk factors for lymph node metastasis from intramucosal gastric carcinoma. Cancer. 1996;77:602–6.
20. Mita T, Shimoda T. Risk factors for lymph node metastasis of submucosal invasive differentiated type gastric carcinoma: clinical significance of histological heterogeneity. J Gastroenterol. 2001;36:661–8.
21. Alvarez Herrero L, Pouw RE, van Vilsteren FG, et al. Risk of lymph node metastasis associated with deeper invasion by early adenocarcinoma of the esophagus and cardia: study based on endoscopic resection specimens. Endoscopy. 2010;42:1030–6.
22. Gotoda T, Yanagisawa A, Sasako M, et al. Incidence of lymph node metastasis from early gastric cancer: estimation with a large number of cases at two large centers. Gastric Cancer. 2000;3:219–25.
23. Nishizawa T, Yahagi N. Long-term outcomes of using endoscopic submucosal dissection to treat early gastric cancer. Gut Liver. 2018;12:119–24.
24. Hirasawa T, Gotoda T, Miyata S, et al. Incidence of lymph node metastasis and the feasibility of endoscopic resection for undifferentiated-type early gastric cancer. Gastric Cancer. 2009;12:148–52.
25. Hanaoka N, Tanabe S, Mikami T, et al. Mixed-histologic-type submucosal invasive gastric cancer as a risk factor for lymph node metastasis: feasibility of endoscopic submucosal dissection. Endoscopy. 2009;41:427–32.
26. Lauren P. The two histological main types of gastric carcinoma: diffuse and so-called intestinal-type carcinoma. An attempt at a histo-clinical classification. Acta Pathol Microbiol Scand. 1965;64:31–49.
27. Sako A, Kitayama J, Ishikawa M, et al. Impact of immunohistochemically identified lymphatic invasion on nodal metastasis in early gastric cancer. Gastric Cancer. 2006;9:295–302.
28. Yonemura Y, Endou Y, Tabachi K, et al. Evaluation of lymphatic invasion in primary gastric cancer by a new monoclonal antibody, D2-40. Hum Pathol. 2006;37:1193–9.
29. del Casar JM, Corte MD, Alvarez A, et al. Lymphatic and/or blood vessel invasion in gastric cancer: relationship with clinicopathological parameters, biological factors and prognostic significance. J Cancer Res Clin Oncol. 2008;134:153–61.
30. Sugai T, Inomata M, Uesugi N, et al. Analysis of mucin, p53 protein and Ki-67 expressions in gastric differentiated-type intramucosal neoplastic lesions obtained from endoscopic mucosal resection samples: a proposal for a new classification of intramucosal neoplastic lesions based on nuclear atypia. Pathol Int. 2004;54:425–35.
31. Ko WJ, Song GW, Kim WH, et al. Endoscopic resection of early gastric cancer: current status and new approaches. Transl Gastroenterol Hepatol. 2016;1:24.
32. Korea ESD Study Group. Clinical outcomes of endoscopic resection for low-grade dysplasia and high-grade dysplasia on gastric pre-treatment biopsy. Gut Liver. 2021;15:225–31.
33. Nishizawa T, Suzuki H, Arano T, et al. Characteristics of gastric cancer detected within 1 year after successful eradication of helicobacter pylori. J Clin Biochem Nutr. 2016;59:226–30.
34. Choi MK, Kim GH, Park DY, et al. Long-term outcomes of endoscopic submucosal dissection for early gastric cancer: a single center experience. Surg Endosc. 2013;27:4250–8.
35. Nakamura K, Honda K, Akahoshi K, et al. Suitability of the expanded indication criteria for the treatment of early gastric cancer by endoscopic submucosal dissection: Japanese multicenter largescale retrospective analysis of short- and long-term outcomes. Scand J Gastroenterol. 2015;50:413–22.
36. Min BH, Kim KM, Park CK, et al. Outcomes of endoscopic submucosal dissection for differentiated-type early gastric cancer with histological heterogeneity. Gastric Cancer. 2015;18:618–26.
37. Abe S, Oda I, Suzuki H, et al. Short- and long-term outcomes of endoscopic submucosal dissection for undifferentiated early gastric cancer. Endoscopy. 2013;45:703–7.
38. Yamamoto Y, Fujisaki J, Miyamoto Y, et al. The long term prognosis of expanded indication lesion of endoscopic submucosal dissection for undifferentiated type early gastric cancer. Stomach Intest. 2014;49:1569–77.
39. Fukunaga S, Nagami Y, Shiba M, et al. Long-term prognosis of expanded-indication differentiated-type early gastric cancer treated with endoscopic submucosal dissection or surgery using propensity score analysis. Gastrointest Endosc. 2017;85:143–52.
40. Kabashima A, Yao T, Sugimachi K, et al. Relationship between biologic behaviour and phenotypic expression in Intramucosal gastric carcinomas. Hum Pathol. 2002;33:80–6.
41. Nakamura K, Sugano H, Takagi K. Carcinoma of the stomach in incipient phase: its histogenesis and histological appearances. Gann. 1968;59:252–8.
42. Tatematsu M, Ichinose M, Miki K, et al. Gastric intestinal phenotypic expression of human stomach cancers as revealed by peptinogen immunohistochemistry and mucin histochemistry. Acta Pathol Jpn. 1990;40:494–504.
43. Egashira Y. Mucin histochemical study of differentiated adenocarcinoma of stomach. Jpn J Gastroenterol. 1994;91:839–48.
44. Yao T, Kabashima A, Kouzuki T, et al. The phenotypes of the gastric carcinoma—evaluation by a new

immunohistochemical method. I To Cho (Stomach Intestine). 1999;34:477–85.
45. Kabashuma A, Yao T, Tsuneyoshi M. Gastric and intestinal phenotypic expression in the carcinomas and background mucosa of multiple early gastric carcinomas. Histopathology. 2000;37:513–22.
46. Endoh Y, Tamura G, Motoyama T, et al. Well-differentiated adenocarcinoma mimicking complete-type intestinal metaplasia in the stomach. Hum Pathol. 1999;30:826–32.
47. Yoshino T, Shimoda T, Saitou A, et al. Macroscopic features of differentiated gastric adenocarcinoma with gastric or intestinal phenotype expression in early gastric cancer. I To Cho (Stomach Intestine). 1999;34:507–25.
48. Kubo K, Yanagisawa A, Ninomiya Y, et al. Characteristics of differentiated-type carcinoma with gastric phenotype of the stomach. I To Cho (Stomach Intestine). 1999;34:487–94.
49. Koseki K, Takizawa T, Koike M, et al. Subclassification of well differentiated gastric cancer with reference to biological behaviour and malignancy, gastric type vs. intestinal type, and papillary carcinoma vs. tubular carcinoma. I To Cho (Stomach Intestine). 1999;34:507–12.
50. Oya M, Yao T, Tsuneyoshi M. A correlation of intramural invasion with mucin histochemistry, and immunohistochemical expressions of oncogene-related proteins in early gastric carcinoma. I To Cho (Stomach Intestine). 1997;32:31–9.

13 Interpretation of Endoscopic Mucosal Biopsy for Gastric Carcinoma

Over the last two decades, there has been gross improvement in the endoscopic technology. These changes have produced a positive impact on daily diagnostic and therapeutic application of the various modalities. Along with the increasing number of biopsies, myriads of gastric epithelial lesions are observed by the practising pathologist in day-to-day routine clinical practice. These are associated with several challenges including a practising pathologist to upkeep with the new entities and diseases. More often, the controversies are related to subtle morphological changes associated with epithelial cells exhibiting either regeneration or early dysplasia [1, 2]. Issues that need to be identified with respect to the probable and hypothetical development of certain conditions like differentiated adenocarcinomas believed to be originated from intestinal metaplasia of gastric mucosa as the result of long-standing *H. pylori* infection; whereas, undifferentiated diffuse type of adenocarcinomas originate from gastric mucosa with no precursor mucosal changes like intestinal metaplasia [3–5]. Sometimes, it is difficult to draw a line between hyperplastic gastric foveolar epithelium and the metaplastic epithelium showing features of microvesicular change, as epithelium with a micro-vesicular morphology may be showing incomplete intestinal metaplasia in special mucin histochemistry.

13.1 Challenging Issues in Interpretation of Pre-neoplastic and Neoplastic Lesions in Gastric Biopsies

The first step in management of a patient who is suspected to have a neoplastic gastric mucosal lesion is to undergo upper GI endoscopy examination and appropriately a mucosal biopsy is to be sampled. Interpreting a mucosal biopsy may have its own challenges that include interpretation and offering a conclusive remark. These can be due to multiple reasons—lack of a standardized criterion for the histological changes observed under the microscope or the biopsy sample may be inadequate as it is too small or maybe non-representative it may be mainly composed of necrotic tissue or mucous fragment or gastric content. The difficulty may be associated with unable to categorize regenerating atypia or dysplasia or malignancy [6]. A malignant tumour like an adenocarcinoma of the stomach is defined as a tumour in which the cells show invasion into lamina propria by penetration of the basement membrane of the native glands. Despite this clear definition, there has been controversy in distinguishing between high-grade dysplasia and carcinoma in endoscopic biopsy specimens of gastric mucosal lesions, especially between the patholo-

K. Vaiphei, *Interpretation of Endoscopic Biopsy - Gastritis, Gastropathies and Beyond*,
https://doi.org/10.1007/978-981-16-6026-9_13

gist based in the east and the west [7]. Pathologist in the West makes a diagnosis of adenocarcinoma only when there are definite histological evidence of destruction of basement membrane associated with single-cell infiltration across the basement membrane, presence of small clusters of atypical cells or buds in the lamina propria, all these changes to be associated with stromal desmoplasia [8, 9]. Contrary to these features practiced by the Europeans and American pathologists, Japanese pathologists put the weightage to extend of cytological atypia and disorganisation of the normal glandular architecture. The associated cytological abnormalities, not specific for gastric pre-neoplastic and neoplastic morphology, are increased nucleocytoplasmic ratio, anisonucleosis, coarse chromatin which may be clumped giving vesicular appearance of the nuclei, irregular nuclear membrane, loss of nuclear polarity, prominent and large nucleoli and atypical mitosis. The glands may look overcrowded, occasionally arranged in gland, and closely packed where the glands are arranged in back-to-back appearances with no intervening basement membrane and stroma, which could also produce abortive glands and cribriform architecture [10–13]. Hence, an intramucosal neoplastic lesion may be in situ carcinoma or intramucosal carcinoma irrespective of the submucosal invasion. Personally, I give importance to every bit of atypical cytological changes exhibited by the epithelial cells; and presence of invasion into lamina propria by the atypical cells across the basement membrane, associated with glandular disarray, branching, atypical shapes and sizes, and glandular buds. Changes of dysplasia, unlike in intestinal preneoplasia, may not be a prominent histological feature in gastric mucosa; rather disorganization of the glandular architecture and individual cell character change acquiring cells with microvesicular character, are more frequently observed features. The labelled of early or intramucosal carcinomas by the pathologists from the East will be unanimously diagnosed by the European and American pathologists as high-grade dysplasia; followed-up ESD in such cases, significant numbers have reportedly shown invasion beyond muscularis mucosae into submucosa suggesting a frank intramucosal carcinoma. Additional histological features that have been documented by the Eastern pathologists to suggest a frankly malignant tumour with submucosal invasion in an endoscopic biopsy are presence of necrotic/apoptotic debris within disorganized and distorted glands, papillary fronds, fused glands, glandular budding and ulceration [11, 14–17]. There are many examples in the Western literature in which a diagnosis of high-grade dysplasia (HGD) was entertained, subsequent submucosal biopsies revealing frank infiltrative tumour to submucosa along with lympho-vascular embolization [18, 19]. Identifying HGD in an endoscopic biopsy is an important predictor for the presence of carcinoma in followed-up resected specimen equally both for gastric and other sites, however, in gastric biopsy, high dysplasia may not be a frequently observed feature [1, 17]. Stromal invasion observed with HGD epithelium used as an indicator for the presence of intramucosal carcinoma or carcinoma per se might prevent negative conversion to lower grade mucosal lesion in a resected specimen as it has been observed to have low specificity [1, 16–19].

13.2 Atypical Epithelium and Diagnosis of Frank Carcinoma

A biopsy exhibiting florid changes of regenerative epithelium or foveolar type dysplasia may easily be misdiagnosed for well-differentiated adenocarcinoma. The difficulties associated with in identifying foveolar type dysplasia may be multifactorial, i.e. (1) may be unawareness of the reporting pathologist for the existence of such type of mucosal lesion and the terminology associated with, (2) morphologic features resemble normal foveolar epithelial cells in a casual look and the nuclear changes like enlargement, hyperchromasia and stratification, though are present, are not prominent features [20, 21]. Reactive changes in the gastric foveolar epithelium in inflammatory conditions may mimic dysplasia as there will be associated relative lack of mucin and nuclear atypia; but in inflamed mucosa, there will be additional mucosal changes in the form of oedema, vascular congestion, lack of nuclear crowding and multilayering and gradual transition to the adjacent non-inflamed mucosa (Fig. 13.1). There are certain useful clues for differentiating reactive atypia from true dysplasia include—presence of vascular congestion and stromal oedema, lack of epithelial cell stratification and transition of atypical glands to adjacent normal epithelium [20, 21]. In true dysplasia, there will be an abrupt transition of the atypical glands with the adjoining normal looking glands and in regenerative changes there will be a gradual transition between the two types of glands (Fig. 13.2a–d). It is also important to note the extent of epithelial atypia present and the degree of inflammation present. In most of the cases, step serial sectioning may solve the problem. In biopsies that are associated with heavy inflammation and epithelial destruction, such controversial issues may be solved with a follow-up biopsy carry out at least a gap of 2 weeks or after the inflammation settles down. And in the follow-up biopsy, if extend of the epithelial atypia exceeds degree of mucosal inflammation, most likely, there is true epithelial atypia, that may be graded appropriately. In routine practice, a pathologist may sometimes be in a critical situation and if interpretation of the morphological features is from a therapeutic viewpoint, discriminating dysplasia from carcinoma may not be important as all are manageable by ESD in the hand of an expert endoscopist. If a borderline mucosal lesion is found to be persistent on repeated endoscopic biopsy, subjecting the patient to ESD will be the preferred method of treatment [1].

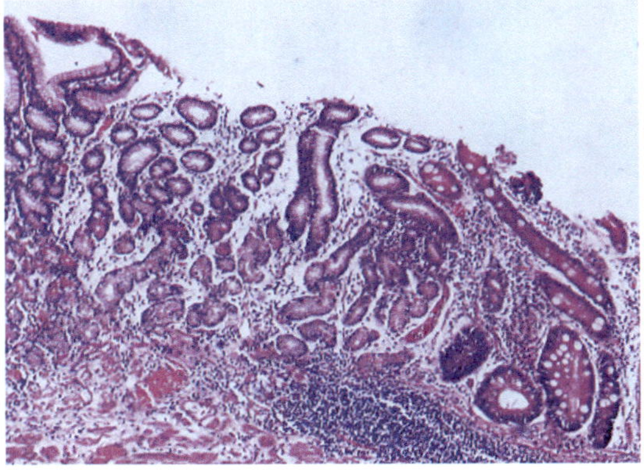

Fig. 13.1 Photomicrograph of gastric antral mucosa to show changes of mucosal atrophy accompanied by chronic inflammation, foveolar hyperplasia and intestinal metaplasia. Some of the glands are showing atypia which will be due to the ongoing inflammation and regeneration (HE, ×200)

13.3 Newer Concepts for Early Mucosal Lesions

Variation in interpretation of dysplasia carcinoma spectrum of gastric epithelium amongst the same and between the pathologists is a longstanding issue, especially between the pathologists in the Eastern and the Western countries [7]. Dysplasia is a term traditionally defined as an obvious, unambiguous morphological changes due to cytologic and architectural alteration of the epithelial cells of the glands and the surface lining having intact basement membrane and no invasion into lamina propria. Mucosal lesions with atypical epithelial cells qualify for diagnosis of carcinoma having the potential to develop frank malignancy regardless of morphologic grade should be labelled as intramucosal neoplasia [22, 23]. Adenoma, a pre-neoplastic lesion, has been described in the West as a raised polypoid mucosal lesion whereas in the East, adenoma has been used for much broader conditions which include besides the polypoidal lesions, flat as well as depressed mucosal lesions [22]. Most gastric mucosal lesions exhibiting epithelial dysplasia or intra-mucosal neoplasia may be divided into many subtypes based on their phenotypic expressions either for stomach (foveolar and pyloric type) (Fig. 13.3a and b) and colonic (adenomatous) (Fig. 13.4a and b) [24–26]. A dysplastic epithelium is conventionally classified into two histological variants of low (LGD) (Fig. 13.5a and b) and high-grade (HGD) (Fig. 13.4a and b) [20].

Adenomatous type is a common type and shares the morphological features of a colonic adenoma [24], and is followed by the foveolar subtype resembling normal foveolar epithelium [6, 24]. Occasionally, a gastric polyp may show

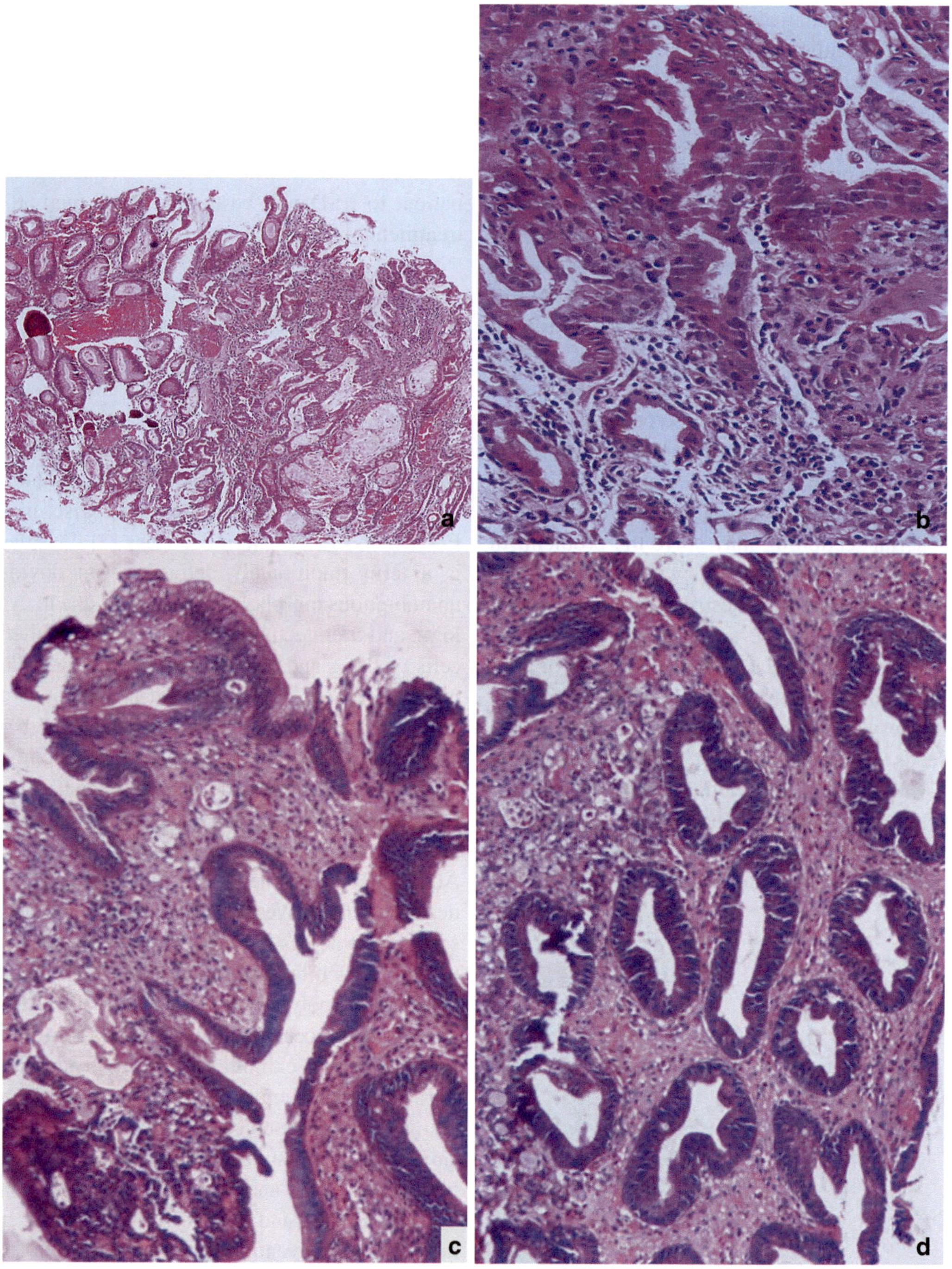

Fig. 13.2 (**a**) A biopsy exhibiting dysplasia, there will be an abrupt transition of the atypical glands (on the right) with the adjoining nondysplastic glands (on the left) as seen in this photomicrograph in contrast to a regenerating epithelium where there will not be any clear cut demarcation. The atypical glands show irregular outline and loss of normal orientation of the glands with respect to surface epithelium, epithelial cell pleomorphism, lack of mucin and stratification (HE, ×200); (**b**) high power view of those abnormal glands to bring out the atypical cellular morphology better (HE, ×350); (**c**) and (**d**) those atypical epithelial cells are showing parietal cell morphology and arranged in tubule-papillary pattern with anisonucleosis, stratification, micropapillary frond and goblet cell metaplasia. No lamina propria invasion or obviously prominent atypical mitosis. In gastric pre-neoplastic lesions, the nuclear changes may not be a prominent feature, i.e. not like the conventional colonic dysplasia but more like the micro-vesicular changes as in a serrated adenoma (HE, ×350)

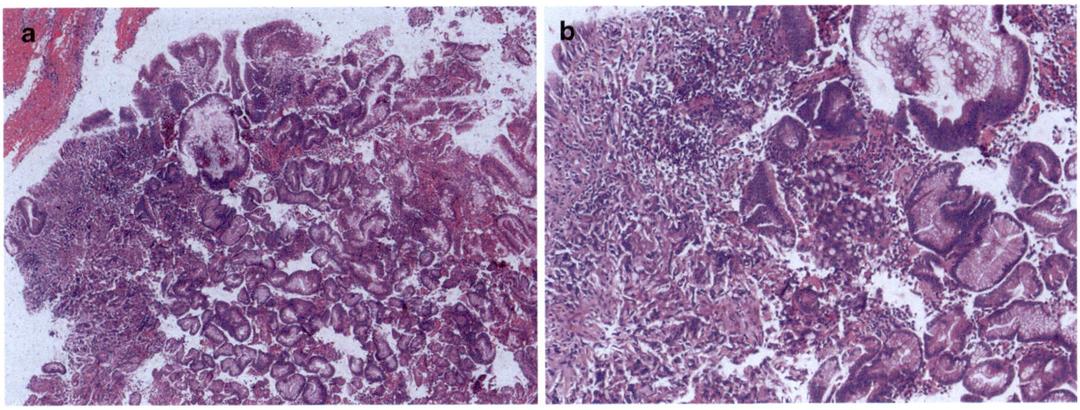

Fig. 13.3 (**a**) and (**b**) Photomicrographs of gastric biopsy to show the intramucosal invasive carcinoma with epithelial dysplasia with foveolar and pyloric phenotype (HE, ×350)

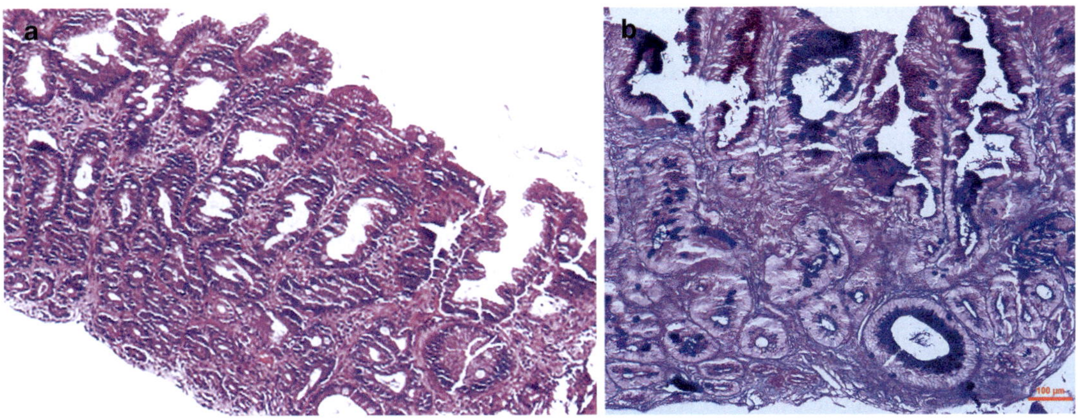

Fig. 13.4 (**a**) Photomicrograph of gastric biopsy to show the intramucosal carcinoma with high-grade epithelial dysplasia of colonic/adenomatous phenotype (HE, ×350). (**b**) Photomicrograph of the same biopsy in alcian blue PAS staining to different patterns of alcian blue and PAS positivity (Alcian blue PAS, ×350)

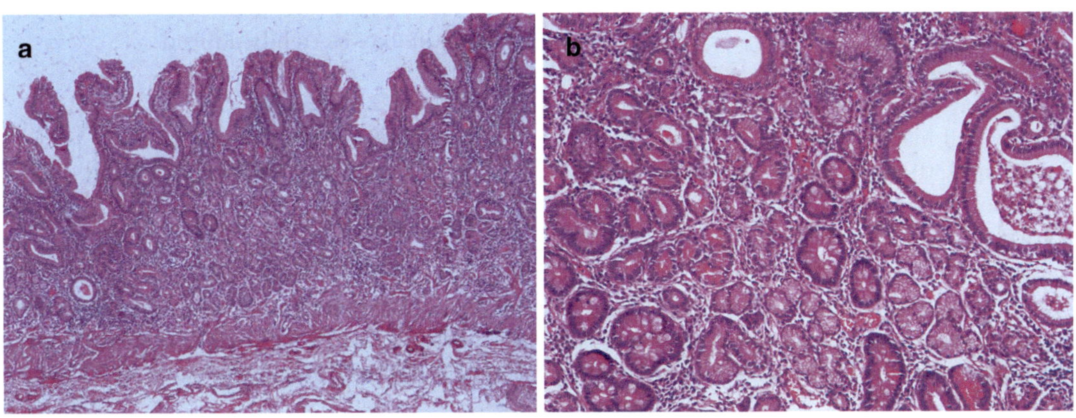

Fig. 13.5 (**a**) and (**b**) Photomicrograph of gastric biopsy to show foci of dysplastic glands that may be in occasional isolated few glands or may be observed in more number clustering in one focus of the mucosa, histological of low dysplasia (LGD) (HE, ×300)

hybrid morphology simulating the two types of epithelial characters that have been described and also expressed distinctive immunohistochemical properties; cells mimicking gastric foveolae expresses MUC5AC and the adenoma cells show positive staining for MUC2, CD10 and CDX2 [24, 27]. Intestinal type of dysplastic epithelium is identified by the presence of nuclear stratification (Fig. 13.4a and b) whereas the cells of foveolar type do not show nuclear stratification maintaining its mono layering (Figs. 13.2a–c and 13.4a and b) [6, 9]. Diagnostic features for LGD are mild nuclear crowding, hyperchromasia and overlapping, cells present in simple tubular structures, increased N:C and mucodepletion. HGD shows glandular crowding which may be showing occasional branching, high N:C, cuboidal and elliptical nuclei with prominent nucleoli [28]. Active cellular proliferation indicated by complex glandular patterns containing necrotic debris are features suggestive of an intramucosal invasive carcinoma [6]. Major issue may sometimes be differentiating LGD from HGD in foveolar type of mucosal lesion. In HGD compared to LGD, nuclear size tends to be double or more than the normal nuclei, prominent and maybe multiple nucleoli, moderate-to-abundant cytoplasm tends to be more eosinophilic, sometimes looking like an oncocytic cell, however, with disorganized glandular architecture (Fig. 13.2b–d) [29].

13.4 Foveolar Type Adenoma

Gastric foveolar type dysplasia (GFTD) like lesions may be present in sites other than stomach like gall bladder, pancreato-biliary tract and duodenum [30]. GFTD is a relatively new entity more recently described. This condition hence is not well recognized and a diagnosis of GFTD is seldom made in routine reporting [31, 32]. WHO (2019) classification mentions this condition as foveolar type adenoma with no dysplasia with no malignant potential [33]. GFTD has not been observed to be associated with inflamed gastric mucosa [32]. The criteria used to diagnose GFTD are variable and have not uniformly been described. It can be found anywhere within the different parts of the stomach though more frequently involving proximal segment. Epithelial cells show enlarged monomorphic nuclei, prominent nucleoli with no stratification [31–33]. GFTD histologically shows less nuclear changes compared to the histological features exhibited by conventional dysplasia of a classic intestinal or colonic type (Fig. 13.6a–e). Even in HGD, the cells do not exhibit prominent anisonucleosis [20, 34]. GFTD had been described mainly from antrum and non-lesser curvature sites and were found to be smaller in size, normal to reddish mucosa and had flat or depressed configuration as well and may show variable grades of mucosal changes [34, 35]. Goblet and Paneth cells are rarely identified and there can be rarely hybrid features of both GFTD and intestinal type of dysplasia (Fig. 13.7a and b) [32, 35]. In the presence of associated mucosal erosions or ulceration, inflammatory atypia is a confounder but shows a gradual transition to normal epithelium usually is observed [31]. Abnormal foveolar epithelium can be seen in confluence with intestinal type of gastric carcinoma having similar looking cells suggesting atypical foveolar epithelium to be the precursor mucosal changes in the pathway of development of such carcinoma (Fig. 13.8a and b). Though the term of foveolar type adenocarcinoma is not in vogue, possibly under certain circumstances with the appropriate histological changes, it may be rightly utilized.

13.5 Pyloric Gland—Pre-neoplastic and Neoplastic Lesions

Pyloric gland adenoma (PGA) is a recently described uncommon entity. This condition has been described in about 3% of patients who presents with upper GI-related problem; its incidence

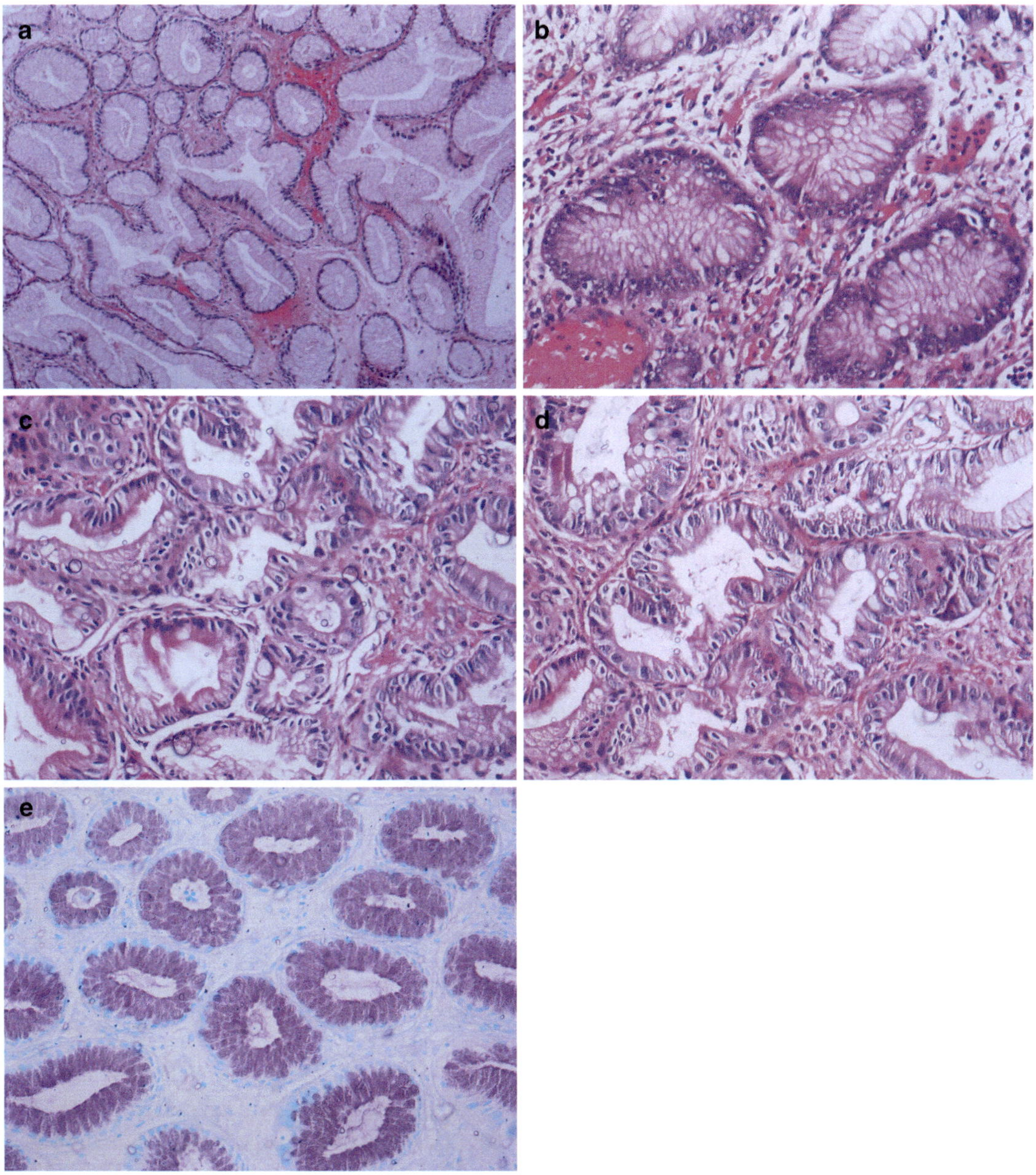

Fig. 13.6 (**a**) Depicts a classic feature of gastric foveolar adenoma composed of cells with abundant pale cytoplasm and uniform basally placed nuclei. The glands are of variable shapes and sizes, some with nice angulated and branched, lamina propria is relatively lack of any inflammatory cell with sparse stromal component (HE, ×200). (**b**) Another photomicrograph of similar lesion, however, the picture is focused on two atypical glands exhibiting mild nuclei stratification and enlargement and bubbly looking cytoplasm (HE, ×350). (**c**) and (**d**) Both the photomicrographs were taken from different areas of one lesion showing tubule-papillary patterns with significant cellular atypia. The cells have a lesser amount of pale cytoplasm, mild-to-moderately enlarged nuclei with anisonucleosis, no feature for a carcinoma (HE, ×350). (**e**) A strong cytoplasmic PAS positivity of the cells as seen in (**a**) (PAS, ×350)

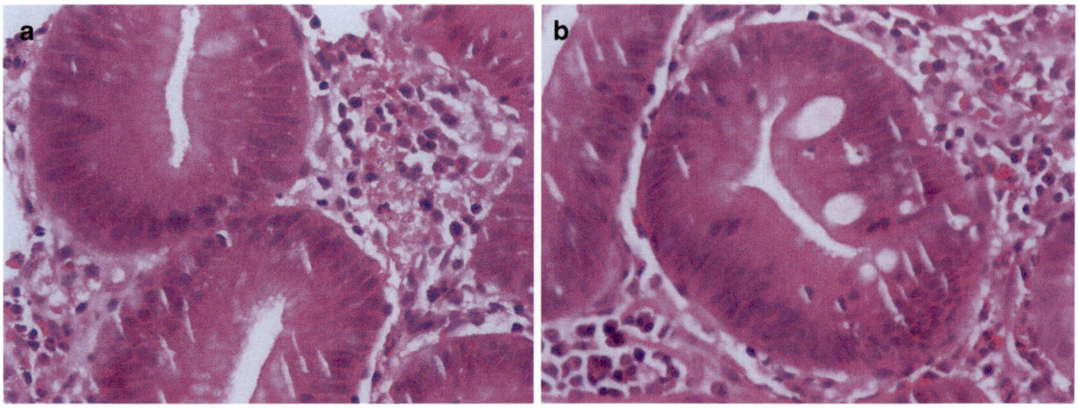

Fig. 13.7 (**a**) and (**b**) Medium power photomicrographs to show a pylori antrum located pyloric gland adenoma with features of low- and high-grade dysplasia of intestinal type along with goblet cells (HE, ×400)

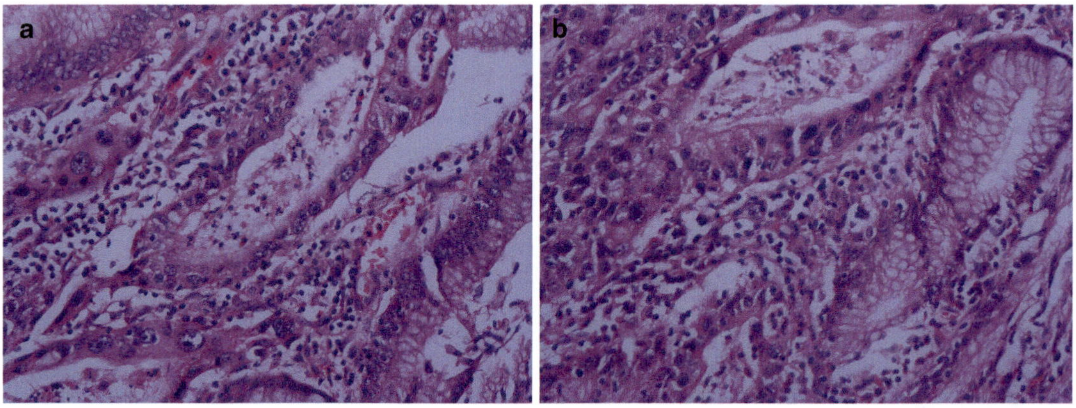

Fig. 13.8 (**a**) and (**b**) In these two photomicrographs, abnormal foveolar epithelium can be seen in confluence with the carcinoma cells forming the glands exhibiting similar morphology suggesting foveolar epithelium to be the cell of origin and the precursor mucosa in the development of such carcinoma (HE, ×350)

is higher in patients having syndromic presentation [36]. In FAP, the patients are older and have shown a predilection for female having proximal location [37–39] and in Lynch syndrome it is more common in young males [37, 40]. PGAs have a similar histologic appearance to normal pyloric glands. The glands in an adenoma usually are made up of closely packed glands and each gland has a lining of cuboidal or columnar cells having apical mucin [38, 39, 41]. Presence of apical mucin helps to differentiate from foveolar type and intestinal type adenomas with no well-formed mucin cap. PGA has cells with eosinophilic to amphophilic cytoplasm with round to oval nuclei occasionally visible nucleoli. Squamous morules have been described [41–44]. The glands tend to be complex and branched lined by cells having nuclear atypia (Fig. 13.9a–c) [39]. Certain number of biopsies exhibiting features of dysplasia will also show focus/foci of malignant transformation in the form of fused and branch glands, however, distinguishing between HGD and carcinomatous transformation or focus may be difficult based only on cytomorphologic features [45]. Histochemical stains and immunohistochemistry may be of help to identify PGAs. Unlike gastric foveolar type adenomas, PGAs can be identified by the presence of neutral

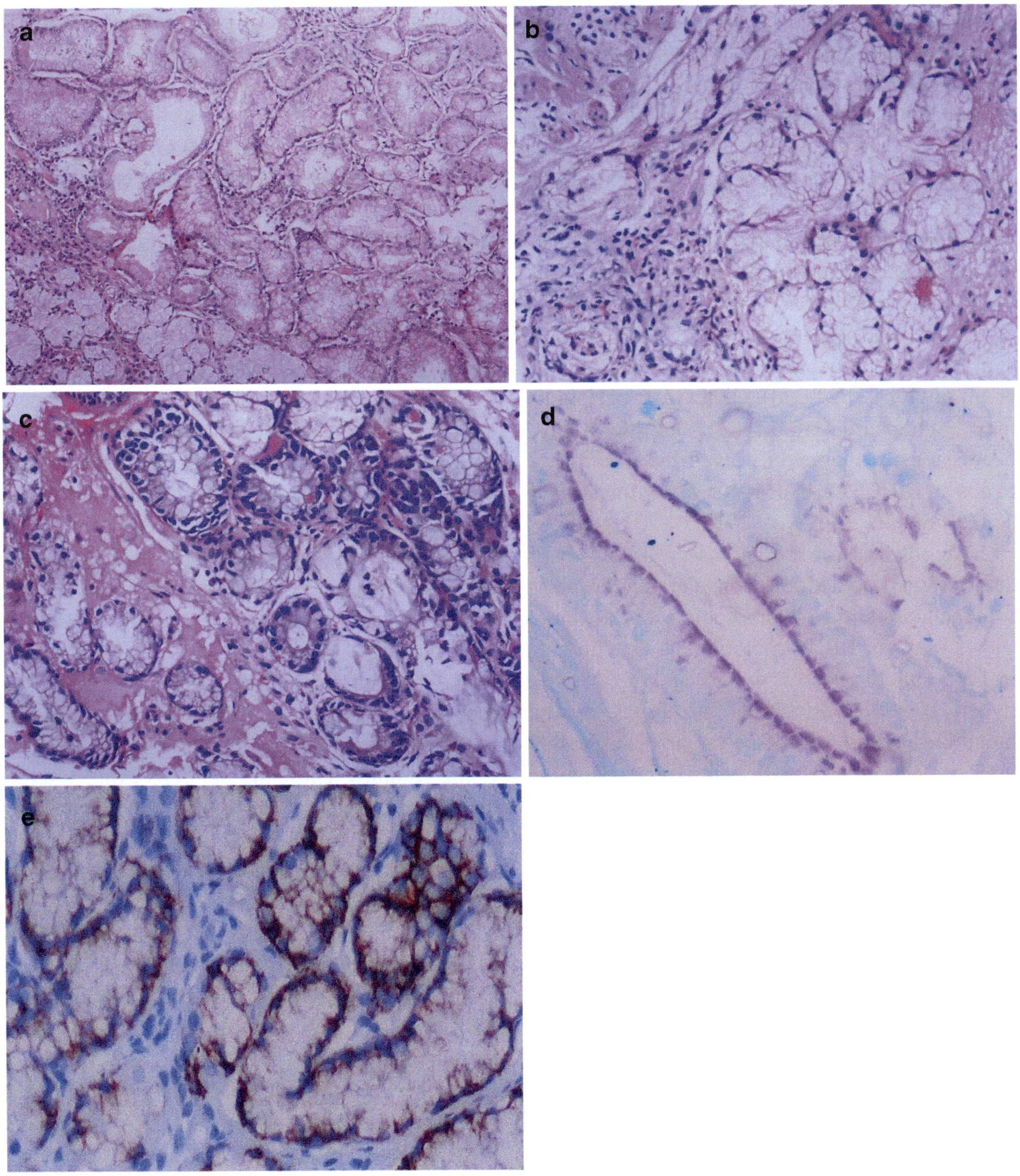

Fig. 13.9 (**a**) Medium power photomicrograph of the adenoma composed of closely packed glands lined by cuboidal to columnar cells with apical mucin. The glands are of variable shapes, occasionally complex and larger than the native pyloric gland seen at the lower portion of the picture (HE, ×300). (**b**) The adenoma in higher power picture to show the character of the individual cells with no nuclei atypia. Focal inflammation and destruction of the glands where the proliferating epithelial cells are seen in cluster (HE, ×500). (**c**) Another picture of pyloric gland adenoma where there are mild nuclei stratification and enlargement and the glands focally almost arranged in back-to-back pattern (HE, ×500). (**d**) Unlike gastric foveolar-type adenoma, PGAs can be identified by the presence of neutral mucin cap in periodic acid–Schiff with few scatter granular cytoplasmic PAS-positive material (AB-PAS, ×350). (**e**) PGA may be further confirmed by IHC by demonstrating positive staining for MUC6 (PAP, ×500)

mucin cap in periodic acid–Schiff/Alcian blue stain (PAS/AB) with granular cytoplasmic PAS-positive material (Fig. 13.9d). Gastric foveolar type adenomas give bright red uniform cytoplasmic staining. PGA may be further confirmed by IHC by demonstrating positive staining for MUC6 (Fig. 13.9e) and negative for MUC5AC. Similar staining patterns have been demonstrated in those PGA located away from the pyloric region. MUC6 expression is considered to be more specific than MUC5AC expression, which may also show focal nuclear positivity for CDX2 ± MUC2. PGA occasionally may show different MUC6 and MUC5AC expressions, strong and diffuse MUC6 with low to absent MUC5AC expression along the surface epithelium [46, 47].

Like other gastric carcinomas, PGA has been demonstrated to exhibit considerable chromosomal abnormalities. Sporadic form of adenomas shows frequent KRAS mutation along with gain in 17pq and 20q, loss of 4q, 5q, and 6q [48, 49]. Lynch syndrome-associated adenomas exhibit mutation in DNA mismatch repair genes with a high potential for malignant transformation. Gastric PGAs express p53 less frequently compared to intestinal-type adenomas. And those gastric PGAs expressing p53 tend to have high-grade dysplastic features or malignant transformation [40, 47, 50]. PGA expressing nuclear p53 may be an indicator of high risk. MMR protein loss has been found to be infrequent involving only about 4.3% loss of MLH1 and PMS2 [49, 51]. This group also studied other gastric adenomas and adenocarcinomas for MMR protein loss 2.9% and 7% of cases, respectively, similar results to PGA, however, the foveolar type was found to have higher loss of MMR proteins in 52% of the cases. There were a couple of conflicting results reported by other studies [51–53]. Two studies conducted amongst the Japanese patients made important conclusions—(1) foveolar type has frequent MSI whereas majority of intestinal type is MS stable; (2) contrary to this conclusion, American patients with intestinal and foveolar type adenomas were microsatellite unstable in one-third of cases. Based on these limited studies with contrasting results between the Western and Eastern patients, future studies in a larger cohort of patients, are indicated.

13.6 Oxyntic (Parietal) Gland Adenoma/Adenocarcinoma

It was in 2003 that J. Muller-Hocker and Rellecke made a case report entitled "Chief cell proliferation of the gastric mucosa mimicking early gastric cancer: an unusual variant of fundic gland polyp" (Fig. 13.10a–c) [54]. Since then there have been a few more case reports and case series. A case report was made in 2007 by Tsukamoto et al. entitled gastric adenocarcinoma with chief cell differentiation (GA-CCD) in 16 mm size gastric fundic polypoidal lesion [55]. This particular tumour showed an adenocarcinoma having a well-differentiated morphology arranged mainly in tubular pattern (Fig. 13.11a–f). It is considered to be a type of gastric cancer with uncertain clinicopathologic features [56]. The tumour cells were columnar or cuboidal having basophilic cytoplasm with a few coarse eosinophilic granules. These tumour cells expressed the characteristic marker for chief cells, i.e. pepsinogens I and II, and RUNX3, and mucus neck cell marker MUC6; tumour cells were negative for parietal cell markers like proton pump alpha subunit and immunomarker for intestinal phenotypes like Cdx2 and defensin-5. Tumour cells expressed chief and mucous neck cell phenotypes like a primitive chief cell in fundic gland. These group tumours show mild nuclear atypia, low Ki67 and p53 indices, no invasive property or recurrence. Further analysis showed GA-CCD to be rare having a distinct clinicopathological characteristic of location, morphologic features and phenotypes. Hence, fundic gland type of adenocarcinoma with chief cell predominance is to be considered as a new entity [57].

Fundic gland polyps (FGPs) are benign involving the body region comprising benign fundic glands arranged disorderly with cystic dilatation (Fig. 13.10a–c) [58–60]. FGP maybe just one focus or many more and incidence in the general population is just about 1.4% and may be a component of FAP [61–63]. Origin of these

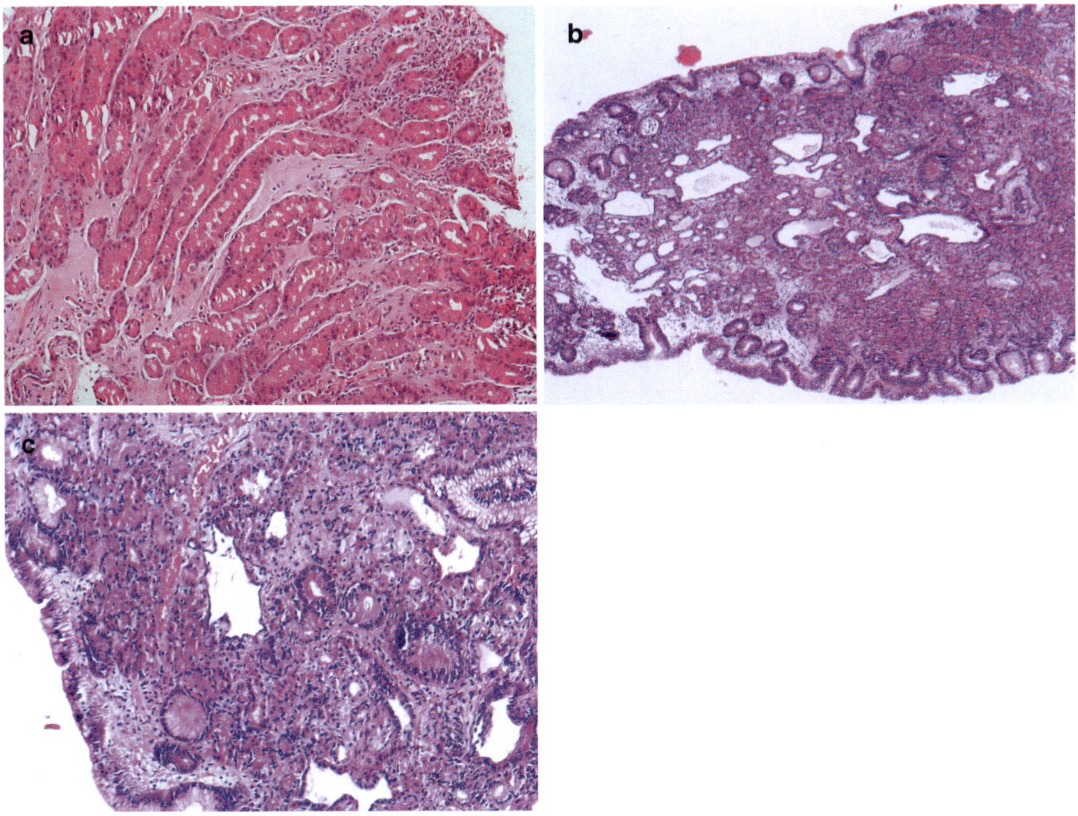

Fig. 13.10 (**a**) Medium power photomicrograph of a body mucosal biopsy showing grossly hyperplastic parietal cells arranged in cords extending up to the denuded surface, separated by fine collagenised stroma. There was no nodular area to suggest a possibility of an adenoma. However, it cannot be definitely excluded for the small endoscopic biopsy in the biopsy sample (HE, ×300). (**b**) A low power view of a biopsy from the fundic polyp covered all around by the foveolar epithelial cells along with component of the inflamed lamina propria. There are many cystically dilated glands lined by flattened cells dispersed in between relatively normal looking fundic glands, which are the characteristic features for this type of adenoma (HE, ×150). (**c**) A higher power photomicrograph of the same adenoma to bring out the described morphology better. In addition, there are features of pyloric metaplasia as well (HE, ×300)

polyps remains controversial. It has been best characterized as either a hyperplastic polyp which may exhibit either a progressive or regressive property [64–67]. Comparing the phenotypic features of FGPs in syndromic and non-syndromic situations, the ones with syndromic presentation displayed distinct mucin histochemical features, younger age of presentation, higher male-to-female ratio, larger and more in number, tends to have more cystic dilation of the glands along with more component of smooth muscle [62, 63, 68]. A study has found that FGPs in FAP are more cystic with more smooth muscle components [66, 69, 70]. FGP, first described in FAP, was thought to be specific [66] but later on it was also observed in non-FAP individuals but of lesser frequency and number; about 70% of FAP patients will develop FGP in their lifetime and prevalence of FGP in the general population is just only about 0.8% to 1.4% [69, 70]. Many pathologists believe that FGPs are an underdiagnosed and underestimated condition [66, 68, 70–72]. Due to its higher prevalence rate in female patients in sporadic cases, hormonal factors are considered to have a role in its pathogenesis [73].

Development of FGPs is believed to be related to long-term omeprazole intake that has a strong inhibitory effect on gastric acid secretion [74,

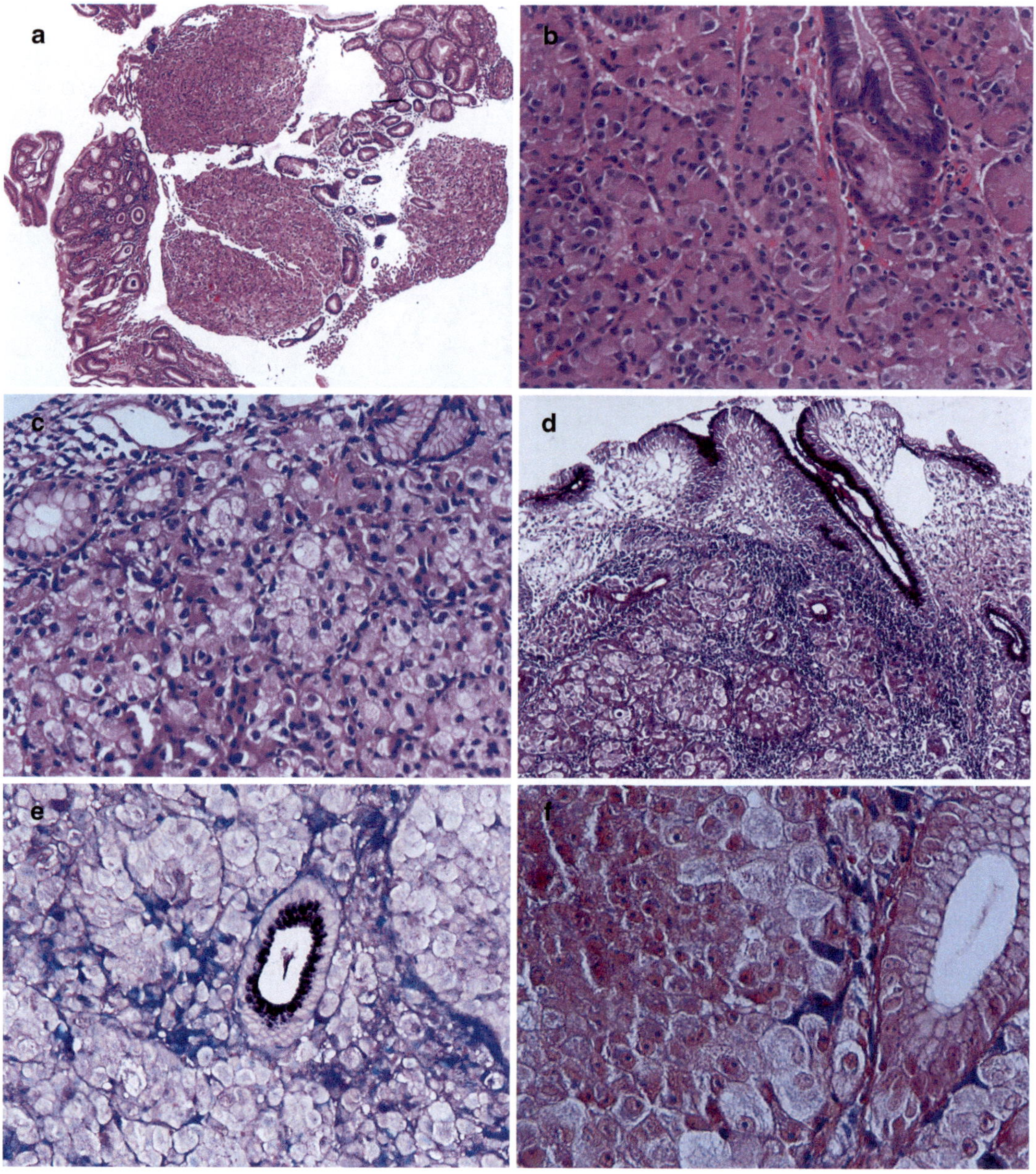

Fig. 13.11 (**a**) A low-power view of the endoscopic biopsy showing multiple tissue pieces. Some of the pieces are more cellular and looking different from the adjacent inflamed and atrophic gastric fundus mucosa (HE, ×150). (**b**) Higher power view of the tumour fragment to show cell morphology better. The tumour cells are arranged in tubular pattern exhibiting minimal anisonucleosis and moderate-to-abundant eosinophilic finely granular cytoplasm, similar to the benign parietal cells (HE, ×350). (**c**) High-power view of a similar tumour with slightly different cellular morphology where the cytoplasm is paler. Besides the tubular pattern, some of the cells are arranged in small groups (HE, ×350). (**d**)–(**f**) Tumour cells are lightly PAS positive, negative on alcian blue staining and strong granular cytoplasmic staining for phosphor tungstic acid haematoxylin stain

75]. However, the underlying pathobiology in the development of the polyp is not well understood, whether FGP represents a localized and morphologically reversible oxyntic cell hyperplasia in response to alteration in gastric acid secretion [74, 75]. Irrespective of its associated background, FGPs are considered as benign polyp with no malignant potential and still so far there are reports of only six GFPs associated with epithelial dysplasia and all were from FAP background; and these are the group of patients who are already having increased risk of dysplastic foci in upper gastrointestinal tract [66, 69, 76–78].

Issues of gastric adenocarcinoma fundic gland (GA-FG) and oxyntic gland polyp/adenoma (OGP) [79]**:** These two conditions are composed of combinations of oxyntic and chief cells [55, 79]. These conditions are newly categorized variants of tumours expressing gastric phenotype exhibiting features of a well-differentiated adenocarcinoma arising from oxyntic mucosa as the tumour cells look alike to fundic glandular cells [80]. These mucosal lesions appear in endoscopic examination as normal pinkish colour or pale mucosa with visible prominent branched vasculature [55, 79–82]. Polyps localized to fundus having chief cell morphology was considered a subtype of FGP [81]. After the first-time report of gastric adenocarcinoma with chief cell differentiation (GA-CCD) [55], later on the term gastric adenocarcinoma—fundic gland type with chief cell predominance (GA-FG-CCP) was proposed as the chief cells with nuclear atypia were believed to have the ability to invade [81]. These lesions are considered to develop directly from normal mucosa without any intestinal metaplasia [54, 83, 84]. This condition has been reported mostly from the Eastern part of the world with only a few from the West [85]. These lesions may be divided into 3 subtypes depending upon the dominant cell type—chief cell type is the dominant type constituting about 99%, and the remaining cases are either parietal cell type and mix type [80, 81, 86]. Later on, Singhi et al. also defined these lesions as chief cell type mucosal lesions without any desmoplasia, necrosis, perineural or lymphovascular and submucosal invasion, but with a certain degree of nuclear atypia [87]. Originally these lesions were described as a variant of fundic gland polyps with parietal or chief cell component [81, 87, 88].

In contrast to previous series, Chan et al. [79] observed a morphological continuum unifying the two concepts. Chan et al. observed in their cases mainly chief cells arranged in glands of varying sizes and shapes resulting in complex morphology including cribriform pattern, clusters and anastomosing cords of cells, and tumour cells had low proliferative activity, which was also observed by Shroff et al. [89]. Shroff et al. further emphasized possible existence of a spectrum where the adenoma at one end and at the opposite end chief cell predominant adenocarcinoma [89]. From a morphological viewpoint, some of the patterns such as clustering of tumour cells arranged in cords and trabeculae may lead to misdiagnosis for a neuroendocrine tumour, tumour cells displayed weak-to-moderate synaptophysin and/or CD56 positivity but chromogranin A negative precluding neuroendocrine origin as foregut neuroendocrine tumours are chromogranin A positive [79, 90–92]. Besides, synaptophysin and CD56 are not specific markers for neuroendocrine differentiation particularly in foregut tumours [79, 92]. Interestingly, majority of patients with this type of tumours had a history of intake of either proton pump inhibitor or H2 receptor antagonist [74, 93, 94]. A possible role of altered Wnt/b-catenin signalling pathway has been put forward in these tumour pathobiology [95]. The tumour cells are believed to accumulate nuclear b-catenin along with CTNNB1 or AXIN gene mutation resulting in disturbance of normal downstream pathway thereby affecting gastrin secretion [96]. MUC5AC and MUC6 are expressed by most of these tumours indicating their gastric phenotype [94].

References

1. Ahn S, Park DY. Practical points in gastric pathology. Arch Pathol Lab Med. 2016;140:397–405.
2. Peixoto A, Silva M, Pereira P. Biopsies in gastrointestinal endoscopy: when and how. GE Port J Gastroenterol. 2015;23:19–27.
3. Nakamura K, Sugano H, Takagi K. Carcinoma of the stomach in incipient phase: its histogenesis and histological appearances. Gan. 1968;59:251–8.
4. Yashima K, Sasaki S, Koda M, et al. Premalignant lesions in gastric cancer. Clin J Gastroenterol. 2010;3:6–12.

5. Kabashima A, Yao T, Sugimachi K, et al. Gastric or intestinal phenotypic expression in the carcinomas and background mucosa of multiple early gastric carcinomas. Histopathology. 2000;37:513–22.
6. Lisovsky M, Lauwers GY. Gastric dysplasia. In: Tan D, Lauwers GY, editors. Advances in surgical pathology: gastric cancer. Baltimore, MD: Lippincott Williams & Wilkins; 2011. p. 325–41.
7. Vieth M, Riddell RH, Montgomery EA. High-grade dysplasia versus carcinoma: east is east and west is west, but does it need to be that way? Am J Surg Pathol. 2014;38:1453–6.
8. Schlemper RJ, Itabashi M, Kato Y, et al. Differences in diagnostic criteria for gastric carcinoma between Japanese and western pathologists. Lancet. 1997;349(9067):1725–9.
9. Kang HJ, Park do Y, Kim KH, et al. Pathologic diagnosis of gastric epithelial neoplasia. Korean J Gastroenterol. 2008;52:273–80.
10. Lauwers GY, Shimizu M, Correa P, et al. Evaluation of gastric biopsies for neoplasia: differences between Japanese and Western pathologists. Am J Surg Pathol. 1999;23:511–8.
11. Sakurai U, Lauwers GY, Vieth M, et al. Gastric high-grade dysplasia can be associated with submucosal invasion: evaluation of its prevalence in a series of 121 endoscopically resected specimens. Am J Surg Pathol. 2014;38:1545–50.
12. Schlemper RJ, Borchard F, Dixon MF, et al. International comparability of the pathological diagnosis for early cancer of the digestive tract: Munich meeting. J Gastroenterol. 2000;35(suppl 12):102–10.
13. Schlemper RJ, Kato Y, Stolte M. Review of histological classifications of gastrointestinal epithelial neoplasia: differences in diagnosis of early carcinomas between Japanese and Western pathologists. J Gastroenterol. 2001;36:445–56.
14. Takahashi T, Iwama N. Atypical glands in gastric adenoma: three dimensional architecture compared with carcinomatous and metaplastic glands. Virchows Arch A Pathol Anat Histopathol. 1984;403:135–48.
15. Lee SM, Yang S, Joo M, et al. Poorly differentiated component in gastric pinch biopsies predicts submucosal invasion. Diagn Pathol. 2014;9:34.
16. Vieth M, Stolte M. Distinction of high-grade intraepithelial neoplasia and tubular gastric adenocarcinoma. In: Kaminishi M, Takubo M, Mafune K, editors. The diversity of gastric carcinoma pathogenesis, diagnosis, and therapy. Tokyo, Japan: Springer-Verlag; 2005. p. 109–16.
17. Lim H, Jung HY, Park YS, et al. Discrepancy between endoscopic forceps biopsy and endoscopic resection in gastric epithelial neoplasia. Surg Endosc. 2014;28:1256–62.
18. Sung HY, Cheung DY, Cho SH, et al. Polyps in the gastrointestinal tract: discrepancy between endoscopic forceps biopsies and resected specimens. Eur J Gastroenterol Hepatol. 2009;21:190–5.
19. Jung MK, Jeon SW, Park SY, et al. Endoscopic characteristics of gastric adenomas suggesting carcinomatous transformation. Surg Endosc. 2008;22:2705–11.
20. Lauwers GY, Riddell RH. Gastric epithelial dysplasia. Gut. 1999;45:784–90.
21. Goldstein NS, Lewin KJ. Gastric epithelial dysplasia and adenoma: historical review and histological criteria for grading. Hum Pathol. 1997;28:127–33.
22. Bosman FT, Carneiro F, Hruban RH, et al. WHO classification of tumours of the digestive system, vol. 3. Lyon, France: IARC Press. World Health Organization Classification of Tumours; 2010.
23. Riddell RH, Goldman H, Ransohoff DF, et al. Dysplasia in inflammatory bowel disease: standardized classification with provisional clinical applications. Hum Pathol. 1983;14:931–68.
24. Park do Y, Srivastava A, Kim GH, et al. Adenomatous and foveolar gastric dysplasia: distinct patterns of mucin expression and background intestinal metaplasia. Am J Surg Pathol. 2008;32:524–33.
25. Ghandur-Mnaymneh L, Paz J, Roldan E, Cassady J. Dysplasia of non-metaplastic gastric mucosa: a proposal for its classification and its possible relationship to diffuse-type gastric carcinoma. Am J Surg Pathol. 1988;12:96–114.
26. Kumarasinghe MP, Lim TK, Ooi CJ, et al. Tubule neck dysplasia: precursor lesion of signet ring cell carcinoma and the immunohistochemical profile. Pathology. 2006;38:468–71.
27. Park do Y, Srivastava A, Kim GH, et al. CDX2 expression in the intestinal type gastric epithelial neoplasia: frequency and significance. Mod Pathol. 2010;23:54–61.
28. Jass JR. A classification of gastric dysplasia. Histopathology. 1983;7:181–93.
29. Mahajan D, Bennett AE, Liu X, et al. Grading of gastric foveolar-type dysplasia in Barrett's esophagus. Mod Pathol. 2010;23:1–11.
30. Brown IS, Whiteman DC, Lauwers GY. Foveolar type dysplasia in Barrett esophagus. Mod Pathol. 2010;23:834–43.
31. Serra S, Ali R, Bateman AC, et al. Gastric foveolar dysplasia: a survey of reporting habits and diagnostic criteria. Anat Pathol. 2017;49:391–6.
32. Stefano S, Rola A, Bateman AC, et al. Gastric foveolar dysplasia: a survey of reporting habits and diagnostic criteria. Pathology. 2017;9:391–6.
33. Nagtegaal ID, Odze RD, Klimstra D, et al. WHO classification of tumours editorial board. The 2019 WHO classification of tumours of the digestive system. Histopathology. 2020;76:182–8.
34. Schlemper RJ, Riddell RH, Kato Y, et al. The Vienna classification of gastrointestinal epithelial neoplasia. Gut. 2000;47:251–5.
35. Baek DH, Kim GH, Park DY, et al. Gastric epithelial dysplasia: characteristics and long-term follow-up results after endoscopic resection according to morphological categorization. BMC Gastroenterol. 2015;15:17. (15th February Online)
36. Oberhuber G, Stolte M. Gastric polyps: an update of their pathology and biological significance. Virchows Arch. 2000;437:581–90.
37. Wood LD, Salaria SN, Cruise MW, et al. Upper GI tract lesions in familial adenomatous polyposis

(FAP): enrichment of pyloric gland adenomas and other gastric and duodenal neoplasms. Am J Surg Pathol. 2014;38:389–93.
38. Vieth M, Kushima R, Borchard F, et al. Pyloric gland adenoma: a clinico-pathological analysis of 90 cases. Virchows Arch. 2003;442:317–21.
39. Chen ZM, Scudiere JR, Abraham SC, et al. Pyloric gland adenoma: an entity distinct from gastric foveolar type adenoma. Am J Surg Pathol. 2009;33:186–93.
40. Lee SE, Kang SY, Cho J, et al. Pyloric gland adenoma in Lynch syndrome. Am J Surg Pathol. 2014;38:784–92.
41. Kushima R, Remmele W, Stolte M, et al. Pyloric gland type adenoma of the gallbladder with squamoid spindle cell metaplasia. Pathol Res Pract. 1996;192:963–9. discussion 961–70
42. Albores-Saavedra J, Sheahan K, O'Riain C, Shukla D. Intraductal tubular adenoma, pyloric type, of the pancreas: additional observations on a new type of pancreatic neoplasm. Am J Surg Pathol. 2004;28:233–8.
43. Adsay V, Jang KT, Roa JC, et al. Intracholecystic papillary-tubular neoplasms (ICPN) of the gallbladder (neoplastic polyps, adenomas, and papillary neoplasms that are ¼1.0 cm): clinicopathologic and immunohistochemical analysis of 123 cases. Am J Surg Pathol. 2012;36:1279–301.
44. Albores-Saavedra J, Chable-Montero F, Gonzalez-Romo MA, et al. Adenomas of the gallbladder: morphologic features, expression of gastric and intestinal mucins, and incidence of high-grade dysplasia/carcinoma in situ and invasive carcinoma. Hum Pathol. 2012;43:1506–13.
45. Borchard F. Forms and nomenclature of gastrointestinal epithelial expansion: what is invasion [in German]? Verh Dtsch Ges Pathol. 2000;84:50–61.
46. Wani Y, Notohara K, Fujisawa M. Aberrant expression of an "intestinal marker" Cdx2 in pyloric gland adenoma of the gallbladder. Virchows Arch. 2008;453:521–7.
47. Vieth M, Kushima R, Mukaisho K, et al. Immunohistochemical analysis of pyloric gland adenomas using a series of Mucin 2, Mucin 5AC, Mucin 6, CD10, Ki67 and p53. Virchows Arch. 2010;457:529–36.
48. Kushima R, Vieth M, Borchard F, et al. Gastric type well-differentiated adenocarcinoma and pyloric gland adenoma of the stomach. Gastric Cancer. 2006;9:177–84.
49. Matsubara A, Sekine S, Kushima R, et al. Frequent GNAS and KRAS mutations in pyloric gland adenoma of the stomach and duodenum. J Pathol. 2013;229:579–87.
50. Kushima R, Muller W, Stolte M, et al. Differential p53 protein expression in stomach adenomas of gastric and intestinal phenotypes: possible sequences of p53 alteration in stomach carcinogenesis. Virchows Arch. 1996;428:223–7.
51. Abraham SC, Park SJ, Lee JH, et al. Genetic alterations in gastric adenomas of intestinal and foveolar phenotypes. Mod Pathol. 2003;16:786–95.
52. Endoh Y, Sakata K, Tamura G, et al. Cellular phenotypes of differentiated type adenocarcinomas and precancerous lesions of the stomach are dependent on the genetic pathways. J Pathol. 2000;191:257–63.
53. Ohmura K, Tamura G, Endoh Y, et al. Microsatellite alterations in differentiated-type adenocarcinomas and precancerous lesions of the stomach with special reference to cellular phenotype. Hum Pathol. 2000;31:1031–5.
54. Muller-Hocker J, Rellecke P. Chief cell proliferation of the gastric mucosa mimicking early gastric cancer: an unusual variant of fundic gland polyp. Virchows Arch. 2003;442:496–500.
55. Tsukamoto T, Yokoi T, Maruta S, et al. Gastric adenocarcinoma with chief cell differentiation. Pathol Int. 2007;57:517–22.
56. Ueyama H, Yao T, Nakashima Y, et al. Gastric adenocarcinoma of fundic gland type (chief cell predominant type): proposal for a new entity of gastric adenocarcinoma. Am J Surg Pathol. 2010;34:609–19.
57. Ushiku T, Kunita A, Kuroda R, et al. Oxyntic gland neoplasm of the stomach: expanding the spectrum and proposal of terminology. Mod Pathol. 2020;33:206–16.
58. Odze RD, Marcial MA, Antonioli D. Gastric fundic gland polyps: a morphological study including mucin histochemistry, stereometry, and MIB-1 immunohistochemistry. Hum Pathol. 1996;27:896–903.
59. Lee RG, Burt RW. The histopathology of fundic gland polyps of the stomach. Am J Clin Pathol. 1986;86:498–503.
60. Marcial MA, Villafafia M, Hernandez-Denton J, et al. Fundic gland polyps: prevalence and clinicopathologic features. Am J Gastroenterol. 1993;88:1711–3.
61. Iida M, Yao T, Watanabe H, et al. Fundic gland polyposis in patients without familial adenomatosis coli: its incidence and clinical features. Gastroenterology. 1984;86:1437–42.
62. Nishiura M, Hirota T, Itabashi M, et al. A clinical and histopathological study of gastric polyps in familial polyposis coll. Am J Gastroenterol. 1984;79:98–103.
63. Watanabe H, Enjoji M, Yao T, et al. Gastric lesions in familial adenomatosis coll. Hum Pathol. 1978;9:269–83.
64. Hanada M, Takami M, Hirata K, et al. Hyperplastic fundic gland polyp of the stomach. Acta Pathol Jpn. 1983;33:1269–77.
65. Sipponen P, Laxen F, Seppla K. Cystic hamartomatous gastric polyps: a disorder of oxyntic glands. Histopathology. 1983;7:727–9.
66. Iida M, Yao T, Itoh H, et al. Natural history of fundic gland polyposis in patients with familial adenomatosis coil/gardner's syndrome. Gastroenterology. 1985;89:1021–5.
67. Iida M, Yao T, Watanabe H, et al. Spontaneous disappearance of fundic gland polyposis: report of three cases. Gastroenterology. 1980;79:725–8.
68. Odze RD, Marcial MA, Antonioli D. Gastric fundic gland polyps: a morphological study including mucin histochemistry, stereometry, and MIB-I immunohistochemistry. Hum Pathol. 1996;27:896–903.

69. Domizio P, Talbot IC, Spigelman AD, et al. Upper gastrointestinal pathology in familial adenomatous polyposis: results from a prospective study of 102 patients. J Clin Pathol. 1990;43:738–43.
70. Kinoshita Y, Tojo M, Yano T, et al. Incidence of fundic gland polyps in patients without familial adenomatous polyposis. Gastrointest Endosc. 1993;39:161–3.
71. Haruma K, Sumii K, Yoshihara M, et al. Gastric mucosa in female patients with fundic glandular polyps. J Clin Gastroenterol. 1991;13:565–9.
72. Eidt S, Stolte M. Gastric glandular cysts: investigations into their genesis and relationship to colorectal epithelial tumors. Gastroenterology. 1989;27:212–7.
73. Odze R, Gallinger S, So K, et al. Immunohistochemical ex-pression of transforming growth factor alpha (TGF-beta) and epidermal growth factor receptor (EGF-R) in gastric fundic gland polyps (FGP). Mod Pathol. 1993;6:50A. (Abstr)
74. Graham JR. Gastric polyposis: onset during long-term therapy with omeprazole. Med J Aust. 1992;157:287–8.
75. Stoke M. Fundic gland polyps: a rare, innocuous, and reversible disturbance. Gastroenterology. 1993;105:1590–1.
76. Burt RW, Berenson MM, Lee RG, et al. Upper gastrointestinal polyps in Gardner's syndrome. Gastroenterology. 1984;86:295–301.
77. Goodman AJ, Dundas SAC, Scholefield JM, et al. Gastric carcinoma and familial adenomatous polyposis (FAP). Int J Color Dis. 1988;3:201–3.
78. Lynch HT, Smyrk TC, Lanspa SJ, et al. Upper gastrointestinal manifestations in families with hereditary flat adenoma syndrome. Cancer. 1993;71:2709–14.
79. Chan K, Brown IS, Kyle T, et al. Chief cell-predominant gastric polyps: a series of 12 cases with literature review. Histopathology. 2016;68:825–33.
80. Chiba T, Kato K, Masuda T, et al. Clinicopathological features of gastric adenocarcinoma of the fundic gland (chief cell predominant type) by retrospective and prospective analyses of endoscopic findings. Dig Endosc. 2016;28:722–30.
81. Ueyama H, Matsumoto K, Nagahara A, et al. Gastric adenocarcinoma of the fundic gland type (chief cell predominant type). Endoscopy. 2013;46:153–7.
82. Yao T, Ueyama H, Kushima R, et al. New type of gastric carcinoma-adenocarcinoma of the fundic gland type: its clinicopathological features and tumor development. Stomach Intest. 2010;45:1192–201.
83. Kushima R, Sekine S, Matsubara A, et al. Gastric adenocarcinoma of the fundic gland type shares common genetic and phenotypic features with pyloric gland adenoma. Pathol Int. 2013;63:318–25.
84. Matsukawa A, Kurano R, Takemoto T, et al. Chief cell hyperplasia with structural and nuclear atypia: a variant of fundic gland polyp. Pathol Res Pract. 2005;200:817–21.
85. Benedict MA, Lauwers GY, Jain D. Gastric adenocarcinoma of the fundic gland type. Am J Clin Pathol. 2018;149:461–73.
86. Fan X, Yang XS, Bai P, et al. Gastric adenocarcinoma of the fundic gland type. A case report. Medicine (Baltimore). 2020;99:e20361.
87. Singhi AD, Lazenby AJ, Montgomery EA. Gastric adenocarcinoma with chief cell differentiation: a proposal for reclassification as oxyntic gland polyp/adenoma. Am J Surg Pathol. 2012;36:1030–5.
88. Park ES, Kim YE, Park CK, et al. Gastric adenocarcinoma of fundic gland type: report of three cases. Korean J Pathol. 2012;46:287–91.
89. Shroff S, Taggart M, Rashid A, et al. Gastric chief cell adenomas: proposal for a new entity[abstract]. Mod Pathol. 2012;25:180A.
90. Al-Khafaji B, Noffsinger AE, Miller MA, et al. Immunohistochemical analysis of gastrointestinal and pulmonary carcinoid tumours. Hum Pathol. 1998;29:992–9.
91. Fahrenkamp AG, Wibbeke C, Winde G, et al. Immunohistochemical distribution of chromogranins A and B and secretogranin II in neuroendocrine tumours of the gastrointestinal tract. Virchows Arch. 1995;426:361–36.
92. Lloyd RV. Practical markers used in the diagnosis of neuroendocrine tumours. Endocr Pathol. 2003;14:293–301.
93. Hongo M, Fujimoto K. Gastric polyps study group. Incidence and risk factor of fundic gland polyp and hyperplastic polyp in long-term proton pump inhibitor therapy: a prospective study in Japan. J Gastroenterol. 2010;45:618–24.
94. Fukuda M, Ishigaki H, Sugimoto M, et al. Histological analysis of fundic gland polyps secondary to PPI therapy. Histopathology. 2019;75:537–45.
95. Hidaka Y, Mitomi H, Saito T, et al. Alteration in the Wnt/b-catenin signalling pathway in gastric neoplasias of fundicgland (chief cell predominant) type. Hum Pathol. 2013;44:2438–48.
96. Koh TJ, Bulitta CJ, Fleming JV, et al. Gastrin is a target of the B-catenin/TCF-4 growth-signal-ling pathway in a model of intestinal polyposis. J Clin Invest. 2000;106:533–9.

Gastric Carcinoma—Early and Advanced Carcinomas

14

Establishing a diagnosis of carcinoma in endoscopic biopsy is of utmost important as further management of the patients relies on a positive or a negative report. In majority of gastric cases, the patient usually presents with non-specific symptoms relating to upper gastrointestinal tract [1, 2]. Specific symptoms of obstructive symptoms of gastric outflow tract are usually associated with pyloric antral growth [3, 4]. Gastric cancer usually remains silent in its early stage and there is no available non-invasive technology to detect early-stage cancer and majority (>70%) present with advanced stage tumour [5]. This is one disease considered to affect elderly, but lately an increasing trend of younger patients is observed [6]. There is a great progress and improvement in medical and surgical technologies in gastric cancer management. Better understanding the pathobiology has resulted in a preventive approach in the management and treatment by developing targeted therapies [7]. Despite all the efforts in improvement of its management, surgery has still so far remained its main treatment modality. Detecting and treating in early stage has remained its main prognostic factor [8–11]. Usually, individuals who found to have lymph node free early gastric cancer (EGC) are the ones who undergo routine endoscopic screening. These are the group of patients suitable for endoscopic submucosal dissection (ESD) [12]. Patients undergoing investigation for upper GI symptoms and who had never undergone previous screening endoscopy have been found to be associated with advanced stage gastric cancer [13, 14]. Interesting observations made amongst the Korean population who undergoes periodic endoscopic examination reported incidences of interval gastric cancer [15]. One important factor that may be considered in optimizing diagnostic yield of gastric cancer by carrying out endoscopy mapping of the entire gastric mucosa [16], is irregular reddish or any abnormal colour, elevated or depressed area which bleeds easily to touch [12]. In addition, lately all patients who are found to have suspicious mucosal lesion are further subjected to more advanced endoscopic examination to confirm the diagnosis and the recent endoscopic techniques routinely used are chromoendoscopy with indigo carmine and narrow band imaging [12] and followed by taking biopsy form the suspicious focus is currently the choice for as an investigative tool [17]. There are limited comparative studies on the topic of diagnostic yield of the advanced endoscopes except few, and majority of the published data are based on the older version endoscopies (fiberscopes) [17–20].

Interpretaiton of small endoscopic biopsy is greatly influenced by the quality of the sample, i.e. a representative sampling from the area of lesion and appropriate bites. There are

K. Vaiphei, *Interpretation of Endoscopic Biopsy - Gastritis, Gastropathies and Beyond*,
https://doi.org/10.1007/978-981-16-6026-9_14

many studies analysing the accuracy of the diagnosis with number of biopsy specimens. Diagnostic accuracy of endoscopic biopsies was found to increase with increasing number of biopsy tissue fragment, though there are variations in the percentages reported in different studies [16, 18]. Accuracy has been reported higher with 92.5% when two biopsies were taken compared to one biopsy group (83.9%); although accuracy was 95.9% in three or more biopsy specimen group with no significant difference with 2 biopsy group [18]. Comparison between size of the lesion, i.e. 10 mm and more with <10 mm size lesions, accuracy was observed with number of biopsy samples increased with increasing number of biopsies, rather than size of the lesion. Similar findings were with type of the lesions, i.e. elevated or non-elevated, and both types revealed a correlation with increasing number of biopsy specimens. Hence, optimal biopsy number required for an accurate diagnosis of gastric carcinoma in different types of lesions irrespective of the tumour stage requires a minimum of two tissue bits [17, 21, 22]. It is obvious that taking more than one biopsy will enhance identifying the mucosal lesion more appropriately by reducing chances of sampling error including small lesions and also it makes the pathologist to be more comfortable to commit for the presence of a carcinoma. Older studies had documented diagnostic accuracy of 97–100% with five or more biopsy tissue pieces when sampled from the suspected lesions [18, 23, 24]. Based on various available published data, recommended different number of biopsies tissue pieces, in Germany it was 8 pieces, in UK it was 6 and in the United States it was 6–8 pieces [25].

GC can be classified in many ways; clinically it is classified into early and advanced stage. Classifications of the tumour according to their location sometimes may be difficult if the tumour is not confined to one anatomical site, like when the tumour is located in the proximal stomach involving lower oesophagus through gastro-oesophageal junction (GEJ). The controversy involved in this type of tumour is due to the similarity in histologic feature and immunophenotype between the gastric cardiac mucosa with the metaplastic epithelium present at lower end of oesophagus due to frequently associated reflux disease [26–28]. Many working groups had tried to solve this issue by modifying several classifications [29]. International Gastric Cancer Association proposed to group tumours according to the sites, i.e. type I, II and III representing lower end of oesophagus, cardia and distal to cardia, respectively, however, defining the criteria for each anatomical location [28, 30–32]. Eighth Edition of TNM classification has redefined the criteria by identifying the epicentre of the tumour location and GEJ status [33, 34]. Determination of the GEJ status is in reference to determine origin of the adenocarcinoma, i.e. oesophagus or stomach. Redefined GEJ according to AJCC/UICC cancer staging is an adenocarcinoma within 2 cms of epicentre in cardia are considered as oesophageal adenocarcinomas and accordingly. And tumours having more than 2 cms extension into proximal stomach are to be considered as primary gastric cancer and to be staged appropriately [34]. Molecular studies of tumours located in these critical areas had demonstrated different molecular profiles amongst the GEJ tumours; hence, categorizing and grouping these tumours depending upon their genetic signature may exactly able to identify the cell of origin of the tumours [35–37]. Huang et al. observed in a retrospective study amongst Chinese patients that cardiac tumours involving GEJ or distal oesophagus had clinical outcome similar to gastric than oesophageal cancers [31]. This observation however needs further confirmation by carrying out studies in larger cohort in different patient population across the globe [38].

14.1 Early and Advanced Gastric Carcinoma

Early gastric cancer (EGC) concept originated in Japan (1962) had a definition of a neoplasm successfully treatable by surgery [38]. It has been redefined as an adenocarcinoma restricted to mucosa or submucosa irrespective of lymph node metastasis (T1, any N) having significantly better outcome with 90% five-year survival rate [39]. The definition of EGC has been adopted universally irrespective of the small number of patients with lymph node involvement [40]. EGC with positive nodes are dealt in two ways—I. patients with T1 and positive nodes likelihood of having larger tumour, configuration and deeper invasion, may not be appropriate candidates for endoscopic resection; gastrectomy with removal of the regional nodes will be the appropriate treatment strategy for such patients. II. patients with node-positive resected EGC are candidates for adjuvant therapy [41]. EGCs are small lesions of 2–5 cm size, often located along lesser curvature including angularis area, rarely may be multifocal. Gross types of EGC—type I or protruding type, type II or plaque lesion, type III or excavating growth and type IV or infiltrative lesion having lateral spread [41]. Type II may be an elevated (IIa) or flat (IIb) or depress (IIc) lesions [41]. Paris classification made certain modifications based on the original classification by the Japanese group [42] based on gross endoscopic appearances of the lesion—type 0-I or polypoid growth, and p and s are added to 0-I for a pedunculated as well as for a sessile growth, respectively; and in type 0-II or nonpolypoid growth, a, b and c are added to signify a slightly elevated, flat and depressed growths, respectively, and type 0-III solely for ones with excavation [42]. Morphological types commonly seen in EGC are well-differentiated carcinoma—tubular and papillary differentiation. Intramucosal carcinoma needs to be differentiated from in situ carcinoma or high-grade dysplasia as the first one usually develops positive lymph nodes, unlike colorectal carcinomas [43, 44]. An intramucosal invasive tumour will show breakage in glandular basement membrane associated with tumour cells in isolation or in clusters will be present in the lamina propria, and also the malignant glands will be of variable shape and sizes [45–47]. Five year survival for carcinoma infiltrating into muscularis propria or beyond is about 60% or less [48–50]. When dealing with EGC, it is important to remember familial gastric cancer group where there can be just few glands showing pagetoid lesions with innocuous looking signet ring cells infiltrating the lamina propria [51]. Age-old gross classification of advanced gastric tumour by Borrmann still holds true and is followed [52]. Gastric cancers have been observed to exhibit cytological heterogeneity, many tumours can show many types of growth patterns together. The distinction between early and advanced gastric carcinomas is differentiated before the major surgery by radiology and this step is important from the perspective of decision for administering a pre-operative neoadjuvant therapy in order to downgrade the tumour for a more favourable outcome [53, 54]. There are many studies proposing different histological classifications depending upon the type of cells identified under microscope and a compilation of the different classifications is given as a Table 14.1.

In addition to the above conditions, there are other rare types of gastric carcinomas added in the latest WHO classification [59]—choriocarcinoma, embryonal, endodermal sinus tumour, malignant rhabdoid tumour, mixed adeno-neuroendocrine, mucoepidermoid, oncocytic adenocarcinoma and paneth cell carcinomas. Over all 5 years survival for gastric carcinoma is 20% or less. The most important parameter for EGC prognosis is the depth of the tumour infiltrate ion, not the nodal involvement. Some of the factors that have been associated with poor outcome are—young patient with diffuse histology, tumour located in proximal half, depth of infiltration, positive margins and the last but not the least is lymph node metastases [60–62].

Table 14.1 Histological classifications of gastric carcinoma [55–58]

Lauren' classification (1965)	Nakamura's classification (1968)	Japanese Gastric Cancer Association (2017)	WHO 5th edition (2018)
Intestinal	Differentiated	Papillary and tubular types—well and moderately differentiated types	Papillary tubular, well-differentiated Tubular, moderately differentiated
Indeterminate	Undifferentiated	Poorly differentiated or solid type.	Tubular, poorly differentiated (solid)
Diffuse	Undifferentiated	Signet ring cell carcinoma (SRC)	Poorly cohesive, SRC type Poorly cohesive, NOS
Intestinal/diffuse/ indeterminate	Differentiated/ undifferentiated	Mucinous	Mucinous
Mixed		Description according to the proportion	Mixed
Not defined	Not defined	**Special type:** Adenosquamous Squamous cell Undifferentiated Carcinoma with lymphoid stroma Hepatoid adenocarcinoma Adenocarcinoma with enteroblastic differentiation Adenocarcinoma of fundic gland type	**Histological variants:** Adenosquamous Squamous cell Undifferentiated Carcinoma with lymphoid stroma Hepatoid carcinoma Adenocarcinoma with enteroblastic differentiation Adenocarcinoma of fundic gland type Micropapillary adenocarcinoma

References

1. Venerito M, Link A, Rokkas T, et al. Gastric cancer—clinical and epidemiological aspects. Helicobacter. 2016;21(Suppl 1):39–44.
2. Shiotani A, Cen P, Graham DY. Eradication of gastric cancer is now both possible and practical. Semin Cancer Biol. 2013;23(6 Pt B):492–501.
3. Shone DN, Nikoomanesh P, Smith-Meek MM, et al. Malignancy is the most common cause of gastric outlet obstruction in the era of H2 blockers. Am J Gastroenterol. 1995;90:1769–70.
4. Misra SP, Dwivedi M, Misra V. Malignancy is the most common cause of gastric outlet obstruction even in a developing country. Endoscopy. 1998;30:484–6.
5. Digklia A, Wagner AD. Advanced gastric cancer: current treatment landscape and future perspectives. World J Gastroenterol. 2016;22:2403–14.
6. Sun Z, Wang Q, Yu X, et al. Risk factors associated with splenic hilar lymph node metastasis in patients with advanced gastric cancer in Northwest China. Int J Clin Exp Med. 2015;8:21358–64.
7. Obermannova R, Lordick F. Insights into next developments in advanced gastric cancer. Curr Opin Oncol. 2016;28:367–75.
8. Kim DG, An JY, Kim H, et al. Clinical implications of microsatellite instability in early gastric cancer. J Gastric Cancer. 2019;19:427–37.
9. Das M. Neoadjuvant chemotherapy: survival benefit in gastric cancer. Lancet Oncol. 2017;8:e307.
10. Kikuchi S, Katada N, Sakuramoto S, et al. Survival after surgical treatment of early gastric cancer: surgical techniques and long-term survival. Langenbeck's Arch Surg. 2004;389:69–74.
11. Kim YI, Kim YW, Choi IJ, et al. Long-term survival after endoscopic resection versus surgery in early gastric cancers. Endoscopy. 2015;47:293–301.
12. Kim SJ, Choi CW. Common locations of gastric cancer: review of research from the endoscopic submucosal dissection era. J Korean Med Sci. 2019;34:e231.
13. Zhang X, Li M, Chen S, et al. Endoscopic screening in Asian countries is associated with reduced gastric cancer mortality: a meta-analysis and systematic review. Gastroenterol. 2018;155:347–354.e9.
14. Hamashima C, Ogoshi K, Okamoto M, et al. A community-based, case-control study evaluating mortality reduction from gastric cancer by endoscopic screening in Japan. PLoS One. 2013;8:e79088.
15. Park MS, Yoon JY, Chung HS, et al. Clinicopathologic characteristics of interval gastric cancer in Korea. Gut Liver. 2015;9:166–73.
16. Yao K. The endoscopic diagnosis of early gastric cancer. Ann Gastroenterol. 2013;26:11–22.
17. Allum WH, Blazeby JM, Griffin SM, et al. Guidelines for the management of oesophageal and gastric cancer. Gut. 2011;60:1449–72.

18. Tatsuta M, Iishi H, Okuda S, et al. Prospective evaluation of diagnostic accuracy of gastrofiberscopic biopsy in diagnosis of gastric cancer. Cancer. 1989;63:1415–20.
19. Misumi A, Mori K, Ikeda T, et al. Evaluation of fiber gastroscopic biopsy in the diagnosis of gastric cancer: a study of 339 cases. Gastroenterol Jpn. 1978;13:255–63.
20. National Comprehensive Cancer Network (NCCN). NCCN clinical practice guidelines in oncology. Gastric Cancer (including cancer in the proximal 5cm of the stomach). Version 2; 2013.
21. Ajani JA, Bentrem DJ, Besh S, et al. Gastric cancer, version 2. 2013: featured updates to the NCCN guidelines. J Natl Compr. Canc Netw. 2013;11:531–46.
22. Gun KW, Jin HW, Hak KJ, et al. Understanding the diagnostic yield of current endoscopic biopsy for gastric neoplasm a prospective single Centre analysis based on tumour characteristics stratified by biopsy number and site. Medicine. 2016;95:e4196.
23. Dekker W, Tytgat GN. Diagnostic accuracy of fiber endoscopy in the detection of upper intestinal malignancy. A follow-up analysis. Gastroenterol. 1977;73:710–4.
24. Sancho-Poch FJ, Balanzó J, Ocaña J, et al. An evaluation of gastric biopsy in the diagnosis of gastric cancer. Gastrointest Endosc. 1978;24:281–2.
25. Moehler M, Al-Batran SE, Andus T, et al. German S3-guideline "diagnosis and treatment of esophagogastric cancer". Z Gastroenterol. 2011;49: 461–531.
26. Chandrasoma PT, Der R, Ma Y, et al. Histology of the gastroesophageal junction: an autopsy study. Am J Surg Pathol. 2000;24:402–9.
27. Genta RM, Huberman RM, Graham DY. The gastric cardia in helicobacter pylori infection. Hum Pathol. 1994;25:915–9.
28. Siewert JR, Stein HJ. Classification of adenocarcinoma of the oesophagogastric junction. Br J Surg. 1998;85:1457–9.
29. Ajani JA, D'Amico TA, Almhanna K, et al. Esophageal and esophagogastric junction cancers, version 1.2015. J Natl Compr Cancer Netw. 2015;13:194–227.
30. Edge SB, Byrd DR, Compton CC, et al. AJCC cancer staging manual. 7th ed. New York: Springer; 2010.
31. Huang Q, Shi J, Feng A, et al. Gastric cardiac carcinomas involving the esophagus are more adequately staged as gastric cancers by the 7th edition of the American joint commission on cancer staging system. Mod Pathol. 2011;24:138–46.
32. Hamilton R, Aatonen LA. Tumors of digestive system. Lyon IARC. 2000:39–52.
33. Rice TW, Patil DT, Blackstone EH. 8th edition AJCC/UICC staging of cancers of the esophagus and esophagogastric junction: application to clinical practice. Ann Cardiothorac Surg. 2017;6:119–30.
34. Hayakawa Y, Sethi N, Sepulveda AR, et al. Oesophageal adenocarcinoma and gastric cancer: should we mind the gap? Nat Rev Cancer. 2016;16:305–18.
35. Xie L, Cai L, Wang F, et al. Systematic review of prognostic gene signature in gastric cancer patients. Front Bioeng Biotechnol. 2020; https://doi.org/10.3389/fbioe.2020.00805.
36. Cancer Genome Atlas Research Network. Comprehensive molecular characterization of gastric adenocarcinoma. Nature. 2014;513:202–9.
37. Hu B, El Hajj N, Sittler S. Gastric cancer: classification, histology and application of molecular pathology. J Gastrointest Oncol. 2012;3:251–61.
38. Murakami T. Patho-morphological diagnosis. Definition and gross classification of early gastric cancer. Gann Monohr Cancer Res. 1971;11:53–5.
39. Gotoda T. Endoscopic resection of early gastric cancer: the Japanese perspective. Curr Opin Gastroenterol. 2006;22:561.
40. Alfaro EE, Lauwers GY. Early gastric neoplasia: diagnosis and implications. Adv Anat Pathol. 2011;18:268.
41. Katai H, Sano T. Early gastric cancer: concepts, diagnosis, and management. Int J Clin Oncol. 2005;10:375–83.
42. The Paris endoscopic classification of superficial neoplastic lesions (2003) esophagus, stomach, and colon: November 30 to December 1, 2002. Gastrointest End 58: supp 6: S3–S43.
43. Kohli Y, Kawai K, Fujita S. Analytical studies on growth of human gastric cancer. J Clin Gastroenterol. 1981;3:129.
44. Maehara Y, Orita H, Okuyama T, et al. Predictors of lymph node metastasis in early gastric cancer. Br J Surg. 1992;79:245.
45. Everett SM, Axon AT. Early gastric cancer in Europe. Gut. 1997;41:142.
46. Yasuda K, Shiraishi N, Suematsu T, et al. Rate of detection of lymph node metastasis is correlated with the depth of submucosal invasion in early stage gastric carcinoma. Cancer. 1999;85:2119.
47. Okada K, Fujisaki J, Yoshida T, et al. Long-term outcomes of endoscopic submucosal dissection for undifferentiated-type early gastric cancer. Endoscopy. 2012;44:122.
48. Kamangar F, Dores GM, Anderson WF. Patterns of cancer incidence, mortality, and prevalence across five continents: defining priorities to reduce cancer disparities in different geographic regions of the world. J Clin Oncol. 2006;24:2137–50.
49. Karpeh M, Kelsen D, Tepper J. Cancer of the stomach. In: De Vita V, Hellman S, Rosenberg S, editors. Cancer principles & practice of oncology. Philadelphia: Lippincott, Williams & Wilkins; 2001. p. 1092–126.
50. Yoshikawa K, Maruyama K. Characteristics of gastric cancer invading to the proper muscle layer--with special reference to mortality and cause of death. Jpn J Clin Oncol. 1985;15:499–503.
51. Oliveira C, Pinheiro H, Figueiredo J, et al. Familial gastric cancer: genetic susceptibility, pathology, and implications for management. Lancet Oncol. 2015;16:e60–70.

52. Borrmann R. Makroskopishe Formen des vorgeschritteten Magenkrebses. In: Henke F, Lubarsch O, editors. Handbuch der speziellen pathologischen Anatomie und Histologie, vol. 4/1. Berlin: Springer; 1926.
53. Cunningham D, Allum WH, Stenning SP, et al. MAGIC trial participants. Perioperative chemotherapy versus surgery alone for resectable gastroesophageal cancer. N Engl J Med. 2006;355: 11–20.
54. Ychou M, Boige V, Pignon JP, et al. Perioperative chemotherapy compared with surgery alone for resectable gastroesophageal adenocarcinoma: an FNCLCC and FFCD multicenter phase III trial. J Clin Oncol. 2011;29:1715–21.
55. Lauren P. The two histological main types of gastric carcinoma: diffuse and so-called intestinal-type carcinoma. An attempt at a histo-clinical classification. Acta Pathol Microbiol Scand. 1965;64:31–49.
56. Nakamura K, Haruo S, Kunio T. Carcinoma of the stomach in incipient phase: its histogenesis and histological appearances. Gann. 1968;59:251–8.
57. Association Japanese Gastric Cancer. Japanese classification of gastric carcinoma. 15th ed. Tokyo: Kanehara Shuppan; 2018.
58. Nagtegaal ID, Odze RD, Klimstra D, et al. WHO classification of tumours editorial board. The 2019 WHO classification of tumours of the digestive system. Histopathol. 2020;76:182–8.
59. Bosman FT, Carneiro F, Hruban RH, et al. WHO classification of tumours of the digestive system, vol. 3. 4th ed. Lyon: International Agency for Research on Cancer; 2010.
60. Siewert JR, Bottcher K, Stein HJ, et al. And the German gastric carcinoma study group. Relevant prognostic factors in gastric cancer, ten-year results of the German gastric cancer study. Annals of Surgery. 1998;228:449–61.
61. Allgayer H, Heiss MM, Schil Dberg FW. Prognostic factors in gastric cancer. Br J Surg. 1997;84:1651–64.
62. Scartozzi M, Galizia E, Freddari F, et al. Molecular biology of sporadic gastric cancer: prognostic indicators and novel therapeutic approaches. Cancer Treat Rev. 2004;30:451–9.

15 Morphological Aspect of Gastric Carcinomas

Biopsy is usually submitted in multiple FPM tissue pieces. Examining every tissue bit that has been submitted for histopathology is of utmost importance not to miss any microscopic focus/foci of tumour cells. Enumerating the number of FPM with the tissue bits and counting them over the histological sections are to be carried out routinely. While examining the biopsy fragments under low power, a visual impression can be made of the different components of the biopsy fragments, i.e. variation from the normal and the abnormal tissue fragments can also be identified. My personal approach is starting with the least involved fragment thereby studying the site of biopsy and the mucosal changes in the least involved surrounding mucosa. Histological changes of gastritis with or without *H. pylori*, atrophy, metaplasia and dysplasia are usually revealed by a relatively uninvolved tissue fragment. Approach from the least involved fragment to gradually more involved fragments not to overlook the lesser degree of mucosal changes. If the maximally involved fragment bearing the malignant fragment, it is easy to overlook with a casual approach for the other tissue fragments with a lesser degree of morphological changes. Except for the hereditary cancers, though not absolute in developing countries, almost all other forms of gastric cancer will have associated mucosal changes of long-standing mucosal inflammation and its consequences.

15.1 Microscopic Features

Gastric carcinomas (GC) are tumours that exhibit mark heterogeneity from one case to another (inter-tumour heterogeneity), and also within the same tumour (intratumor heterogeneity). This is due to the different types of cellular components existing within the tumour mimicking its cell of origin, i.e. gastric and intestinal type of epithelium [1–3]. Intratumor heterogeneity refers to an inherent difference between distinctive subpopulations of tumour cells within same tumour by either germline or acquired mutations or both [4, 5]. Studies utilizing molecular techniques enable identification of different regions of a tumour having subtypes of distinct genetic and epigenetic features [6]. The microenvironment of the tumour, i.e. the inflammatory cells, stroma and endothelial cells, interacts with the cancerous population of cells and forms the regional microenvironments [7]. GCs heterogeneity has been shown both at molecular level and also by the diversities of the phenotypes expressed by the tumour cells, which can be explainable by the interactions between the gastric tumour initiating cells at genetic/epigenetic levels with microenvironments [8, 9]. As the tumour evolves from early to advanced stages, there is postinduction mutations resulting in production of divergent clonality of the tumour cells [10]. The histological types of the tumour will be evident by the

K. Vaiphei, *Interpretation of Endoscopic Biopsy - Gastritis, Gastropathies and Beyond*,
https://doi.org/10.1007/978-981-16-6026-9_15

characteristic morphology in HE stain sections, which may be intestinal type characterized by the tall columnar cells, goblet cells or Paneth cells, or it may also show neuroendocrine differentiation. All these characteristics of morphological differentiations may be further confirmed by special histochemistry and immunohistochemistry stains, and ultrastructural study. Some of the tumours may have characteristic gastric type of morphology as the tumour develops from gastric mucosa or the intestinal metaplastic epithelium may revert back to gastric phenotype [11]. Intestinal type of gastric cancer is defined as the result of long-lasting infection by *Helicobacter pylori* (HP); however, the outcome of HP eradication in the prevention of cancer development has not yet been proven [12–14]. Besides these sporadic forms of GCs, a small number of GC (1 to 3%) are known to be associated with clearly identifiable inherited syndromic conditions like—(a) Familial adenomatous polyposis, (b) Hereditary non-polyposis colon cancer, (c) Peutz-Jeghers syndrome, (d) Cowden's syndrome and (e) Li-Fraumeni syndrome [15–17]. Since 1800s, after documentation of multiple gastric cancers in Bonaparte family, existence of the familial form of GC is known [18].

15.2 Morphological Classification of Gastric Carcinoma

The morphological aspect of gastric carcinoma brings out the marked heterogeneity in the cellular architectural patterns and the tumour cell types, and different types of architecture and cell types coexist [2]. Lauren classification published in the 1960s still holds true in gastric cancer histological classifications and it is based microscopic morphology of the tumour cells [19]. This is a most used system for gastric cancer still so far and gastric adenoCa is classified into two types, i.e. diffuse (32%) (Fig. 15.1a) and intestinal type (54%) (Fig. 15.1b), and the third type also known as the indeterminate type (15%) (Fig. 15.1c) has a combination of diffuse and intestinal types. Intestinal type is composed of clusters of cohesive cells arranged in glandular patterns showing a well-differentiated cellular characters and grows slowly. This type involves more often males than females and occurs more often in older people. They constitute about 60% of the GCs. These tumours are usually seen in the pylori antrum and arise from intestinalized mucosa. They frequently associate with discrete distant metastasis as they likely show lymphatic or vascular invasion. Diffuse type is composed of poorly differentiated tumour cells in a background of desmoplastic stroma, behaves aggressively and tends to scatter or infiltrate throughout the stomach involving the muscular wall. The tumour cells which are dominantly composed of signet ring cells are dominantly present towards the upper portion of the mucosa or involved part of the stomach, and density of the signet ring cells are lesser in the deeper portion of the tumour. Tumour cells become more pleomorphic, singly scattered. A few abortive singly scattered glands may be seen. The tumour cells exhibit little differentiation and sometimes they may look very innocuous simulating histiocytes where immunostaining for cytokeratin may be required to confirm the carcinoma cell, not a macrophage. These special stains are required and should be carried out to differentiate from another condition like a healed peptic ulcer with abundant collagenized stroma and scattered chronic inflammatory cells including histiocytes. A diffuse GC seldom forms discrete tumour focus, it tends to infiltrate transmurally up to the serosa with transperitoneal spread. Due to the diffuse infiltration of the wall of the stomach, stomach wall becomes stiff and less distensible and is known as the linitis plastica or old leather water bottle. If the spread involves the mesentery and peritoneum, the cells may become inconspicuous and difficult to identify cancer cells unless special stains like alcian blue PAS and cytokeratin are being carried out. This tumour type is responsible for most of the cases that present with ascites and Krukenberg ovarian tumour. Equal distribution has been seen in diffuse type of cancer with no sex predilection and it has been observed more frequently in the younger age group.

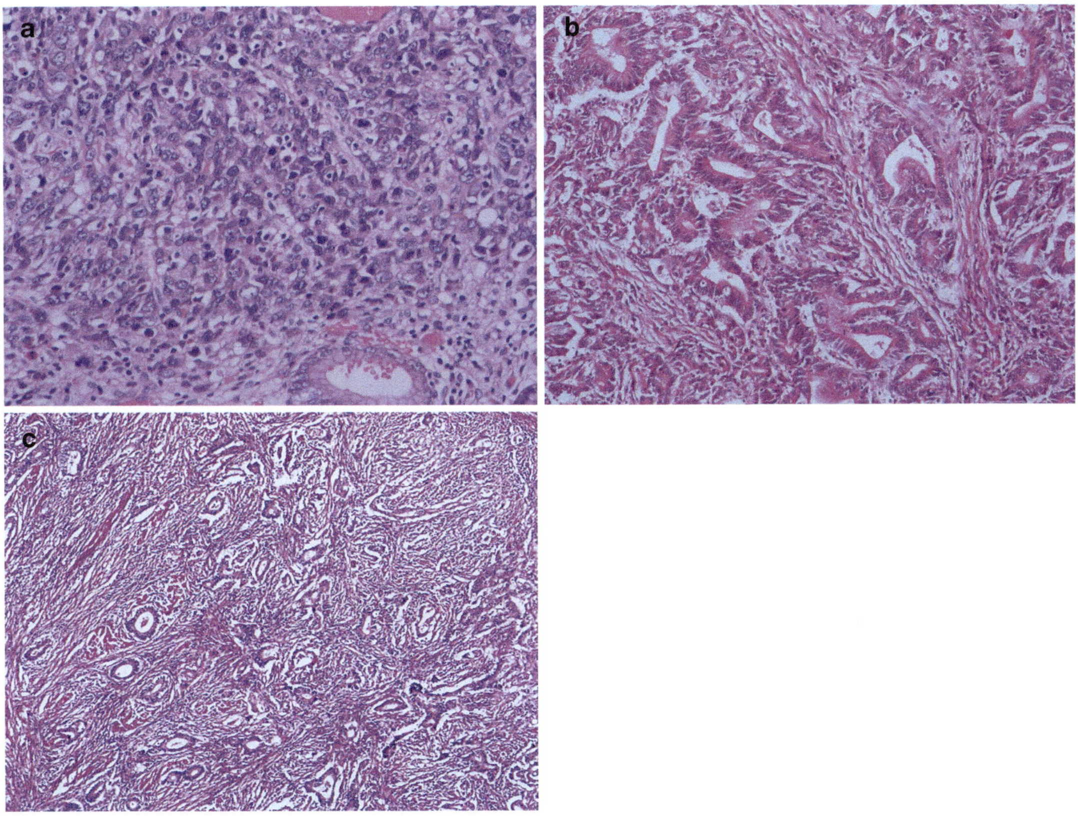

Fig. 15.1 Photomicrographs of three different types of gastric carcinomas. (**a**) Diffuse type, (**b**) intestinal type and (**c**) indeterminate or mixed type (HE, ×300)

GC with diffuse type morphology has been shown to carry mutation in E-cadherin (CDH1) gene in 25%, has been named as hereditary diffuse gastric cancer (HDGC) and was demonstrated for the first time in the year 1994 [20–23]. CDH1 mutations have been documented in 40–83% in sporadic diffuse cancers as well [24, 25]. The cancer cells in diffuse form develop aberrant cell-to-cell adhesion due to abnormal E-cadherin expression which is demonstrated as loss of its expression in immunohistochemistry [23, 26] (Fig. 15.2). Till date, only one record of E-cadherin germline mutation in an apparently sporadic gastric cancer exists in the English literature [27]. Diffuse GCs may arise due to germline mutation in E-cadherin gene. A genetic syndrome may be suspected especially when such type of tumour is seen in a very young individual and show multiple foci of intramucosal signet ring cell carcinoma. Diffuse GC has been associated with β-catenin/APC genes mutations apart from CDH1 gene [28, 29]. Germline mutation of CDH1 gene in HDGC syndrome was confirmed in studies using gastric cancer cell lines and tumour tissue form gastric carcinomas [30, 31]. These observations were further supported by evidence obtained from the families with a history of aggregation of diffuse gastric cancer—3 mutations in CDH1 gene detected in Maori family members of New Zealand with diffuse cancer and mutation were substitution in donor splice consensus sequence of exon 7, frameshift mutation in exon 15 and premature stop codon interrupting exon 13 [32]. Since then, many different ethnic groups were found to have germline mutations [33–36]. HDGC exhibits little or no E-cadherin immunoreactivity and it is believed that loss of heterozygosity does not happen rather an epigenetic allelic inactivation takes place due to hypermethylation of CDH1 gene

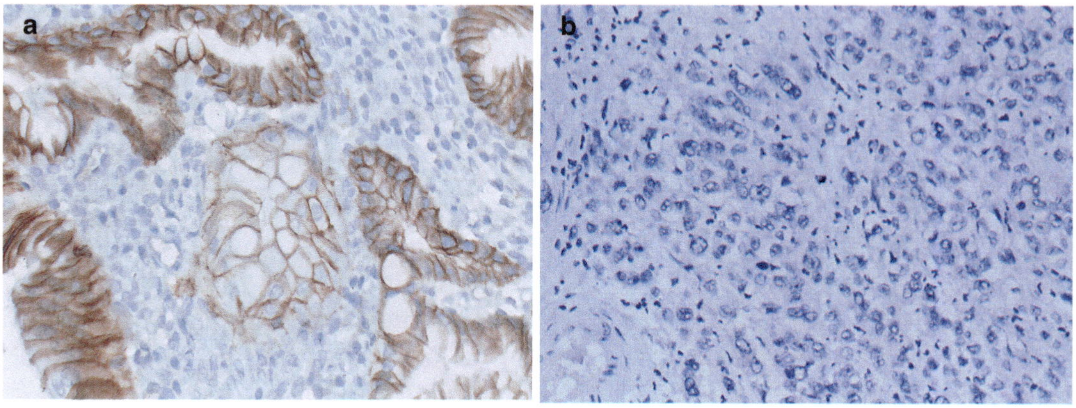

Fig. 15.2 Photomicrographs of E-cadherin immunohistochemistry sections. (**a**) Epithelial cells of the glands showing membranous positivity and (**b**) diffuse gastric carcinoma showing diffuse negativity (PAP, ×500)

promoter [36–38]. Tumours with CDH1 gene mutation have in situ carcinoma characterized by presence of signet ring cells along the basement membrane of gastric foveolae and glands, which may be easily overlooked in routine biopsy specimens and may be mistaken for macrophages. This can be confirmed by carrying out histochemistry stain like alcian blue PAS and also immunohistochemistry like CK to confirm the epithelial cells are not a macrophage or by excluding histiocytic cells by using CD68. And the gastric glands and foveolae may also show pagetoid spread whereby the signet ring cells spread in single layer in continuous or discontinuous manner in between the benign lining epithelial cells and the basement membrane. Also, these tumour cells will lose their membrane staining for E-cadherin, unlike many other diffuse signet ring cells will have to retain E-cadherin in immunohistochemistry stained section [39–41].

Diagnostic criteria for HDGC [42, 43] are—(a) two or more cases of diffuse gastric cancer in 1st-or 2nd-degree relatives, one being diagnosed <50 years of age, or (b) three or more cases of DGC in 1st/2nd-degree relatives, independent of the age of onset. Inactivation of CDH1 gene is also known to result in lobular breast cancer as the 2nd most common epithelial neoplasm. Women with CDH1 gene mutation having a family history of HDGC have an estimated 20–40% lifetime risk for lobular breast cancer. Best approach to detect such women is unknown and possibly following the standard recommendations for BRCA1 and BRCA2 screening protocol is advisable [44, 45].

Popularity of Lauren classification is due to its simplicity and can be used easily for large epidemiological studies. But it is of less significance to predict tumour outcome. WHO Classification of gastric cancer [11] has graded intestinal type of gastric cancer on the presence of recognizable glands ranging from well to moderately differentiated tumours, and some with poorly differentiated morphology along advancing margin. Well-differentiated carcinomas are recognizable with well-formed glands. Poorly differentiated tumours have poorly formed glands composed of very pleomorphic cells arranged in small clusters or solid sheets. Moderately differentiated tumours are intermediate between these two extremes. These adenocarcinomas typically have a background of intestinal metaplasia. The mucinous phenotype of intestinal type of these carcinoma subsets may be of intestinal, gastric and gastrointestinal morphology [11]. In 2019, WHO classification of tumours [46] further subclassifies GCs into papillary, tubular, mucinous and mixed types. In addition, many other rarer histological types have been added. To name the carcinoma subtypes are adenosquamous, squamous cell, undifferentiated, carcinoma with lymphoid stroma, hepatoid, adenocarcinoma with enteroblastic differentiation, adenocarcinoma of fundic gland type and micropapillary adenocarcinoma.

Gradings primarily apply to tumours with tubular and papillary carcinomas and not to other subtypes of GC.

Small pieces of endoscopic biopsy usually get the superficial tissue component, i.e. a part of the polypoidal growth, edges of fungating mass, margins of ulcerated growth, nodular and granular mucosa or an indurated mucosal lesion. Every fragment of the multiple tissue pieces may reveal different morphology. There can be tumorous fragments, non-neoplastic inflammatory fragments or the necrotic neutrophil exudate. Amongst the fragments bearing the tumour tissue may show variable morphology but the most important thing that requires attention is the character of the tumour—is it malignant or benign, if malignant then is it a carcinoma or something else. If it is a carcinoma, efforts have to be made to categorize the type of carcinoma. Most of the time, gastric carcinomas tend to be adenocarcinomas and their variants and subtypes. Most frequently tumour cells show tubular or papillary pattern of arrangement and in such carcinoma, grading of the tumour must be carried out. Presence of pools of mucin should be looked into and presence of signet ring cells in the mucin pools to qualify for the diagnosis of signet ring cell carcinoma. Signet ring cells in GC have its own importance, as have been discussed in the previous chapter. Sometimes some may come across the rare variants of gastric carcinoma and any unusual morphological features should be a guiding feature to consider the rarer variants of gastric cancer. In the non-carcinomatous fragments, it is important to look for the premalignant changes and presence of dysplasia and intestinal metaplasia, and *H. pylori*. Infrequently, some of the lymphatics in the lamina propria may be bearing a small cluster of carcinoma cells. In such situation, the best way to deal is to get step serial sections and it may be a rewarding effort as there can be many more foci having the tumour cells. Simple special stains like alcian blue PAS sometimes help to bring out the small microscopic clusters of tumour cells in the background of the unhealthy and heavily inflamed mucosa. If need be, it is worthwhile to utilize appropriate immunohistochemistry to highlight the carcinoma cells. A close differential diagnosis of carcinoma in routine endoscopic biopsy form gastric mucosal lesion is lymphoid neoplastic lesions like MALT (mucosa-associated lymphoid tissue) lymphoma. As the name suggest, this group of lymphoma is different from the conventional non-Hodgkin lymphoma. Similar to gastric adenocarcinomas, MALT lymphomas also arise from a background of chronically inflamed gastric mucosa and are associated with *H. pylori* infection.

15.3 Histological Subtypes

Tubular adenocarcinoma. This is the commonest subtype amongst the GCs with different frequencies in different parts of the world. Among the different countries, Japan recorded the highest frequency of 64% [47] and European countries report a frequency of 45% [48]. However, more recently much higher frequency of 72.4% of GC has been reported amongst the Japanese elderly patients [49]. This subtype is composed of branching tubules of variable sizes, some with slit-like spaces, acinar structure may also be a component of this tumour subtype. Individual tumour cells may be columnar to cuboidal to flattened with variable amounts of luminal mucin and necrotic cellular debris (Fig. 15.3a–d). There can be areas of clear cell change, which possibly has been seen frequently in the proximal stomach including gastroesophageal tumours. Some of the tumours may be more solid with minimal glandular or tubular structures and these solid tumours are classified as poorly differentiated tubular carcinoma [46, 50].

Papillary adenocarcinoma. This is a relatively uncommon subtype of GC accounting for about 3–10%. This subtype of GC tends to be a protruding exophytic mucosal growth. Histologically majority of these tumours have well-differentiated morphology and show finger-like processes with central fibrovascular core and lined by columnar or cuboidal cells. Despite being well differentiated, these tumours tend to have a pushing or an invading margin, frequently infiltrated by inflammatory cells [2, 51]

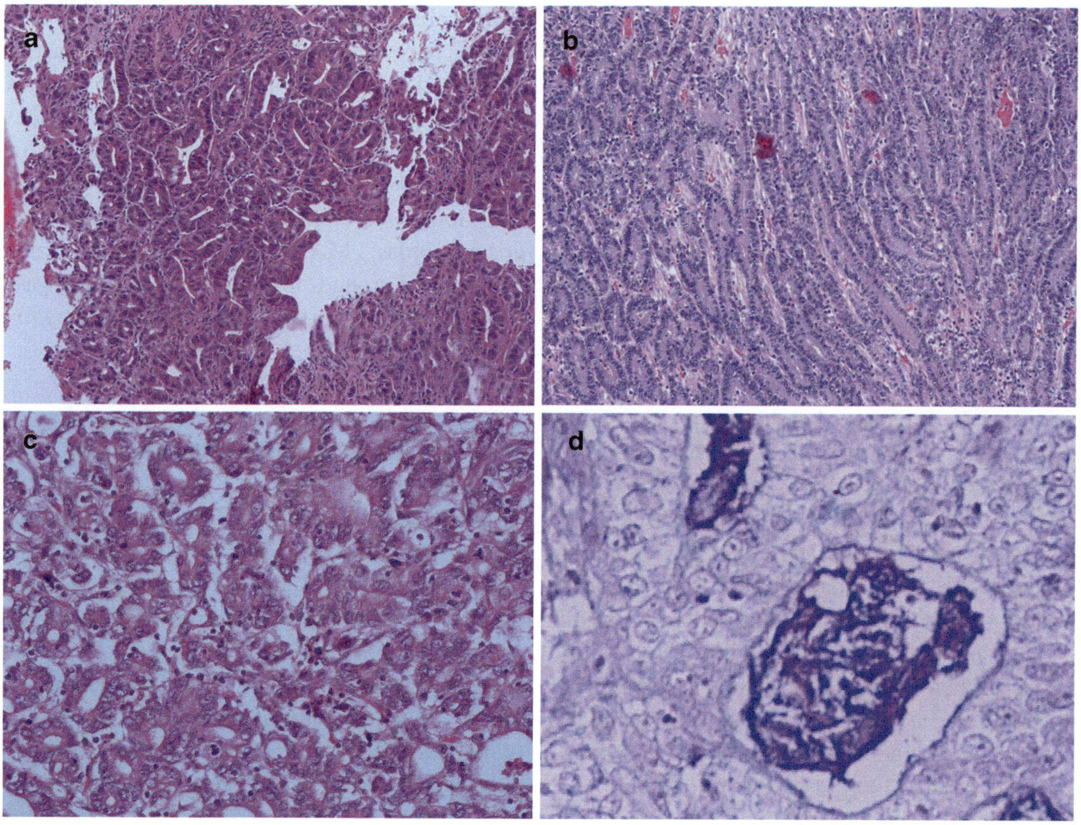

Fig. 15.3 (**a–c**) Photomicrographs show different patterns of tubular differentiation by gastric carcinomas (HE, ×300). (**d**) Highlights the luminal mucin as alcian blue positivity (AB-PAS, ×500)

(Fig. 15.4a–c). There may also be a component of micropapillary where there is reverse polarity as inside out pattern with apical surface placed towards the stroma, or the tumour may also show a combination of the two patterns. This type of tumour is frequently seen in elderly individuals, proximal tumour location, higher rate of LN involvement, frequent liver metastasis and associates with poor patient outcome [52, 53].

Signet ring cell (SRC) carcinoma and other subtypes. This group of tumours is also known as poorly cohesive carcinoma (PCC), accounts for 20–54% of GCs and incidence of these subtypes of Lauren's diffuse type has increased in the recent past [54–56]. PCCs are composed of poorly cohesive malignant cells present as singly or in small clusters with no glandular differentiation. PCC tumours may be of SRC type or non-signet ring cell type. SRCs are round cells having a central optically clear droplet of mucin with peripherally located nuclei with sickle or round to oval shaped giving the cell a signet ring appearance (Fig. 15.5a, b). These cells are arranged in interconnected cords and lace-like patterns giving appearance of glands, or may be arranged in delicate micro-trabecular patterns, especially in the superficial portion of the tumour mainly in the mucosal component. The other components of the PCCs are non-signet ring cells having bland appearance resembling histiocytes with moderate amount of pale eosinophilic cytoplasm. Tumour cells may also have hyperchromatic nuclei with deeply eosinophilic cytoplasm, significant pleomorphism and bizarre nuclei (Fig. 15.5c). Mixture of these different looking cells may be seen in some including signet ring cells. There may be desmoplastic reaction specially in deeper portion of tumour like in submucosal or beyond [57]. PCC tumours were further subclassified into three subtypes in a consensus

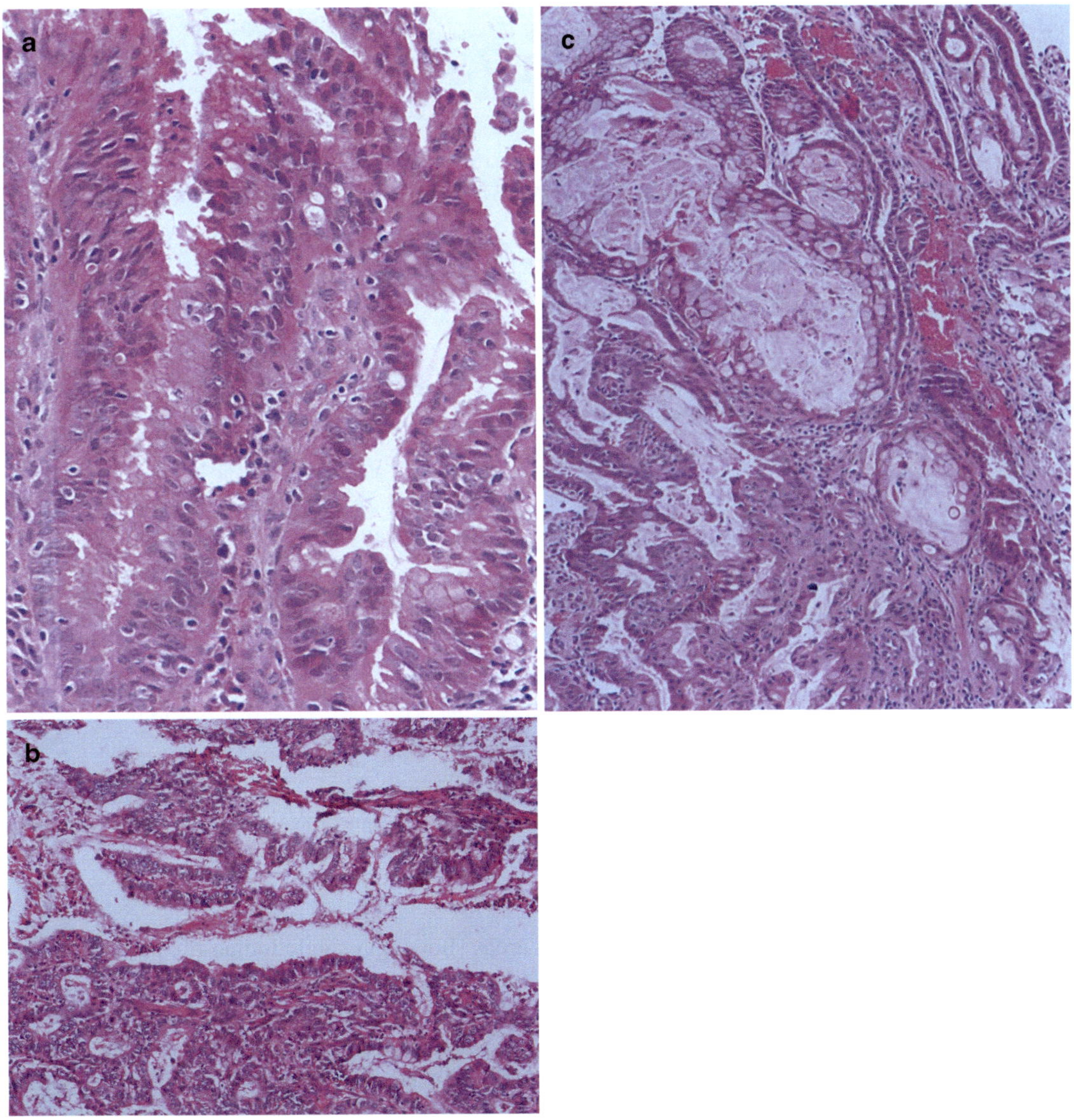

Fig. 15.4 Photomicrographs showing different cell types and papillary fronds in papillary carcinomas in (**a**) to (**c**). In (**b**), the central area shows almost a micropapillary pattern and in (**c**) there is a focus on glandular differentiation with mucin production (HE, ×300)

held in Verona in 2017 into—(a) class of signet ring cell (SRC) carcinoma if SRC component constitutes >90% of tumour; (b) all other PCC are further classified into non-SRC PCC subtype if the SRC component constitutes <90% but >10% of tumour and (c) third subtype of PCC not otherwise specified if SRC component constitutes <10% of tumour cells. SRC tumours are less sensitive to chemoradiation and are associated with poorer outcome [58, 59]. PCCs have been analyzed using panels of several genes. Certain genes have been found to be associated with particular tumour properties, i.e. HDCA9 and IGF1R with perineural invasion, PIK3CA, CTNNB and KRAS with lymphovascular emboli and PIK3CA, CDH1, PTEN, RHOA, HDCA9, KRAS and ATM with a diffuse infiltrative growth pattern. Tumours having PDGFRB mutation

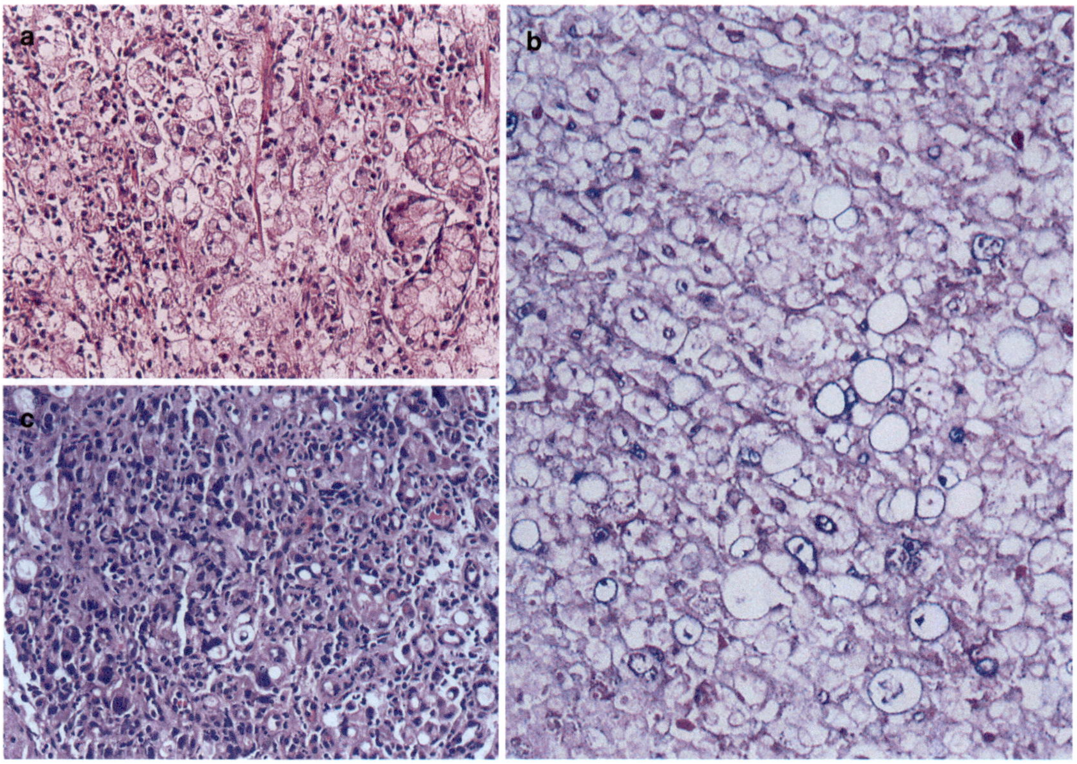

Fig. 15.5 (**a–c**) Poorly cohesive carcinoma may dominantly be of signet ring cells as in (**a**), showing intracellular rim of alcian blue positive mucin as in (**b**). The third picture, i.e. (**c**) shows a tumour showing both signet ring as well as non-signet ring type of cells, many with pleomorphic nuclei

showed favourable prognosis and MET mutation indicated an aggressive tumour. PCC-NOS type had a greater tendency for deeper invasion and more lymph node involvement than SRC dominant type, and these tumour types also had mutations in TP53, BRAF, PI3CA, SMAD4 and RHOA. RHOA mutated PCC tumour tends to be more of superficial SRC with limited tubular component [57, 60, 61].

Mucinous adenocarcinoma. Mucinous gastric adenocarcinoma / carcinoma (MGC) is rare constitutes about 3.3% to 7.1% of gastric carcinomas and to qualify for the diagnosis of mucinous tumour, pools of mucin should form at least 50% of the total tumour volume histologically [62–64]. A diagnosis of MGC can be excluded if the mucin component is dominantly intracellular with little or no extracellular mucin. In MGC, floating tumour cells may have columnar morphology arranged in glands and tubules with areas showing a single Indian file pattern, chain-like fashion, small groups or nests and singly scattered signet ring cells (Fig. 15.6a–d). Occasionally, the mucin pool maybe lack of tumour cells and WHO had classified it under poorly differentiated [65] or undifferentiated type by Japanese pathologists [62, 66]. Pathobiology of MGC is still not well defined and a typical adenocarcinoma is believed to be the precursor lesion. Comparison clinicopathological features of MGC with non-mucinous carcinoma (NMGC) has remained inconsistent as NMGC group is heterogenous frequently containing well as well as poorly differentiated or undifferentiated cases [67, 68]. Comparing the outcome of MGC with NMGC of intestinal and diffuse subtypes, MGC cases were found to be more aggressive having more advanced-stage disease associated with deeper invasion and poor survival outcomes as their response to adjuvant intraperitoneal perfu-

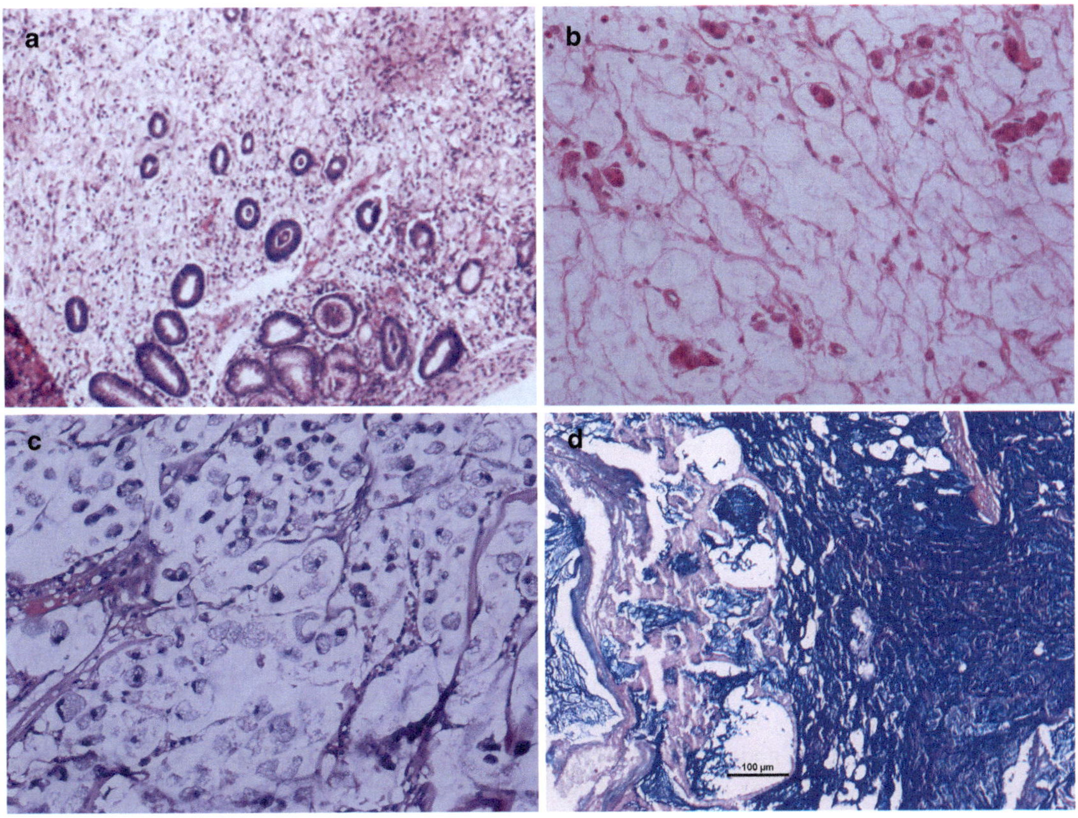

Fig. 15.6 (**a**, **b**) Photomicrographs show tumours having a pale background with scanty number of floating tumour cells, which is a very characteristic appearance for mucinous carcinoma; (**c**) similar looking tumour with many singly scattered signet ring cells floating in the abundant extracellular mucin (HE, ×250). (**d**) Medium power photomicrograph to show pools of extracellular mucin highlighted as blue colour in special stain (Alcian blue at 2.5 pH, ×250)

sion chemotherapy is also less satisfactory [62, 67]. MGCs have been with higher HER-2 gene amplification and EGFR protein overexpression than NMGCs and associated with poorer prognosis [68, 69].

Mixed adenocarcinoma. This terminology has been under-recognized and under-reported by the pathologists, ignoring the different components of the tumour mass. Any patient suspected to have malignancy, endoscopic examination followed by biopsy from suspicious site is a routine practice before the patient is subjected to further definitive treatment. Gastric carcinomas with mixed patterns are more aggressive than pure forms [70, 71]. Reported incidence of mixed gastric carcinoma is 6 to 22%. Mixed-type (MT) gastric cancer may demonstrate histological components of a well differentiated type (DT) and undifferentiated type (UDT) [72, 73]. Stelzner and Emmrich observed different behaviour by the mixed type carcinomas and accordingly, the tumours could be grouped into four distinct categories, i.e. (a) a combination of intestinal and diffuse features, (b) more diffuse structures with a nodular growth pattern, (c) both a glandular pattern and signet ring cells and (d) tumour reveals an excessive production of mucin [74] (Figs. 15.1c and 15.7a, b). According to Japanese guidelines, UDT-predominant MT (M-UDT) is to be considered UDT [72]. Another large series had analyzed tumour associated factors like size, presence tumour associated ulcer and requirement for re-surgery between pure and mixed type UDT. The study concluded that mixed

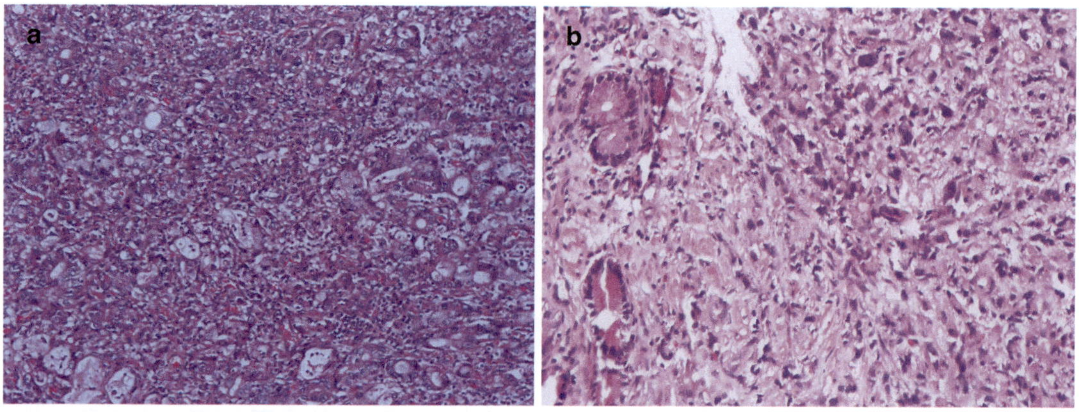

Fig. 15.7 (**a**, **b**) Photomicrographs showing a mixture of tumour cells arranged in glandular as well as in singly scattered pleomorphic cells indicating presence of a better differentiated carcinoma cells along with higher grade poorly differentiated carcinoma (HE. ×250)

type UDT had positive predictive values for all the three parameters indicating its more aggressive behaviour [75]. In addition, mixed UDT type showed higher frequency of lymphovascular invasion and risk of lymph node metastasis [76, 77]. Mixed carcinomas having isolated cells and glandular components, both types of cells showed overexpression and amplification of ERBB2 as an early genetic event [78–80]. Mixed carcinoma with differentiated type shows divergent phenotypes associated with somatic mutation in CDH1 by mixed tumour showing diffuse and signet ring cell type [24]. CDH1 gene mutation is one important event in initiation and/or progression in majority of diffuse cancer, however, normal E-cadherin expression has been observed in sporadic and familial forms [40–43]. These mixed tumours have also found to show similar patterns of chromosomal aberrations by array comparative genomic hybridization technique [79].

Gastric (adeno)carcinoma with lymphoid stroma (GCLS). It is known as gastric lymphoepithelioma-like carcinoma (Fig. 15.8a, b). It is comprising of undifferentiated carcinoma and heavy lymphoid cell component and constitutes 1–4% of all gastric cancer and >80% is associated with EBV infection [81–84]. Like in breast cancer, similar lymphoid-rich stroma in gastric cancer was reported way back in 1922 [85]. The terms which were used to denote were "blue cell carcinoma" and "medullary carcinoma with lymphoid infiltration" and was regarded to be a different group of tumours with a pathologic entity that should be separated from gastric carcinomas of a common type. GCLS has a better prognosis than any other gastric cancers [86, 87]. Different terminology had been used initially emphasizing the histologic and distinct prognosis observed in these carcinoma groups. The histologic criteria proposed by Hamazaki for distinguishing this carcinoma were (a) intercellular oedema and lymphoid cell infiltration of the tumour parenchyma, (b) lymphoid feature of the tumour stroma and (c) uniformity in distribution of these elements within the tumour [88]. GCLS tumours were observed more frequently in males, proximal location, protruding growth, submucosal involvement and lesser lymph node metastasis [81, 89]. These tumours are typically well-circumscribed consisting of diffuse sheet-like growth of syncytial cells intimately associated with dense lymphoid cells obscuring interface between tumour cells and stroma. Glandular differentiation is conspicuously absent and tumour cells have large nuclei with opened-up chromatin along with one or more prominent nucleoli. Tumour infiltrating lymphocytes are the defining feature and their numbers can be quite variable within the tumour itself and from one case to another. Gastric carcinomas with lym-

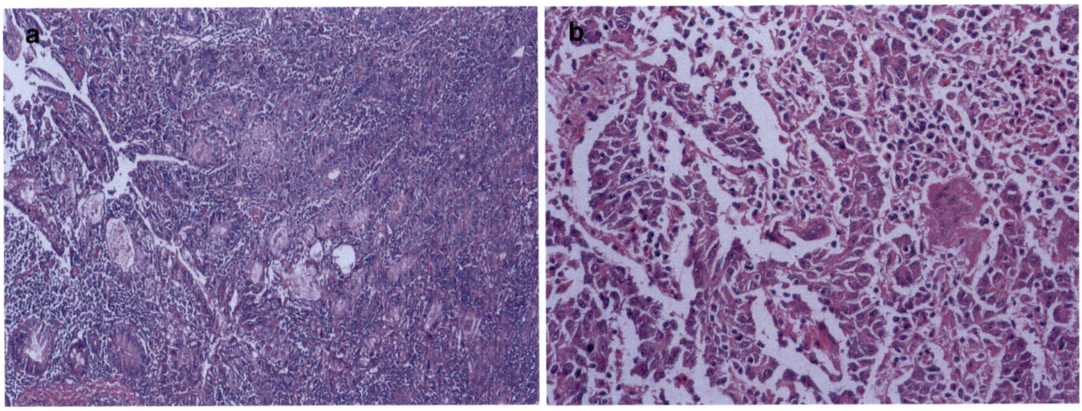

Fig. 15.8 (**a**, **b**) Both photomicrographs show carcinoma cells in diffuse clusters and in trabeculae intermixed closely with lymphomononuclear cells. In (**b**) there are also few scattered multinucleated non-malignant giant cells

phoid stroma frequently harbour EBV encoded RNAs particularly in Asian countries in up to 80% of cases may show EBV positivity. In western countries EBV positivity rates in this tumour type have been reported to be lower. Relatively favourable prognosis may be related to tumour infiltrating lymphocytes, EBV positivity or MMR gene deficiency and all of these parameters have been found to be independent factors for predicting the prognosis [87, 90, 91]. GCLS exhibits frequent PD-L1 expression suggesting its possible susceptibility to checkpoint inhibitor and/or agent targeting receptor tyrosine kinase-mediated signalling [92].

Hepatoid adenocarcinoma of stomach (HAS). This subtype is aggressive cancer associates with a tendency for liver metastasis [93, 94]. Tumour cells are arranged in trabeculae or solid clusters with intervening fine fibrous stroma. The stroma tends to be enriched with many thin wall vascular spaces mimicking sinusoidal spaces. Tumour cells are cuboidal to polygonal, moderate to abundant amount of pale to eosinophilic cytoplasm occasionally with pinkish hyaline globules. Nuclei are large and ovoid shape containing one or more nucleoli (Fig. 15.9a, b). The characteristic histology of this tumour is its resemblance to hepatocellular carcinoma (HCC). Criteria in the diagnosis of HAC are the presence of distinct hepatoid area irrespective of its proportion within the tumour or irrespective of the amount of alpha foetal protein. In addition, HAS are also positive for many immunohistochemical markers similar to HCC of liver origin such as AFP, GPC-3, SALL4, and Hep-Par 1, and this tumour is also associated with increase serum levels of AFP [95, 96]. HAS has more aggressive outcome than other gastric cancers and gastric cancer irrespective of the morphology of the tumour, α-feto protein producing tumours has higher incidence of liver metastasis than tumours not producing α-feto protein [97, 98]. Bourreille et al. reported the 1st α-fetoprotein producing gastric cancer metastasizing to liver [99] and later on the concept of hepatoid adenocarcinoma was proposed constituting just about 0.3% of all gastric carcinomas amongst all the AFP positive gastric cancer of 2.6. to 5.4 [100, 101]. Gastric carcinomas expressing AFP may have two histological types, i.e. medullary type simulating HCC and papillary or tubular type. Other AFP-positive gastric carcinomas are adenocarcinoma with enteroblastic differentiation and yolk sac tumour-like carcinoma [102–104].

Gastric adenocarcinoma with enteroblastic differentiation (GAED). Gastric carcinoma with a clear cell is relatively an uncommon type. The term GAED is not yet well documented except for a few small series or single case reports [105, 106]. Histologically it is characterized to be a primitive intestine-like morphology composed of cuboidal or columnar cells with clear cytoplasm and is found arising from cardia or pylorus accounting for 2.24% of gastric carcinomas [107,

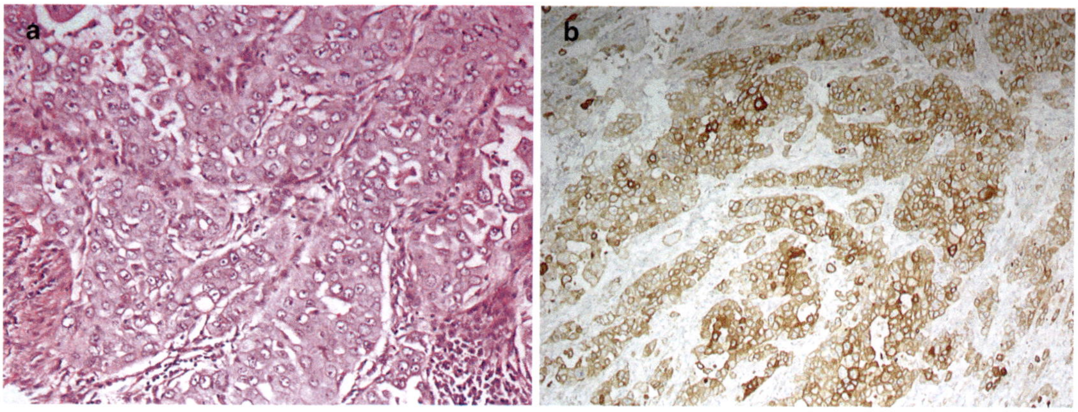

Fig. 15.9 (**a**) Tumour cells are arranged in trabeculae and islands, individual cells are polygonal with moderate to abundant pale to eosinophilic cytoplasm, occasionally with pinkish hyaline globules. Nuclei are large round to oval, vesicular and with one or more nucleoli (HE, ×300). (**b**) Immunohistochemistry staining using Hepar primary antibody showing granular cytoplasmic positivity (PAP, ×300)

108]. Histologically, it is a well-differentiated adenocarcinoma exhibiting tubulo-papillary pattern dominant comprising of clear cells with eosinophilic secretion. More compact areas show larger cells having hyperchromatic nuclei with PAS positive droplets resembling a clear cell component in hepatoid variant tumours (Fig. 15.10a, b). GAEDs also exhibit cytoplasmic AFP staining that may associate with serology AFP. Association between GAED and AFP positivity remains unclear as a few of GAED may be negative AFP [101–104]. HACs have also been observed to show component of cells showing varying degrees of clear cells mimicking foetal gut epithelium but these tumours tend to lack the vascularized stromal component [96, 108]. AFP negative hepatoid or enteroblastic tumours may show positive staining for glypican 3 and SALL4 [109–111]. Glypican 3, expressed by foetal hepatocytes, overlaps with AFP in AFP producing gastric cancer. Glypican 3 and SALL4 have been suggested to be sensitive markers for AFP-producing gastric cancer and related tumours [110, 111].

Micropapillary carcinoma. This relatively rare variant of gastric cancer has been reported in advanced stage tumours and clinicopathological features in early gastric carcinoma have remained elusive [112]. Studies on early gastric carcinomas with small ≥5% focus of micropapillary component were found to have a high frequency of lymph node metastasis [112–114]. The micropapillary component in the tumour for the diagnosis of this tumour subtype has not been stratified but based on the report of ≥5% micropapillary component for increased risk of lymph node metastasis, a cut of 5% has been taken for the diagnosis of micropapillary carcinoma [115–117]. In a small endoscopic biopsy micropapillary pattern may be easily overlooked. The micropapillary growth pattern in gastric tumours has the same distinctive histology as in other organs, comprising of small clusters of epithelial cells exhibiting papillary fronds within empty spaces without any fibrovascular core (Fig. 15.11). The atypical epithelial cells facing the stroma may have apical secretion [116, 117]. In early gastric cancer, micropapillary component may coexists with predominant papillary and/or tubular, occasionally mucinous and poorly differentiated components. Spaces around the epithelial cells may sometimes be confused with tissue retraction artefacts but tumour cells with retraction artefacts will retain the conventional histomorphology of an adenocarcinoma without the apical secretions. Inside-out pattern of micro-

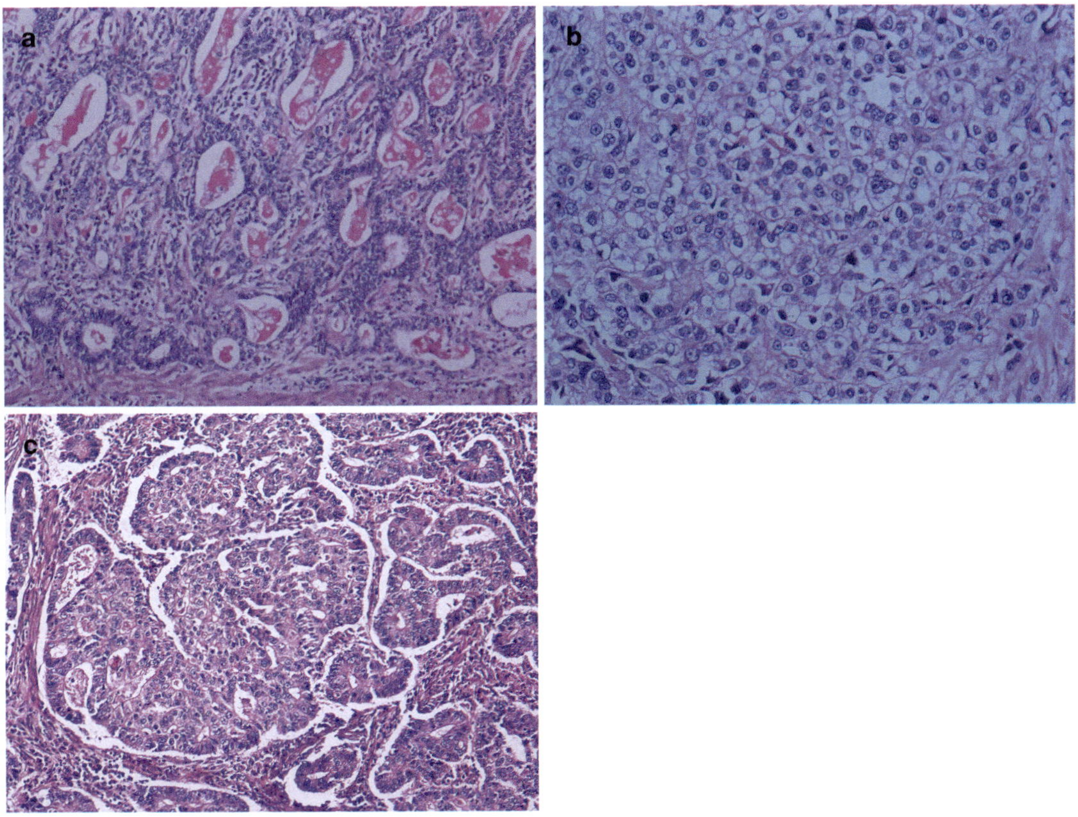

Fig. 15.10 Photomicrographs showing a well-differentiated adenocarcinoma exhibiting (**a**) tubulo-papillary pattern dominant comprising of clear cells with eosinophilic secretion. (**b**, **c**) More compact areas showing larger cells having hyperchromatic nuclei with clear to lightly eosinophilic cells, almost looking like a hepatoid variant tumour (HE, ×300)

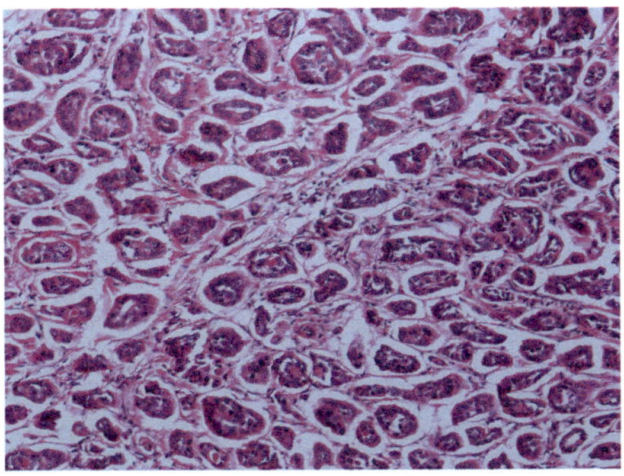

Fig. 15.11 Photomicrograph showing micropapillary growth pattern comprising of small clusters of epithelial cells exhibiting papillary fronds within empty spaces without any obvious fibrovascular core (HE, ×300)

papillary carcinoma can be confirmed with the help of IHC using epithelial membrane antigen or MUC1, which will give linear immunoreactivity on the outer membrane of neoplastic cells [118, 119]. The most important differential diagnosis of micropapillary variant of gastric cancer in a small endoscopic biopsy will be tumour emboli in lymphatics along the biopsy edge, conveniently can be ruled out by immunostainings like D2-40 and CD34 for lymphatics and blood vessels, also metastasis from other sites with micropapillary configuration needs to be differentiated from a primary gastric tumour and the distinctive morphological features should help to distinguish primary from metastatic tumours.

Gastric adenocarcinoma of fundic gland type (GA-FG). A relative new condition and alternative term being well-differentiated gastric adenocarcinoma of chief cell or fundic gland type (GA-FG) [120]. These rare mucosal lesions may exhibit varieties of endoscopic features and histology shows tightly packed to dilated glands of oxyntic cells with weekly basophilic cytoplasm exhibiting mild nuclear pleomorphism with no mitotic activity, giving a seemingly innocuous profile of an adenoma like morphology (Fig. 15.12a, b). The term was proposed first proposed by Tsukamoto et al in 2007 [121]. These lesions may exhibit three distinct subgroups, i.e. (a) chief cell predominant, which is the commonest group; (b) parietal cell predominant and (c) mixed type [122–125]. This tumour occurs in non-metaplastic and non-atrophic mucosa. In spite of its innocuous morphology, these tumour subtypes reported have shown invasion of submucosa and muscularis mucosae with fibroblastic stroma, with rare lymphovascular emboli [124–126]. In addition to gastric phenotype, the cells of the glandular component show overlapping features between fundic mucous neck cells and chief cells [127, 128]. There appears to be a relatively lack of awareness as majority of reported cases are from Japan and Korea, only very few are from the West comprising of tumours with well differentiated and mixed phenotypes. It may also be suggested that less differentiated neoplasms could have been underrecognized due to lack of appropriate immunohistochemical evaluation [129]. Superficial nonneoplastic foveolar cells are stained with Muc-5AC, chief and parietal cells are negative. Neoplastic cells are usually positive for Muc 6, cells having chief cell morphology express pepsinogen I and RUNX3, pepsinogen II is less specific. Parietal cells are positively stained for H+/K+-ATPase. These lesions have invariably normal foveolar type epithelium along the surface and deeper part comprising of mixture of cells normally present in oxyntic glands forming anas-

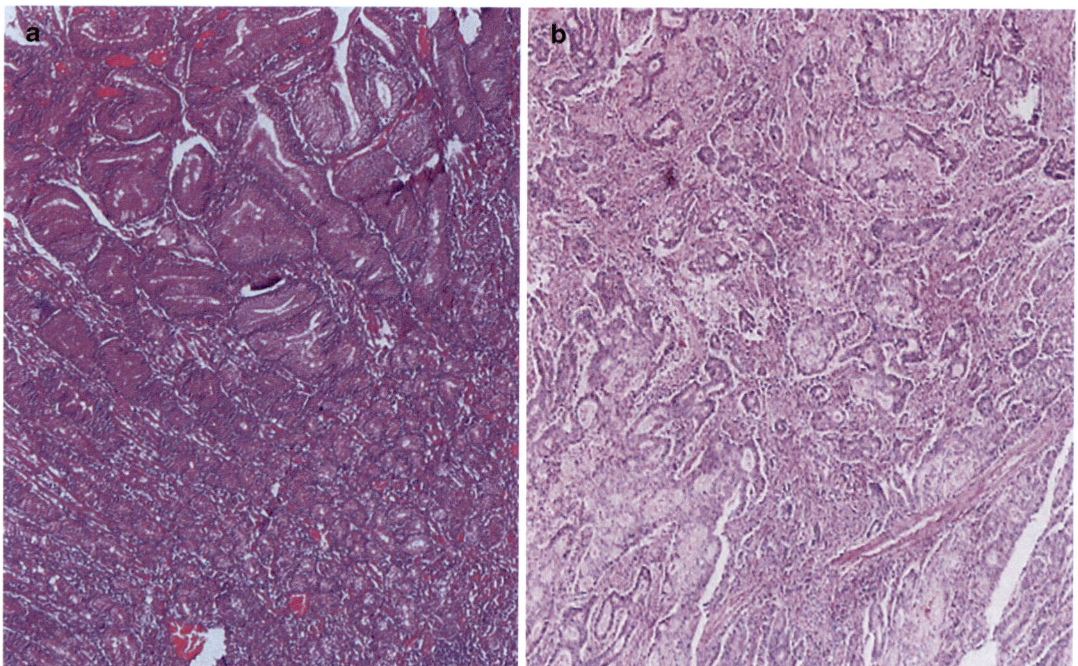

Fig. 15.12 (**a**, **b**) Photomicrographs showing tightly packed to dilated glands of oxyntic cells with weekly basophilic cytoplasm exhibiting mild nuclear pleomorphism, bland nuclei morphology giving an innocuous profile of an adenoma (HE, ×200)

tomosing cords producing endless gland patterns, rarely producing cribriform pattern, multilayering and stratification of the nuclei. These anastomosing cords of glands may have a predominance of either chief cell or parietal cell, or mixture of both cell types. Necrosis is seldom present. Neoplastic cells may show mildly enlarged nuclei with opened up chromatin and inconspicuous nucleoli, mitosis is rare, Ki-67 index is usually less than 5%. Stroma or lamina propria may be normal, oedematous or myxoid change. Rarely there can be desmoplasia, even when the tumour cells are showing submucosal invasion [126, 130]. These tumours are not associated with atrophic mucosa and are usually not positive for *H. pylori* [120]. Pathogenesis is not well understood, maybe a different pathway from conventional gastric cancer. A study reported accumulation of nuclear beta-catenin with CTNNB1 and or AXIN gene mutations suggesting Wnt/beta-catenin pathway activation [131]. A small number of these tumours showed GNAS mutation suggesting an alternative activation of Wnt/beta-catenin pathway [123].

Gastric small cell carcinoma, like other small cell carcinomas, is an aggressive tumour showing neuroendocrine differentiation. More than 200 cases have been reported till the early part of 2021. It was first described by Matsusaka et al as oat cell carcinoma of stomach [132] (Fig. 15.13a, b). Majority of the reports are from Asian continents [133–137] and have been as oat cell carcinomas or atypical carcinoid accounting for <1% of total gastric cancers and constitutes about 15 to 20% of all gastric neuroendocrine tumours, 0.1% of extra-pulmonary small cell carcinomas and <0.1% of all gastric cancer cases. This tumour is primarily seen in males (M:F = 5.4:1) in older age groups ranging from 42 to 84 years [138–142]. It has a similar clinical presentation to patients with conventional gastric adenocarcinoma and these tumours tend to be in an advanced stage by the time the patient comes with the clinical symptoms. Occasionally these

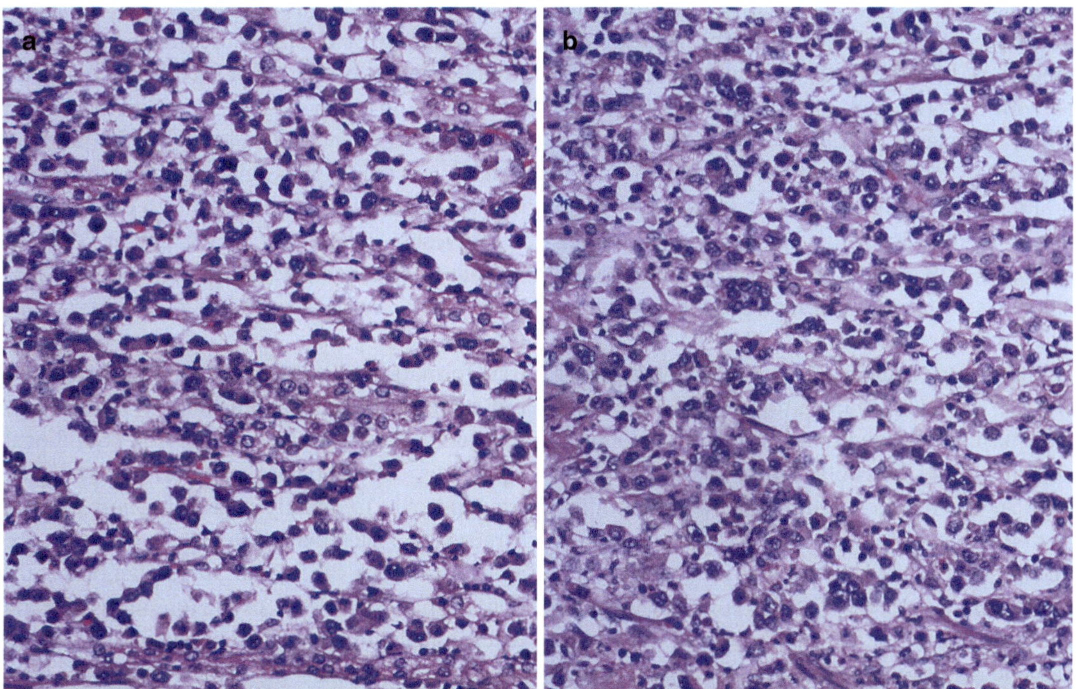

Fig. 15.13 (**a**, **b**) Photomicrographs showing small round to oval cells with scanty pale eosinophilic cytoplasm and hyperchromatic round to oval nuclei, arrange din single cord and small clusters; a few multinucleated tumour cells are also noted (HE, ×350)

tumours have been observed to secret vasoactive peptides resulting in paraneoplastic syndrome [135, 143–146]. These tumours show early metastasis to regional lymph nodes and liver, directly involves surrounding organs including liver, transverse colon, pancreas, spleen and diaphragm even at presentation [147, 148]. Macroscopically, these tumours are large bulking protruding ulcerative lesions invading deeper structures. Histologically these tumours can be grouped into purely composed of similar small cells, or mixed type where small cells intermixed with neuroendocrine cells and diagnostic criteria are similar to tumours seen in other systems. Tumour cells are arranged in sheets, trabeculae, cords and large clusters with focal nesting patterns, and separated by fine fibrovascular septa. In a small endoscopic biopsy, the classic patterns may not present but there may be clusters of primitive or undifferentiated cells with the morphology of blue round cell infiltrating lamina propria replacing gastric glands. Individual cells have a high nuclear-cytoplasmic ratio, hyperchromatic and fine granular chromatin with inconspicuous small nucleoli frequently with moulding. These features of small cell may coexist with the area showing low-grade neuroendocrine neoplasm. Tumour necrosis and a high-grade tumour marker as indicated by high proliferative index with >10 mitoses/10 high power fields. More than half of these tumours may coexist with conventional gastric adenocarcinoma, sarcomatoid carcinoma, adenosquamous and squamous carcinoma [148–154]. The background gastric mucosa may exhibit changes of chronic gastritis with atrophy and intestinal metaplasia. These tumours require immunohistochemistry and possibly Grimelius staining to confirm the diagnosis and also to differentiate from it closed differential diagnoses like lymphomas [155]. Cell of origin for these tumours is a pluripotent stem cell with the potential to grow and differentiate [156]. In addition to exhibiting variable grades of positivity for neuroendocrine markers, gastric oat cell carcinomas are positive for keratin AE1/AE3 and CEA but not for high molecular cytokeratin CK34βE but low molecular weight cytokeratin CK8 [157]. Ki-67 index is high and is an important predictor for tumour aggressiveness and patient outcome [149, 157, 158].

15.4 Other Rare Gastric Carcinomas

Squamous cell and adenosquamous carcinomas reported incidences of <1% in elderly individuals with M:F of 5:1. Clinical manifestations are similar to conventional gastric cancer. These tumours may have mildly elevated serum squamous cell carcinoma antigen and associate with a long history of smoking and alcohol abuse [159–161]. These tumours are seen frequently at advanced stages and show poor response to treatment [162]. To differentiate between gastric and oesophageal squamous carcinoma, Parks et al. have proposed diagnostic criteria, i.e. (a) tumour must not be located in cardia and must not extend into oesophagus and (b) no evidence of squamous cell carcinoma (Fig. 15.14a, b) anywhere else in the body [163]. Criteria by Japanese Classification of Gastric Carcinoma include (a) tumour must consist only of squamous cell carcinoma with no component of adenocarcinoma and (b) any tumour near esophago-gastric junction must be excluded unless evidence for supporting the tumour originated from stomach exists [164]. Hypotheses concerning development of this tumour in stomach are (a) nests of ectopic squamous cells in gastric mucosa, (b) squamous metaplasia of gastric mucosa before malignant transformation, (c) squamous differentiation in a pre-existing adenocarcinoma and (d) multipotential stem cells in gastric mucosa [165, 166]. Focal squamous differentiation in intestinal-type gastric cancer is frequently a phenomenon. Hence, Straus et al. stated that for the diagnosis of gastric adenosquamous carcinoma, the squamous component should be >25% of the tumour as it is the determinant factor for outcome [167] (Fig. 15.14c, d).

Gastric choriocarcinoma was first described in 1905 as a highly aggressive and rare gastric cancer [167]. Male-female ratio is 2.3:1 observed in 5th and 6th decades of life, located in distal

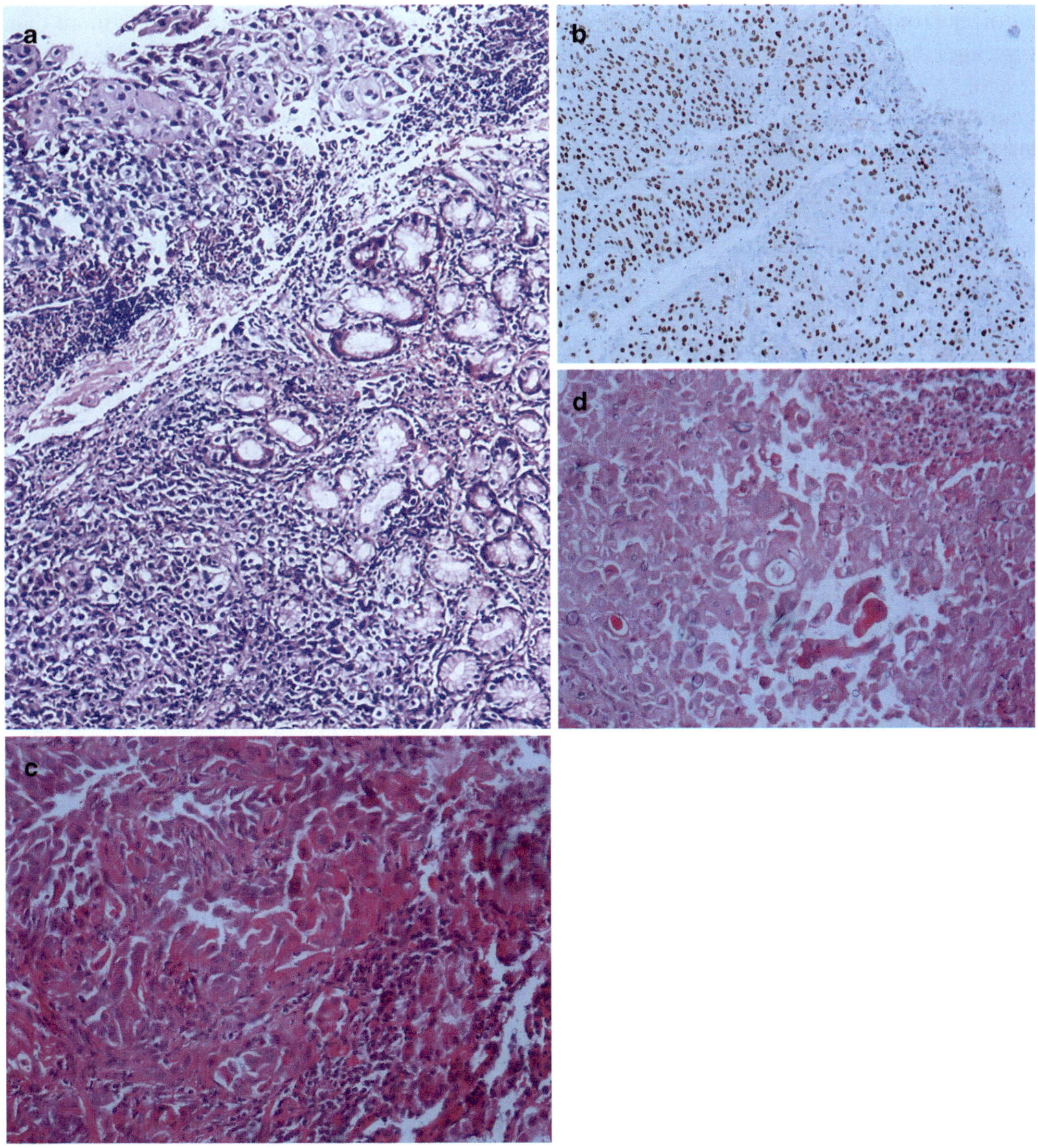

Fig. 15.14 (**a**) Photomicrograph showing a tumour with the features of a moderately differentiated squamous cell carcinoma infiltrating the gastric mucosa (HE, ×300). (**b**) Medium power photomicrograph of an immunostain section using p63 primary antibody showing strong and diffuse nuclear positivity by the tumour cells (PAP, ×300). Photomicrographs from an adenosquamous carcinoma, (**c**) cells showing intracytoplasmic keratinization along with glandular and papillary fronds and (**d**) another focus of the same tumour showing keratin perl formation (HE, ×300)

stomach like a large grossly necrotic tumour [168, 169]. Primary gastric choriocarcinomas coexist as a composite or a mixed tumour with variable degree of adenocarcinoma. These tumours may also have a component of yolk sac component, small cell or hepatoid carcinomas [170–173]. These tumours have tendency for haematogenous dissemination, frequently involving liver [168]. Serum β-HCG level tends to be very high and declines significantly to baseline several months after surgeries. Immunohistochemistry biomarkers for trophoblastic tumours help in confirming the diagnosis, however, some tumours may be negative for β-HCG [174, 175]. Few studies had reported a high level of serum β-HCG to be associated with poorer prognosis. Elevated β-HCG levels in blood and tumour tissue have been reported in about 10% of conventional gastric carcinomas with no histological choriocarcinoma component [176, 177]. In the pathogenesis of this tumour, the most accepted hypothesis is dedifferentiation theory of primary gastric adenocarcinoma proposed by Pick in 1926, supported by Liu et al. [178, 179]. It is reportedly associated with gain of chromosome 12, 2q, 7pq, 8pq, 13q, 17q, 18q, 20pq and deletions in 17p [179].

Undifferentiated gastric carcinoma is composed of anaplastic cells with no specific cytological or architectural differentiation, known as anaplastic or pleomorphic carcinomas (Fig. 15.15a, b) [73]. Tumour subtypes that are included under this terminology are large cell undifferentiated carcinoma with rhabdoid phenotype, pleomorphic carcinomas, sarcomatoid carcinomas and carcinomas with osteoclast-like giant cells. These gastric tumours may involve any segment of the stomach and tends to be large ulcerated growth, which may involve more than segmental areas of the stomach. The tumour frequently shows transmural infiltration with extensive regional lymph node involvement. It has an aggressive course, majority of the patients dying within one year of the diagnosis of the disease. In addition to the morphological subtypes include in the current WHO (2019) classification [73], there are other classifications of gastric cancer which has defined undifferentiated carcinomas differently. Nakamura et al considered that intestinal-type carcinoma is similar to differentiated carcinoma and diffuse-type to undifferentiated-type [180]. Differentiated-type gastric carcinomas have a gastric phenotype in 30% of cases, and are more aggressive compared to ones with intestinal phenotype [181–185]. Undifferentiated type gastric carcinomas have also been reported to have intestinal phenotype, which is considered to be the result of a phenotypic shift from gastric to intestinal type [186–188].

Grossly, undifferentiated gastric carcinomas are large ulceroproliferative lesions with large areas of necrosis and more than one segment may be involved, extending transmurally with multiple regional lymph node metastasis. Histologically, it shows diffuse sheets of anaplastic large to medium sized polygonal cells interspersed frequently with tumour giant cells. Frequently these tumour cells may be

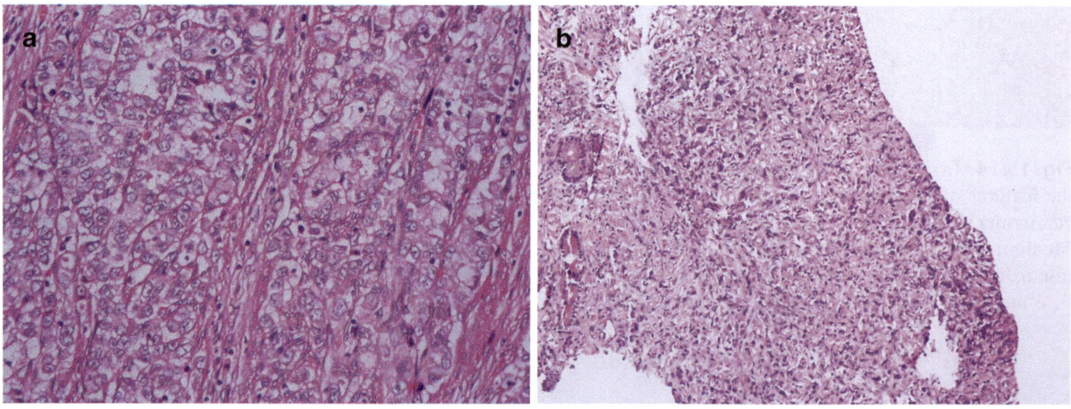

Fig. 15.15 Photomicrographs showing (**a**) round-to-oval undifferentiated cells with pale eosinophilic moderate cytoplasm arranged in trabeculae, cords and nest with vague glandular patterns and vesicular irregular nuclei with more than one nucleoli (HE, ×300); (**b**) diffusely scattered tumour cells with a moderate amount of eosinophilic cytoplasm and grossly pleomorphic nuclei (HS, ×250)

intermixed with other types of tumour cells which may be spindle and sarcomatoid pleomorphic cells, undifferentiated carcinoma with osteoclast-like tumour giant cells, undifferentiated carcinoma with lymphoepithelial like component, and a variable amount of bi- and multinucleated rhabdoid cell components [189, 190]. In the above described histological features, any of these cell types may be intermixed with variable glandular components that may be well formed to ill formed conventional adenocarcinoma components. The adenocarcinoma component may range from small focus to large areas. These variable types of tumour cells may be interspersed with variable stromal components, which tends to be more myxoid and mucinous, and may be intermixed with variable degree of mononuclear inflammatory cells. These undifferentiated cells may show positive staining for pancytokeratin and/or EMA. Vimentin expression is consistent by these undifferentiated tumour cells and produces a perinuclear dot-like pattern [191, 192]. In the differential diagnosis, many conditions including rhabdomyosarcomas and other pleomorphic sarcomas may be considered depending upon the component of the sarcoma and the kind of tissue sample available. In routine endoscopic biopsies, it may be almost impossible to establish a definitive diagnosis. However, with the available immunomarkers, it may be possible to narrow down the differential diagnosis, Other conditions that need to be considered in routine practice are—high-grade lymphomas including anaplastic large cell lymphoma, pleomorphic plasma cell tumours, metastatic melanoma, EBV associated carcinomas with lymphoid stroma, germ cell neoplasms and PEComas [73].

References

1. Gullo I, Carneiro F, Oliveira C, et al. Heterogeneity in gastric cancer: from pure morphology to molecular classifications. Pathobiology. 2018;85:50–63.
2. Hu B, El Hajj N, Sittler S, et al. Gastric cancer: classification, histology and application of molecular pathology. J Gastrointest Oncol. 2012;3:251–61.
3. Gao JP, Xu W, Liu WT, et al. Tumour heterogeneity of gastric cancer: from the perspective of tumour-initiating cell. World J Gastroenterol. 2018;24:2567–81.
4. Welch DR. Tumor heterogeneity – a 'contemporary concept' founded on historical insights and predictions. Cancer Res. 2016;76:4–6.
5. Ho SWT, Tan P. Dissection of gastric cancer heterogeneity for precision oncology. Cancer Sci. 2019;110:3405–14.
6. Gerlinger M, Rowan AJ, Horswell S, et al. Intratumor heterogeneity and branched evolution revealed by multi-region sequencing. N Engl J Med. 2012;366:883–92.
7. Junttila MR, de Sauvage FJ. Influence of tumour micro-environment heterogeneity on therapeutic response. Nature. 2013;501(7467):346–54.
8. Tatematsu M, Tsukamoto T, Inada K. Stem cells and gastric cancer: role of gastric and intestinal mixed intestinal metaplasia. Cancer Sci. 2003;94:135–41.
9. Li K, Dan Z, Nie YQ. Gastric cancer stem cells in gastric carcinogenesis, progression, prevention and treatment. World J Gastroenterol. 2014;20:5420–6.
10. Nakamura T, Yao T, Kabashima A, et al. Loss of phenotypic expression is related to tumour progression in early gastric differentiated adenocarcinoma. Histopathol. 2005;47:357–67.
11. Fenoglio-Preiser CM, Carneiro F, Correa P, et al. Gastric carcinoma. In: Hamilton SR, Aaltonen LA, editors. World Health Organization classification of tumors. Pathology and genetics of tumours of the digestive system. Lyon: IARC Press; 2000. p. 37–68.
12. Parsonnet FG, Vandersteen DP. Helicobacter pylori infection and the risk of gastric carcinoma. N Engl J Med. 1991;325:1127–271.
13. Group IARC (1994) Monographs on the evaluation of the carcinogenic risks to humans. Scistosomes Liver Flukes and Helicobacter pylori. pp 177–241
14. Danesh J. Is Helicobacter pylori infection a cause of gastric neoplasia. Cancer Surv. 1999;33:263–89.
15. Keller G, Rudelius M, Vogelsang H, et al. Microsatellite instability and loss of heterozygosity in gastric carcinoma in comparison to family history. Am J Pathol. 1998;152:1281–9.
16. Varley JM, McGown G, Thorncroft M, et al. An extended Li-Fraumeni kindred with gastric carcinoma and a codon 175 mutation in TP53. J Med Genet. 1995;32:942–5.
17. La Vecchia C, Negri E, Franceschi S, et al. Family history and the risk of stomach and colorectal cancer. Cancer. 1992;70:50–5.
18. Sokoloff B. Predisposition to cancer in the Bonaparte family. Am J Surg. 1938;40:673–8.
19. Lauren P. The two histologic main types of gastric carcinoma: diffuse and so-called intestinal type carcinoma. An attempt at a histo-clinical classification. Acta Pathol Microbiol Scand. 1965;64:31–49.
20. Fitzgerald RC, Caldas C. E-cadherin mutations and hereditary gastric cancer: prevention by resection? Dig Dis. 2002;20:23–31.

21. Guilford P, Hopkins J, Harraway J, et al. E-cadherin germline mutations in familial gastric cancer. Nature. 1998;392:402–5.
22. Guilford P, Humar B, Blair V. Hereditary diffuse gastric cancer: translation of CDH1 germline mutations into clinical practice. Gastric Cancer. 2010;13:1–10.
23. Becker KF, Atkinson MJ, Reich U, et al. E-cadherin gene mutations provide clues to diffuse type gastric carcinomas. Cancer Res. 1994;54:3845–52.
24. Machado JC, Soares P, Carneiro F, et al. E-cadherin gene mutations provide a genetic basis for the phenotypic divergence of mixed gastric carcinomas. Lab Invest. 1999;79:459–65.
25. Perl AK, Wilgenbus P, Dahl U, et al. A causal role for E-cadherin in the transition from adenoma to carcinoma. Nature. 1998;392:190–3.
26. Yoshiura K, Kanai Y, Ochiai A, et al. Silencing of the E-cadherin invasion-suppressor gene by CpG methylation in human carcinomas. Proc Natl Acad Sci U S A. 1995;92:7416–9.
27. Guilford PJ, Hopkins JB, Grady WM, et al. E-cadherin germline mutations define an inherited cancer syndrome dominated by diffuse gastric cancer. Hum Mutat. 1999;14:249–55.
28. Ghatak S, Chakraborty P, Sarkar SR, et al. Novel APC gene mutations associated with protein alteration in diffuse type gastric cancer. BMC Med Genet. 2017;18:61–72.
29. Clements WM, Wang J, Sarnaik A, et al. β-catenin mutation is a frequent cause of Wnt pathway activation in gastric cancer. Cancer Res. 2002;62:3503–6.
30. Berx G, Becker KF, Hofler H, et al. Mutations of the human E-cadherin (CDH1) gene. Hum Mutat. 1998;2:226–37.
31. Chan AO, Luk JM, Hui WM, et al. Molecular biology of gastric carcinoma: from laboratory to bedside. J Gastroenterol Hepatol. 1999;4:1150–60.
32. Guilford P, Blair V, More H, et al. A short guide to hereditary diffuse gastric cancer. Hered Cancer Clin Pract. 2007;5:183–94.
33. Gayther SA, Gorringe KL, Ram SJ, et al. Identification of germ-line E-cadherin mutations in gastric cancer families of European origin. Cancer Res. 1998;58:4086–9.
34. Richards FM, McKee SA, Rajpar MH, et al. Germline E-cadherin gene (CDH1) mutations predispose to familial gastric cancer and colorectal cancer. Hum Mol Genet. 1999;8:607–10.
35. Salahshor S, Hou H, Diep CB, et al. A germline E-cadherin mutation in a family with gastric and colon cancer. Int J Mol Med. 2001;8:439–43.
36. Lee TL, Leung WK, Chan MW, et al. Detection of gene promoter hypermethylation in the tumour and serum of patients with gastric carcinoma. Clin Cancer Res. 2002;8:1761–6.
37. Grady WM, Willis J, Guilford PJ, et al. Methylation of the CDH1 promoter as the second genetic hit in hereditary diffuse gastric cancer. Nat Genet. 2000;26:16–7.
38. Machado JC, Oliveira C, Carvalho R, et al. E-cadherin gene (CDH1) promoter methylation as the second hit in sporadic diffuse gastric carcinoma. Oncogene. 2001;20:1525–8.
39. Wilcox R, Perpich M, Noffsinger A, et al. Hereditary diffuse gastric cancer: multidisciplinary case report with review of the literature. Patholog Res Int. 2011; https://doi.org/10.4061/2011/845821
40. Barber M, Murrell A, Ito Y, et al. Mechanisms and sequelae of E-cadherin silencing in hereditary diffuse gastric cancer. J Pathol. 2008;216:295–306.
41. Graziano F, Humar B, Guilford P. The role of the E-cadherin gene (CDH1) in diffuse gastric cancer susceptibility: from the laboratory to clinical practice. Ann Oncol. 2003;14:1705–13.
42. Caldas C, Carneiro F, Lynch HT, et al. Familial gastric cancer: overview and guidelines for management. J Med Genet. 1999;36:873e80.
43. Oliveira C, Bordin MC, Grehan N, et al. Screening E-cadherin in gastric cancer families reveals germline mutations only in hereditary diffuse gastric cancer kindred. Hum Mutat. 2002;19:510e17.
44. Pharoah PD, Guilford P, Caldas C. Incidence of gastric cancer and breast cancer in CDH1 (E-cadherin) mutation carriers from hereditary diffuse gastric cancer families. Gastroenterology. 2001;121:1348–53.
45. Chan JK, Wong CS. Loss of E-cadherin is the fundamental defect in diffuse-type gastric carcinoma and infiltrating lobular carcinoma of the breast. Adv Anat Pathol. 2001;8:165–72.
46. WHO Classification of Tumours Editorial Board (2019) WHO classification of tumours: digestive system tumours, 5th ed., vol 1. pp 85–92
47. 90th Annual Meeting of the Japanese Gastric Cancer Association, Kyoto, Japan (2018) Reports of national registration analysis results: surgical cases 2009
48. Dawson H, Novotny A, Becker K, et al. Macroscopy predicts tumour progression in gastric cancer: a retrospective patho-historical analysis based on Napoleon Bonaparte's autopsy report. Dig Liver Dis. 2016;48:1378–85.
49. Arai T, Sakurai U, Sawabe M, et al. Frequent microsatellite instability in papillary and solid-type, poorly differentiated adenocarcinomas of the stomach. Gastric Cancer. 2013;16:505–12.
50. Ghotli ZA, Serra S, Chetty R. Clear cell (glycogen rich) gastric adenocarcinoma: a distinct tubulo-papillary variant with a predilection for the cardia/gastro-oesophageal region. Pathology. 2007;39:466–9.
51. Japanese Gastric Cancer Association (2011) Japanese classification of gastric carcinoma: 3rd English ed. Gastric Cancer 14:101–112
52. Huang Q, Zou X. Clinicopathology of early gastric carcinoma: an update for pathologists and gastroenterologists. Gastrointest Tumours. 2017;3:115–24.
53. Yu H, Fang C, Chen L, et al. Worse prognosis in papillary, compared to tubular, early gastric carcinoma. J Cancer. 2017;8:117–23.

54. Marrelli D, Pedrazzani C, Morgagni D, et al. Changing clinical and pathological features of gastric cancer over time. Bri J Surg. 2011;98:1273–83.
55. Wu H, Rusiecki JA, Zhu K, et al. Stomach carcinoma incidence patterns in the United States by histologic type and anatomic site. Cancer Epidemiol Biomarkers Prev. 2009;18:1945–52.
56. Lauwers GY, Carneiro F, Graham DY, et al. Gastric carcinoma. In: Bosman FT, Carneiro F, Hruban RH, Theise ND, editors. WHO classification of tumours of the digestive system. 4th ed. Lyon: IARC Press; 2010. p. 48–58.
57. Kwon CH, Kim YK, Lee S, et al. Gastric poorly cohesive carcinoma: a correlative study of mutational signatures and prognostic significance based on histopathological subtypes. Histopathol. 2018;72:556–68.
58. Mariette C, Carneiro F, Grabsch HI, et al. Consensus on the pathological definition and classification of poorly cohesive gastric carcinoma. Gastric Cancer. 2019;22(1):1–9.
59. Liu K, Wan J, Bei Y, et al. Prognostic impact of different histological types on gastric adenocarcinoma: a surveillance, epidemiology, and end results database analysis. Pathol Oncol Res. 2017;23:881–7.
60. Voron T, Messager M, Duhamel A, et al. Is signet-ring cell carcinoma a specific entity among gastric cancers? Gastric Cancer. 2015;19:1027–40.
61. Jiang H, Zhang H, Tian L, et al. The difference in clinic-pathological features between signet ring cell carcinoma and gastric mucinous adenocarcinoma. Tumor Biol. 2013;34:2625–31.
62. Jian-Hui C, Shi-Rong C, Hui W, et al. Gastric mucinous cancer histology: clinicopathological characteristics and prognostic value. Gastroenterol Res Pract. 2016;2016:8947505. (Open access)
63. Yin C, Li D, Sun Z, et al. Clinicopathologic features and prognosis analysis of mucinous gastric carcinoma. Med Oncol. 2012;29:864–70.
64. Jass JR, Sobin LH, Watanabe H. The World Health Organization's histologic classification of gastrointestinal tumors. A commentary on the second edition. Cancer. 1990;66:2162–7.
65. Bosman FT, Carneiro F, Hruban RH. WHO classification of tumours of the digestive system, vol. 4. Lyon: International Agency for Research on Cancer; 2010.
66. Hsu JT, Wang CW, Le PH, et al. Clinicopathological characteristics and outcomes in stage I-III mucinous gastric adenocarcinoma: a retrospective study at a single medical center. World J Surg Oncol. 2016;14:123.
67. Shi C, Yang B, Chen Q, et al. Retrospective analysis of adjuvant intraperitoneal chemotherapy effect prognosis of resectable gastric cancer. Oncology. 2011;80:289–95.
68. Choi JS, Kim MA, Lee HE, et al. Mucinous gastric carcinomas: clinicopathologic and molecular analyses. Cancer. 2009;115:3581–90.
69. Albarello L, Pecciarini L, Doglioni C. HER2 testing in gastric cancer. Adv Anat Pathol. 2011;18:53–9.
70. Japanese Gastric Cancer Association. Japanese gastric cancer treatment guidelines 2018 (5th ed.). Gastric Cancer. 2020; https://doi.org/10.1007/s10120-020-01042-y. Online ahead of print
71. Thrumurthy SG, Chaudry MA, Hochhauser D, et al. The diagnosis and management of gastric cancer. BMJ. 2013;347:f6367.
72. Japanese Gastric Cancer Association. Japanese classification of gastric carcinoma. 15th ed. Kanehara Shuppan; 2017.
73. Nagtegaal ID, Odze RD, Klimstra D, et al. The 2019 WHO classification of tumours of the digestive system. Histopathol. 2020;76:182–8.
74. Stelzner S, Emmrich P. The mixed type in Laurén's classification of gastric carcinoma. Histologic description and biologic behaviour. Gen Diagn Pathol. 1997;143:39–48.
75. Horiuchi Y, Fujisaki J, Yamamoto N, et al. Undifferentiated-type predominant mixed-type early gastric cancer is a significant risk factor for requiring additional surgeries after endoscopic submucosal dissection. Sci Rep. 2020;10:6748.
76. Horiuchi Y, Ida S, Yamamoto N, et al. Feasibility of further expansion of the indications for endoscopic submucosal dissection in undifferentiated-type early gastric cancer. Gastric Cancer. 2020;23:285–92.
77. Yamada T, Yoshikawa T, Taguri M, et al. The survival difference between gastric cancer patients from the UK and Japan remains after weighted propensity score analysis considering all background factors. Gastric Cancer. 2016;19:479–89.
78. Barros-Silva J, Leitão D, Afonso L, et al. Association of ERBB2 gene status with histopathological parameters and disease-specific survival in gastric carcinoma patients. Br J Cancer. 2009;100:487–93.
79. Carvalho B, Buffart TE, Reisc RM, et al. Mixed gastric carcinomas show similar chromosomal aberrations in both their diffuse and glandular components by microarray – comparative genomic hybridisation (array CGH). Cell Oncol. 2006;28:283–94.
80. Kim MA, Jung EJ, Lee HS, et al. Evaluation of HER-2 gene status in gastric carcinoma using immunohistochemistry, fluorescence in situ hybridization, and real-time quantitative polymerase chain reaction. Hum Pathol. 2007;38:1386–93.
81. Lim H, Park YS, Lee JH, et al. Features of gastric carcinoma with lymphoid stroma associated with Epstein–Barr virus. Clin Gastroenterol Hepatol. 2015;13:1738–44.
82. Watanabe H, Enjoji M, Imai T. Gastric carcinoma with lymphoid stroma: its morphologic characteristics and prognostic correlations. Cancer. 1976;38:232–443.
83. Burke AP, Yen TS, Shekitka KM, et al. Lymphoepithelial carcinoma of the stomach with Epstein-Barr virus demonstrated by polymerase chain reaction. Mod Pathol. 1990;3:377–80.

84. Nakamura S, Ueki T, Yao T, et al. Epstein-Barr virus in gastric carcinoma with lymphoid stroma. Special reference to its detection by the polymerase chain reaction and in situ hybridization in 99 tumours, including a morphologic analysis. Cancer. 1994;73:2239–49.
85. MacCarty WC, Mahle AE. Relation of differentiation and lymphocytic infiltration to postoperative longevity in gastric carcinoma. J Lab Clin Med. 1922;6:473–80.
86. Song HJ, Srivastava A, Lee J, et al. Host inflammatory response predicts survival of patients with Epstein-Barr virus-associated gastric carcinoma. Gastroenterol. 2010;139:84–92.e82.
87. Grogg KL, Lohse CM, Pankratz VS, et al. Lymphocyte-rich gastric cancer: associations with Epstein-Barr virus, microsatellite instability, histology, and survival. Mod Pathol. 2003;16:641–51.
88. Hamazaki M, Sawayama K, Kuriya T. Stomach cancer with lymphoid stroma. J Karyopathol. 1968;12:115–20.
89. Lee JH, Kim SH, Han SH, et al. Clinicopathological and molecular characteristics of Epstein–Barr virus-associated gastric carcinoma: a meta-analysis. J Gastroenterol Hepatol. 2009;24:354–65.
90. Cheng N, Hui DY, Liu Y, et al. Is gastric lymphoepithelioma-like carcinoma a special subtype of EBV-associated gastric carcinoma? New insight based on clinicopathological features and EBV genome polymorphisms. Gastric Cancer. 2015;18:246–55.
91. Oliveira C, Seruca R, Seixas M, et al. The clinicopathological features of gastric carcinomas with microsatellite instability may be mediated by mutations of different "target genes": a study of the TGFbeta RII, IGFII R, and BAX genes. Am J Pathol. 1998;153:1211–9.
92. Hissong E, Ramrattan G, Zhang P, et al. Gastric carcinomas with lymphoid stroma: an evaluation of the histopathologic and molecular features. Am J Surg Pathol. 2018;42:453–62.
93. Liu X, Cheng Y, Sheng W, et al. Analysis of clinicopathologic features and prognostic factors in hepatoid adenocarcinoma of the stomach. Am J Surg Pathol. 2010;34:1465–71.
94. Lin CY, Yeh HC, Hsu CM, et al. Clinicopathological features of gastric hepatoid adenocarcinoma. Biom J. 2015;38:65–9.
95. Zhao M, Sun L, Lai JZ, et al. Expression of RNA-binding protein LIN28 in classic gastric hepatoid carcinomas, gastric fetal type gastrointestinal adenocarcinomas, and hepatocellular carcinomas: an immunohistochemical study with comparison to SALL4, alpha-fetoprotein, glypican-3, and Hep Par1. Pathol Res Pract. 2018;214:1707–12.
96. Ushiku T, Shinozaki A, Shibahara J, et al. SALL4 represents fetal gut differentiation of gastric cancer, and is diagnostically useful in distinguishing hepatoid gastric carcinoma from hepatocellular carcinoma. Am J Surg Pathol. 2010;34:533–40.
97. Liu X, Sheng W, Wang Y. An analysis of clinicopathological features and prognosis by comparing hepatoid adenocarcinoma of the stomach with AFP-producing gastric cancer. J Surg Oncol. 2012;106:299–303.
98. Chang YC, Nagasue N, Abe S, et al. Comparison between the clinicopathologic features of AFP-positive and AFP-negative gastric cancers. Am J Gastroenterol. 1992;87:321–5.
99. Bourreille J, Metayer P, Sauger F, et al. Existence d'alpha-foetoproteine au cours d'un cancer secondaire du foie d'origine gastrique. Presse Méd. 1970;78:1277–8.
100. Ishikura H, Kirimoto K, Shamoto M, et al. Hepatoid adenocarcinoma of the stomach: an analysis of seven cases. Cancer. 1986;58:119–26.
101. Bozkaya Y, Demirci NS, Kurtipek A, et al. Clinicopathological and prognostic characteristics in patients with AFP-secreting gastric carcinoma. Mol Clin Oncol. 2017;7:267–74.
102. Matsunou H, Konishi F, Jalal RE, et al. Alpha-fetoprotein-producing gastric carcinoma with enteroblastic differentiation. Cancer. 1994;73:534–40.
103. Murakami T, Yao T, Mitomi H, et al. Clinicopathologic and immunohistochemical characteristics of gastric adenocarcinoma with enteroblastic differentiation: a study of 29 cases. Gastric Cancer. 2016;19:498–507.
104. Kodama T, Kameya T, Hirota T, et al. Production of alpha-fetoprotein, normal serum proteins, and human chorionic gonadotropin in stomach cancer: histologic and immunohistochemical analyses of 35 cases. Cancer. 1981;48:1647–55.
105. Govender D, Ramdial PK, Clarke B, et al. Clear cell (glycogen-rich) gastric adenocarcinoma. Ann Diagn Pathol. 2004;8:69–73.
106. Ghotli ZA, Serra S, Chetty R. Clear cell (glycogen rich) gastric adenocarcinoma: a distinct tubulo-papillary variant with a predilection for the cardia/gastro-oesophageal region. Pathol. 2007;39:466–9.
107. Lauwers GY, Carneiro F, Graham DY, et al. Gastric carcinoma. In: Bosman FT, Carneiro F, Hruban RH, Theise ND, editors. WHO classification of tumours of the digestive system. 4th ed. Lyon: International Agency for Research on Cancer; 2010.
108. Kumashiro Y, Yao T, Aishima S, et al. Hepatoid adenocarcinoma of the stomach: histogenesis and progression in association with intestinal phenotype. Hum Pathol. 2007;38:857–63.
109. Akazawa Y, Saito T, Hayashi T, et al. Next-generation sequencing analysis for gastric adenocarcinoma with enteroblastic differentiation: emphasis on the relationship with hepatoid adenocarcinoma. Hum Pathol. 2018;78:79–88.
110. Kinjo T, Taniguchi H, Kushima R, et al. Histologic and immunohistochemical analyses of α-fetoprotein-producing cancer of the stomach. Am J Surg Pathol. 2012;36:56–65.
111. Ushiku T, Uozaki H, Shinozaki A, et al. Glypican 3-expressing gastric carcinoma: distinct subgroup unifying hepatoid, clear-cell, and α-fetoprotein-

producing gastric carcinomas. Cancer Sci. 2009;100:626–32.
112. Cheng Y, Du M, Wang Y, et al. Micropapillary early gastric carcinoma with distinct Clinicopathologic features, high risk for lymph node metastasis, and dismal prognosis: a multicenter Clinicopathologic study of 29 cases identified in 1890 early gastric carcinoma radical surgery. Human Path. 2019;83:149–58.
113. Huang Q, Fang C, Shi J, et al. Differences in clinicopathology of early gastric carcinoma between proximal and distal location in 438 Chinese patients. Sci Rep. 2015;5:13439.
114. Fang C, Shi J, Sun Q, et al. Risk factors of lymph node metastasis in early gastric carcinomas diagnosed by WHO criteria in 379 Chinese patients. J Dig Dis. 2016;17:526–37.
115. Eom DW, Kang GH, Han SH, et al. Gastric micropapillary carcinoma: a distinct subtype with a significantly worse prognosis in TNM stages I and II. Am J Surg Pathol. 2011;35:84–91.
116. Zhang Q, Ming J, Zhang S, et al. Micropapillary component in gastric adenocarcinoma: an aggressive variant associated with poor prognosis. Gastric Cancer. 2015;18:93–9.
117. Fujita T, Gotohda N, Kato Y, et al. Clinicopathological features of stomach cancer with invasive micropapillary component. Gastric Cancer. 2012;15:179–87.
118. Ohtsuki Y, Kuroda N, Yunoki S, et al. Immunohistochemical analysis of invasive micropapillary carcinoma pattern in four cases of gastric cancer. Med Mol Morphol. 2013;46:114–21.
119. DobriĐoiu M, Stepan AE, Vere CC, et al. Study of histopatological parameters of gastric carcinomas with micropapillary component. Curr Health Sci J. 2018;44:225–30.
120. Lewin E, Daroca P, Sikka S, et al. Gastric adenocarcinoma of the fundic gland type treated by endoscopic mucosal resection: a case report and review of the literature. Case Rep Pathol. 2016;2016:8646927.
121. Tsukamoto T, Yokoi T, Maruta S, et al. Gastric adenocarcinoma with chief cell differentiation. Pathol Int. 2007;57:517–22.
122. Ueyama H, Yao T, Nakashima Y, et al. Gastric adenocarcinoma of fundic gland type (chief cell predominant type): proposal for a new entity of gastric adenocarcinoma. Am J Surg Pathol. 2010;34:609–19.
123. Kushima R, Sekine S, Matsubara A, et al. Gastric adenocarcinoma of the fundic gland type shares common genetic and phenotypic features with pyloric gland adenoma. Path Int. 2013;63:318–25.
124. Ueo T, Yonemasu H, Ishida T. Gastric adenocarcinoma of fundic gland type with unusual behaviour. Dig Endosc. 2014;26:293–4.
125. Miyazawa M, Matsuda M, Yano M, et al. Gastric adenocarcinoma of fundic gland type: five cases treated with endoscopic resection. World J Gastroenterol. 2015;21:8208–14.
126. Tohda G, Osawa T, Asada Y. Gastric adenocarcinoma of fundic gland type: endoscopic and clinicopathological features. World J Gastrointest End. 2016;8:244–51.
127. Singhi AD, Lazenby AJ, Montgomery EA. Gastric adenocarcinoma with chief cell differentiation: a proposal for reclassification as oxyntic gland polyp/adenoma. Am J Surg Pathol. 2012;36:1030–5.
128. Terada T. Well differentiated adenocarcinoma of the stomach composed of chief cell-like cells and parietal cells (Gastric adenocarcinoma of fundic gland type). Int J Clin Exp Path. 2011;4:797–8.
129. Benedict MA, Lauwers GY, Jain D. Gastric adenocarcinoma of the fundic gland type: update and literature review. Am J Clin Pathol. 2018;149:461–73.
130. Ueyama H, Matsumoto K, Nagahara A, et al. Gastric adenocarcinoma of the fundic gland type (chief cell predominant type). Endoscopy. 2014;46:153–7.
131. Hidaka Y, Mitomi H, Saito T, et al. Alteration in the Wnt/β-catenin signalling pathway in gastric neoplasias of fundic gland (chief cell predominant) type. Hum Pathol. 2013;44:2438–48.
132. Matsusaka T, Watanabe H, Enjoji M. Oat-cell carcinoma of the stomach. Fukuoka Igaku Zasshi. 1976;67:65–73.
133. Wu QQ, Qiang WG, Wang F, et al. Management of primary gastric small cell carcinoma in China. Int J Clin Exp Med. 2015;8:1589–97.
134. Takaku H, Oka K, Naoi Y, et al. Primary advanced gastric small cell carcinoma: a case report and review of the literature. Am J Gastroenterol. 1999;94:1402–4.
135. Murakami H, Rino Y, Yamanaka S, et al. Paraneoplastic neurological syndrome in a patient with gastric cancer. Gastric Cancer. 2010;13:204–8.
136. Fukuda T, Ohnishi Y, Nishimaki T, et al. Early gastric cancer of the small cell type. Am J Gastroenterol. 1988;83:1176–9.
137. Bakogeorgos M, Kalkanis D, Katsaounis P, et al. Small cell carcinoma of the stomach: a report of two cases and a review of the literature. Mol Clin Oncol. 2018;9:11–6.
138. Kim KO, Lee HY, Chun SH, et al. Clinical overview of extrapulmonary small cell carcinoma. J Korean Med Sci. 2006;21:833–7.
139. Matsubayashi H, Takagaki S, Otsubo T, et al. Advanced gastric glandular-endocrine cell carcinoma with 1-year survival after gastrectomy. Gastric Cancer. 2000;3:226–33.
140. Hassan MM, Phan A, Li D, et al. Risk factors associated with neuroendocrine tumors: a U.S.-based case-control study. Int J Cancer. 2008;123:867–73.
141. Kusayanagi S, Konishi K, Miyasaka N, et al. Primary small cell carcinoma of the stomach. J Gastroenterol Hepatol. 2003;18:743–7.
142. Namikawa T, Kobayashi M, Okabayashi T, et al. Primary gastric small cell carcinoma: report of a case and review of the literature. Med Mol Morphol. 2005;38:256–61.

143. O'Byrne KJ, Cherukuri AK, Khan MI, et al. Extrapulmonary small cell gastric carcinoma. A case report and review of the literature. Acta Oncol. 1977;36:78–80.
144. Chejfec G, Gould VE. Malignant gastric neuroendocrinomas. Ultrastructural and biochemical characterization of their secretory activity. Hum Pathol. 1977;8:433–40.
145. Okita NT, Kato K, Takahari D, et al. Neuroendocrine tumors of the stomach: chemotherapy with cisplatin plus irinotecan is effective for gastric poorly-differentiated neuroendocrine carcinoma. Gastric Cancer. 2011;14:161–5.
146. Hirata Y, Sakamoto N, Yamamoto H, et al. Gastric carcinoid with ectopic production of ACTH and beta-MSH. Cancer. 1976;37:377–85.
147. Arai K, Matsuda M. Gastric small-cell carcinoma in Japan: a case report and review of the literature. Am J Clin Oncol. 1998;21:458–61.
148. Matsui K, Kitagawa M, Miwa A, et al. Small cell carcinoma of the stomach: a clinicopathologic study of 17 cases. Am J Gastroenterol. 1991;86:1167–75.
149. Matsui K, Jin XM, Kitagawa M, et al. Clinicopathologic features of neuroendocrine carcinomas of the stomach: appraisal of small cell and large cell variants. Arch Pathol Lab Med. 1998;122:1010–7.
150. Travis WD, Brambilla E, Nicholson AG, et al. On behalf of the WHO panel. The 2015 World Health Organization classification of lung tumors impact of genetic, clinical and radiologic advances since the 2004 classification. J Thorac Oncol. 2015;10:1243–60.
151. Tsuneyama K, Sasaki M, Sabit A, et al. A case report of gastric carcinosarcoma with rhabdomyosarcomatous and neuroendocrinal differentiation. Pathol Res Pract. 1999;195:93–7.
152. Yamazaki K. A gastric carcinosarcoma with neuroendocrine cell differentiation and undifferentiated spindle-shaped sarcoma component possibly progressing from the conventional tubular adenocarcinoma; an immunohistochemical and ultrastructural study. Virchows Arch. 2003;442:77–81.
153. Kuroda N, Oonishi K, Iwamura S, et al. Gastric carcinosarcoma with neuroendocrine differentiation as the carcinoma component and leiomyosarcomatous and myofibroblastic differentiation as the sarcomatous component. APMIS. 2006;114:234–8.
154. Haratake J, Horie A, Inoshita S. Gastric small cell carcinoma with squamous and neuroendocrine differentiation. Pathology. 1992;24:16–20.
155. Brenner B, Tang LH, Klimstra DS, et al. Small-cell carcinomas of the gastrointestinal tract: a review. J Clin Oncol. 2004;22:2730–9.
156. Bartley AN, Rashid A, Fournier KF, et al. Neuroendocrine and mucinous differentiation in signet ring cell carcinoma of the stomach: evidence for a common cell of origin in composite tumors. Hum Pathol. 2011;42:1420–9.
157. Li AF, Li AC, Hsu CY, et al. Small cell carcinomas in gastrointestinal tract: immunohistochemical and clinicopathological features. J Clin Pathol. 2010;63:620–5.
158. Rindi G, Azzoni C, La Rosa S, et al. ECL cell tumor and poorly differentiated endocrine carcinoma of the stomach: prognostic evaluation by pathological analysis. Gastroenterol. 1999;116:532–42.
159. Won OH, Farman J, Krishnan MN, et al. Squamous cell carcinoma of the stomach. Am J Gastroenterol. 1978;69:594–8.
160. Lim SM, Jung ES, Shin SK, et al. A case of synchronous squamous cell carcinoma in the esophagus and stomach. Gut Liver. 2012;6:118–21.
161. Dursun M, Yaldiz M, Işikdoğan A, et al. Primary squamous cell carcinoma of the stomach: a case report and review of the literature. Eur J Gastroenterol Hepatol. 2003;15:329–30.
162. González-Sánchez JA, Vitón R, Collantes E, et al. Primary Squamous Cell Carcinoma of the Stomach. Clin Med Insights Oncol. 2017; https://doi.org/10.1177/1179554916686076.
163. Parks RE. Squamous neoplasms of the stomach. Am J Roentgenol Radium Ther Nucl Med. 1967;101:447–9.
164. Japanese classification of gastric carcinoma (2011) 3rd English ed. Gastric Cancer 14:101–112
165. Mingazzini PL, Barsotti P, Albedi FM. Adenosquamous carcinoma of the stomach: histological, histochemical and ultrastructural observations. Histopathology. 1983;7:433–43.
166. Straus R, Heschel S, Fortmann DJ. Primary adenosquamous carcinoma of the stomach. A case report and review. Cancer. 1969;24:985–95.
167. Davidson C. Chorioepithelium and Magekrebs, eine seltene Verschmelzung zweier bosartiger Geschwulste. Charite Ann. 1905;29:12.
168. Kobayashi A, Hasebe T, Endo Y, et al. Primary gastric choriocarcinoma: two case reports and a pooled analysis of 53 cases. Gastric Cancer. 2005;8:178–85.
169. Yoon JH, Kim MS, Kook EH, et al. Primary gastric choriocarcinoma: two case reports and review of the literatures. Cancer Res Treat. 2008;40:145–50.
170. Satake N, Chikakiyo M, Yagi T, et al. Gastric cancer with choriocarcinoma and yolk sac tumor components: case report. Pathol Int. 2011;61:156–60.
171. Hirano Y, Hara T, Nozawa H, et al. Combined choriocarcinoma, neuroendocrine cell carcinoma and tubular adenocarcinoma in the stomach. World J Gastroenterol. 2008;14:3269–72.
172. Motoyama T, Aizawa K, Fujiwara T, et al. Coexistence of choriocarcinoma and hepatoid adenocarcinoma in the stomach. Pathol Int. 1994;44:716–21.
173. Garcia RL, Ghali VS. Gastric choriocarcinoma and yolk sac tumour in a man: observations about its possible origin. Hum Pathol. 1985;16:955–8.
174. Gurzu S, Copotoiu C, Tugui A, et al. Primary gastric choriocarcinoma – a rare and aggressive tumor with multilineage differentiation: a case report. World J Clin Cases. 2019;7:1837–43.

175. Masuda R, Isoyama T, Bandou T, et al. A primary choriocarcinoma of the stomach with a review of 45 cases in Japan. Gan No Rinsho. 1990;36:1025–30.
176. Tomita K, Kuwajima M. Chorionic gonadotropin in gastric cancer tissue, especially its relation to the patient's prognosis. Gan No Rinsho. 1981;27:2.
177. Yakeishi Y, Mori M, Enjoji M. Distribution of beta-human chorionic gonadotropin-positive cells in non-cancerous gastric mucosa and in malignant gastric tumours. Cancer. 1990;66:695–701.
178. Pick L. Uber die chorioepthelahnlich metastsierende from desmagencarcinomas. Klin Wochenscher. 1926;5:1.
179. Liu AY, Chan WY, Ng EK, et al. Gastric choriocarcinoma shows characteristics of adenocarcinoma and gestational choriocarcinoma: a comparative genomic hybridization and fluorescence in situ hybridization study. Diagn Mol Pathol. 2001;10:161–5.
180. Nakamura K, Sugano H, Takagi K. Carcinoma of stomach in incipient phase: its histogenesis and histological appearances. Gann. 1968;59:251–8.
181. Tatematsu M, Ichinose M, Miki K, et al. Gastric intestinal phenotypic expression of human stomach cancers as revealed by pepsinogen immunohistochemistry and mucin histochemistry. Acta Pathol Jpn. 1990;40:494–504.
182. Kabashima A, Yao T, Tsuneyoshi M. Gastric and intestinal phenotypic expression in the carcinomas and background mucosa of multiple early gastric carcinomas. Histopathol. 2000;37:513–22.
183. Yoshino T, Shimoda T, Saitou A, et al. Macroscopic features of differentiated gastric adenocarcinoma with gastric or intestinal phenotype expression in early gastric cancer. Stomach and Intestine. 1999;34:507–25.
184. Koseki K, Takizawa T, Koike M, et al. Subclassification of well differentiated gastric cancer with reference to biological behavior and malignancy, gastric type vs intestinal type, and papillary carcinoma vs tubular carcinoma. Stomach and Intestine. 1999;34:507–12.
185. Oya M, Yao T, Tsuneyoshi M. A correlation of intramural invasion with mucin histochemistry, and immunohistochemical expressions of oncogene-related proteins in early gastric carcinoma. Stomach and Intestine. 1997;32:31–9.
186. Fiocca R, Villani L, Tenti P, et al. Widespread expression of intestinal markers in gastric carcinoma: a light and electron microscopic study using BD-5 monoclonal antibody. J Clin Pathol. 1988;41:178–87.
187. Yao T, Kajiwara M, Kuroiwa S, et al. Malignant transformation of gastric hyperplastic polyps: alteration phenotypes, proliferative activity, and p53 expression. Hum Pathol. 2002;33:1016–22.
188. Kabashima A, Yao T, Maehara Y, et al. Relationship between biological behavior and phenotypic expression in undifferentiated-type gastric carcinomas. Gastric Cancer. 2005;8:220–7.
189. Jing H, Geng M, Meng Q, et al. Sarcomatoid carcinoma of the stomach with osteoclast-like giant cells. Tumori. 2012;98:82e–5e.
190. Willems S, Carneiro F, Geboes K. Gastric carcinoma with osteoclast-like giant cells and lymphoepithelioma-like carcinoma of the stomach: two of a kind? Histopathol. 2005;47:320–34.
191. Agaimy A, Daum O, Markl B, et al. SWI/SNF complex–deficient undifferentiated/rhabdoid carcinomas of the gastrointestinal tract: a series of 13 cases highlighting mutually exclusive loss of SMARCA4 and SMARCA2 and frequent co-inactivation of SMARCB1 and SMARCA2. Am J Surg Pathol. 2016;40:544–53.
192. Agaimy A, Rau TT, Hartmann A, et al. SMARCB1 (INI1)-negative rhabdoid carcinomas of the gastrointestinal tract: clinicopathologic and molecular study of a highly aggressive variant with literature review. Am J Surg Pathol. 2014;38:910–20.

Helicobacter pylori Negative Gastric Cancer

16

Helicobacter pylori, the organism related to gastroduodenal ulcer, has been classified as a mutagen by World Health Organization [1, 2]. This pathogen related to chronic persistent gastritis that may result in gastric preneoplastic lesions like gastric atrophy, intestinal metaplasia and dysplasia and eradication of HP results in reduction of development of cancer by preventing development of preneoplastic lesions [3–6]. However, contrary to these reports, there are documented studies reporting gastric cancer in individuals with no evidence of HP infection and these patients are grouped as *H. pylori*-negative gastric cancer (HpNGC) [3, 7, 8]. The described aetiological factors for this special group of patients are rather related to lifestyle, viruses like Epstein-Barr virus [9], collagen vascular disorders [10] and genetic susceptibility [3, 11]. One important group of gastric cancer that does not have an association with HP infection is cardia cancers and incidence of this group of cancer is reportedly increasing, especially in the Western countries [3, 12]. Gastric cancers have also been reported to have familial clustering and are associated with germline mutation in 10% of the cases [3, 13–15]. The gene that has been identified to be involved in germline mutation CDH1 gene and this gene encodes adhesion protein E-cadherin and its mutation is observed in diffuse and familial variants of gastric cancer. Hereditary diffuse gastric cancer (HDGC) has also been associated with CDH1 gene mutation [3, 16, 17]. Mutation is identified in about 70% of the specified group of patients and in 40% of these CDH1 mutant-bearing female patients will get lobular carcinoma of the breast [3, 18]. Criteria for the diagnosis of HDGC by International group are—diffuse type of GC in $<$ 40 years of age with or without family history, to be included amongst the genetic testing for CDH1 gene [3, 19] and these patients may also exhibit mutation in adenomatous polyposis coli gene and associated with death at younger age [3, 20, 21]. Gastric carcinoma of the fundic gland having a predominance of chief cell is believed to originate from the deeper portion of gastric mucosa with no evidence of chronic gastritis or other precursor mucosal changes and this tumour has also been classified as a type of HpNGC [3, 22]. The underlying aetiology of HpNGC is not well understood, possibly this condition is associated with a germline mutation in some specified gene, which requires further research in this aspect [3].

K. Vaiphei, *Interpretation of Endoscopic Biopsy - Gastritis, Gastropathies and Beyond*,
https://doi.org/10.1007/978-981-16-6026-9_16

References

1. Warren J, Marshall B. Unidentified curved bacilli on gastric epithelium in active chronic gastritis. Lancet. 1983;1:1273–5.
2. Schistosomes, liver flukes and Helicobacter pylori. IARC Working Group on the evaluation of carcinogenic risks to humans. Lyon, 7–14 June 1994. IARC Monogr Eval Carcinog Risks Hum. 1994;61:1–241.
3. Yamamoto Y, Fujisaki J, Omae M, et al. Helicobacter pylori-negative gastric cancer: characteristics and endoscopic findings. Dig Endosc. 2015;27:551–61.
4. Uemura N, Okamoto S, Yamamoto S, et al. Helicobacter pylori infection and the development of gastric cancer. N Engl J Med. 2001;345:784–9.
5. Fukase K, Kato M, Kikuchi S, et al. Effect of eradication of Helicobacter pylori on incidence of metachronous gastric carcinoma after endoscopic resection of early gastric cancer: an open-label, randomised controlled trial. Lancet. 2008;372:392–7.
6. Shiota S, Murakawi K, Suzuki R, et al. Helicobacter pylori infection in Japan. Expert Rev Gastroenterol Hepatol. 2013;7:35–40.
7. Kato S, Matsukura N, Tsukada K, et al. Helicobacter pylori infection-negative gastric cancer in Japanese hospital patients: incidence and pathological characteristics. Cancer Sci. 2007;98:790–4.
8. Kakinoki R, Kushima R, Matsubara A, et al. Re-evaluation of histogenesis of gastric carcinomas: a comparative histopathological study between Helicobacter pylori-negative and H. pylori-positive cases. Dig Dis Sci. 2009;54:614–20.
9. Zamcheck N, Grable E, Ley A, et al. Occurrence of gastric cancer among patients with pernicious anemia at the Boston City Hospital. N Engl J Med. 1955;252:1103–10.
10. Watanabe H, Enjoji M, Imai T. Gastric carcinoma with lymphoid stroma. Its morphologic characteristics and prognostic correlations. Cancer. 1976;38:232–43.
11. Cisco RM, Ford JM, Norton JA. Hereditary diffuse gastric cancer: implications of genetic testing for screening and prophylactic surgery. Cancer. 2008;113:1850–6.
12. Kamangar F, Dawsey SM, Blaser MJ, et al. Opposing risks of gastric cardia and noncardia gastric adenocarcinomas associated with Helicobacter pylori seropositivity. J Natl Cancer Inst. 2006;98:1445–52.
13. Setia N, Clark JW, Duda DG, et al. Familial gastric cancers. Oncologist. 2015;20:1365–77.
14. Assumpção P, Araújo T, Khayat A, et al. Hereditary gastric cancer: three rules to reduce missed diagnoses. World J Gastroenterol. 2020;26:1382–93.
15. Oliveira C, Pinheiro H, Figueiredo J, et al. Familial gastric cancer: genetic susceptibility, pathology, and implications for management. Lancet Oncol. 2015;16:e60–70.
16. Oda T, Kanai Y, Oyama T, et al. E-cadherin gene mutations in human gastric carcinoma cell lines. Proc Natl Acad Sci U S A. 1994;91:1858–62.
17. Guilford P, Hopkins J, Harraway J, et al. E-cadherin germline mutations in familial gastric cancer. Nature. 1998;392:402–5.
18. Pharoah PD, Guilford P, Caldas C. Incidence of gastric cancer and breast cancer in CDH1 (E-cadherin) mutation carriers from hereditary diffuse gastric cancer families. Gastroenterology. 2001;121:1348–135.
19. Fitzgerald RC, Hardwick R, Huntsman D, et al. Hereditary diffuse gastric cancer: updated consensus guidelines for clinical management and directions for future research. J Med Genet. 2010;47:436–44.
20. Wood LD, Salaria SN, Cruise MW, et al. Upper GI tract lesions in familial adenomatous polyposis (FAP): enrichment of pyloric gland adenomas and other gastric and duodenal neoplasms. Am J Surg Pathol. 2014;38:389–93.
21. Inoue M, Tsugane S. Epidemiology of gastric cancer in Japan. Postgrad Med J. 2005;81:419–24.
22. Yao T, Ueyama H, Ueo T, et al. Two types of neoplasia in fundic-gland mucosa without Helicobacter pylori infection: gastric carcinoma and polyp with dysplasia. Stom Int. 2014;49:874–80.

17 Primary Gastric Lymphoma: Pathobiology, MALT Lymphoma, Diffuse Large B Cell Lymphoma and Burkitt Lymphoma

Incidence of extra-nodal lymphoma is on the rise in the last two decades. GIT lymphoma is the second commonest type [1–3]. Gastric lymphoma represents one third of extra-nodal lymphomas and more than half are seen in stomach [4]. Otherwise, primary gastric lymphoma (PGL) is not frequently observed disease constituting just about 4 to 20% of all lymphoma cases and just about 5% of primary malignant tumours of stomach [4]. It is a disease frequently seen in individuals above 50 years of age and male gender at least 2 to 3 times more than females [5–7]. About 90% are B cell type and almost one third of PGL are marginal zone B cell lymphoma of mucosa associated lymphoid tissue (MALT) and more than half are diffuse large B cell lymphoma (DLBCL) [8, 9]. World Health Organization (WHO) simply classifies it into pure DLBCL with no histological evidence of MALT lymphoma and DLBCL with histological evidence of MALT lymphoma [10–12]. Distinction between DLBCL and gastric DLBCL(MALT) is not as straightforward, hence WHO (2008) has proposed not to use the term "high-grade MALT lymphoma" rather to label DLBCL for all high-grade B cell lymphomas even in the presence of lymphoepithelial lesion [11, 13]. DLBCLs are non-*Helicobacter pylori* (HP) related and are treated with systemic chemotherapy over the years [14, 15]. There are many literature reporting an association between pure DLBCL with HP infection and early-stage gastric lymphomas with or without MALT component cured by HP eradication alone [16–19]. All these observations suggest importance of HP antigenic genes in HP dependent lymphomagenesis. In addition, many other factors associated with PGL are Epstein–Barr virus and human T cell lymphotropic virus 1. Patients with coeliac disease, inflammatory bowel disease and who on immunosuppressive therapy are prone to develop PGL. *Campylobacter jejuni* is another factor implicated with MALT lymphoma specifically in the pathogenesis of immunoproliferative small intestinal disease [20, 21]. Amongst the treatment modalities for PGL, gastrectomy is carried out for rare selected cases. Other routine practice of treatments includes anti-*H. pylori* eradication, immune and chemotherapy, and radiation. Response to treatment and outcome is influenced by histological subtype and tumour stage, age of patient and patient performance status. Clinical profiles are nonspecific, and patient may present with upper GI symptoms like dyspepsia, indigestion, abdominal fullness, indigestion, post prandial discomfort, vomiting and pain, hunger pain, epigastric discomfort and other functional gastric disorders; less common features include weight loss, night sweat, weakness, haematemesis and melena, jaundice and outlet obstruction and acute abdominal pain due to perforation [22, 23]. These patients may also be found to have hepatomegaly, splenomegaly, lymphadenopathy

K. Vaiphei, *Interpretation of Endoscopic Biopsy - Gastritis, Gastropathies and Beyond*,
https://doi.org/10.1007/978-981-16-6026-9_17

and a palpable epigastric mass [24, 25]. Oesophagogastroduodenoscopy is to be performed in every patient and mucosal biopsy will help to establish the diagnosis and endoscopic examination per se cannot differentiate between the various histological types of lesions [4, 26]. Endoscopic mucosal characters for PGL are ulceration, diffuse infiltration and polypoidal growth. While carrying out endoscopy, it is essential to obtain adequate number of mucosal biopsy specimens from the lesion and surrounding area [26]. Status of *H. pylori* in the endoscopy room may be completed the principle of rapid urease test [27]. Radiology may be of help in determining disease stage. Endoscopic ultrasonography and MRI may be useful to comment on extent of mucosal fold thickness, submucosal involvement, annular constricting lesion, exophytic or endophytic tumour and mesenteric/retroperitoneal lymphadenopathy [28, 29]. Ultrasound may sometimes over stage the tumour specially in a post treatment patient [30]. Fluorodeoxyglucose-positron emission tomography projects an increased and variable uptake as the result of different physiologic activity executed by different segments of gastric mucosa. There will also be variable uptake executed by different tumour types and hence is considered to be an inadequate technique for a definitive diagnosis of a particular gastric neoplasm [31, 32].

Pathobiology of PGL. Conventional histological lymphoma type in stomach is MALTOMA. Mantle cell lymphoma (MZL) conventionally can involve the whole length of intestine, jejunum and duodenum are selectively tend to be involved by enteropathy associated T cell lymphoma and follicular lymphoma, respectively [1, 33, 34]. MALT lymphoma and DLBCL are predominant subtypes that involve stomach. Hypothetical mechanism for extra-nodal lymphoma depends on recirculation of mature lymphocyte between blood and lymphoid tissue. Lymphocytes undergoes activation and uncontrolled proliferation by interacting with endothelial cell of venules via lymphocytic specific receptors and integrins [35, 36]. One an old concept that still holds true is ongoing chronic infections and inflammatory conditions resulting in persistent immune stimulation and other autoimmune disorders that may lead on resulting in epigenetic aberrations resulting in lymphoid cell transformation [37]. About 25% of MZL carry specific chromosomal translocations in certain genes like MALT1 and BCL10 activating NF-κB signalling pathways [38]. In MALT lymphoma, marginal zone B lymphocyte is involved and is characterized by heterogeneous cells predominantly small lymphocytes and monocytoid lymphocytes intermixed with larger cells like immunoblast and centroblast. A diagnostic challenge occurs when number of large cell predominates suggesting transformation into DLBCL [39, 40]. PGL is a B cell neoplasm with aggressive clinical course. Recently WHO categorizes large cell type gastric lymphoma to DLBCL [41]. Pathobiology pathway in the development of DLBCL still is a matter of conjecture i.e. either a de-novo tumour or transformed tumour from low-grade lymphoma. Cytogenetic studies demonstrate gastric MALT lymphomas have different profiles from typical primary gastric DLBCL [42–44]. In addition, MALT lymphomas express membrane monoclonal immunoglobulins, pan-B markers (CD19, CD20 and CD79a) and, CD35 and CD21 which are the markers for marginal zone lymphocytes [4]. DLBCL positive for CD45, CD5 and CD10 are immunophenotypically different, and are prognostic indicators [4, 40–42]. A diagnosis of MALT lymphoma should be made in the presence of characteristic histological features [43, 44].

Pathogenesis of Gastric MALTOMA. To understand the development of this group of lymphoma lies in the fact that 75% of early-stage tumour associated with *H. pylori* infection are treated with antibiotics [1, 45, 46]. The pathobiology of this B cell lymphoma resulted from long-standing antigenic stimulation supported by local T cells and macrophages [47, 48]. Early-stage proliferation is monoclonal yet remains in the local site of antigenic stimulation. With time, additional mutations are acquired spreading beyond local site. Role of *H. pylori* in lymphomagenesis holds true in cases harbouring *H. pylori*. Alternatively, theory of long-standing antigenic stimulation loses its validity in *H. pylori* negative cases suggesting existence of an alternative pathway. MALT lymphoma has been postulated to arise from post-germinal centre memory B cells having the properties of marginal zone and plasmacytic cell types [4, 49]. Chromosomal translocations observed are 11;18 (q21;q21), 14;18(q32;q21), 1;14(p22;q32) and 3;14(p13;q32) and interaction between bcl-10 and MALT1 activates nuclear factor (NF)-kB [4, 50, 51]. 1;14(p22;q32) translocation and bcl-10 overexpression produce transformation and survival advantage to neoplastic B cells [4, 50–53]. Nuclear expression of Bcl-10 or NF-kB is associated with non-responsiveness to antibiotic therapy in early-stage MALTOMAs [54].

Pathogenesis of Gastric DLBCL is a high-grade gastric lymphoma. Origin of DLBCL remains unclear—a de-novo tumour or transformed from a low-grade MALT lymphoma [53, 54]. Bcl-6 is frequently expressed by this tumour and alteration in the promoter region of bcl6 may be translocation, somatic hypermutation or deregulation. Bcl6 overexpression predicts a better prognosis [55]. However, bcl-2 is significantly low in DLBCL or high-grade MALToma than primary extra-nodal high-grade B cell lymphomas. DLBCL and MALTOMA express p53 protein uniformly [23, 56].

Immunohistochemistry. DLBCL are molecularly heterogenous tumour. As a consequence of which there is a shift towards personalized evaluation and therapies. Lymphoma with double-hit pattern has c-Myc and Bcl-2, and/or Bcl6 gene rearrangement, and a lymphoma with double-protein expressor shows co-expression of 2 oncogenes like MYC and Bcl-2 [1, 4, 57, 58]. Prognostic implication of double hit and double expressed gastric lymphoma is uncertain unlike other sites DLBCL [59] and gastric lymphoma having this phenotype has been rarely reported [60]. Rare cases of primary double-hit gastric lymphomas with multiple gene amplifications and/or copy gains of c-Myc, Bcl-2 and Bcl-6, and double-protein phenotype are associated with poor disease outcome [4, 61].

Prognostic Factors. A low-grade and surgically resectable tumour in female patient are the indicators for better outcome [1, 57]. In addition to tumour stage, poor prognostic indicators are elderly individual >60 years of age and an elevated LDH level [4, 57, 62]. Depending upon these three factors, patients can be grouped into 3, i.e. low, intermediate and high risk with a score of 0, 1 or >2 depending upon the presence of these factors. Accordingly, the 5-year disease free survival rates reportedly are 70%, 56% and 29%, respectively [4, 57, 62, 63]. These prognostic indices were applicable to both gastric and non-gastric lymphomas.

17.1 Microscopic Description of Gastric MALT Lymphoma

MALT concept. Isaacson and Wright (1983) were the first to suggest the relationship between histology and clinical behaviours of non-nodal lymphomas to mucosa associated lymphoid tissue (MALT), after observing similarity between immunoproliferative small intestinal disease and primary low-grade gastric B cell lymphoma [64]. Unlike nodal lymphomas, both have indolent course and remain localized for long periods. The indolent properties of these tumours may be attributed to its characteristic homing character and having a specific in vivo pathway. Histologically these cells bear morphological similarities with Peyer's patches [65, 66]. According to WHO, MALT lymphomas are classified as extra-nodal marginal zone lymphomas of MALT type [67]. MALTOMA is defined as extra-nodal lymphoma of small B cells comprising of marginal zone centrocyte or monocytoid like cell, small lymphocytes, immature cells resembling immunoblast and centroblast. These cells may show plasma cell differentiation. MALTOMA cells start in marginal zone extending into inter-follicular region. Neoplastic cells (both mature and immature) typically show propensity to infiltrate gastric epithelial cells with destruction forming lymphoepithelial lesion. Lymphoepithelial lesions are to be differentiated from intra-epithelial lymphocytes which do not associate with epithelial cell destruction. In florid cases, there may be extensive destruction of epithelial cells resulting in only few identifiable epithelial cells in remnant of the partly destroyed glands amongst the sheets atypical lymphoid cells. In such setting utilizing special stains like AB-PAS may be helpful to highlight the epithelial cell component and also the basement membrane of the destroyed glands. Help of immunohistochemistry may also be utilized, CD20 or 45 will highlight the lymphoid cell component and any epithelial cell marker will highlight the epithelial cells including the remnant cells in a destroyed gland. Presence of isolated small lymphocytes within epithelium not sufficient to label as a lymphoepithelial lesion. Lymphoepithelial lesions may also be seen in other lymphomas, not specific for MALT lymphoma. Lymphoepithelial lesions may be frequently observed histology in inflammatory conditions of stomach including florid gastritis [44, 68, 69]. Possibility of MALT lymphoma may be considered in condition with heavy or dense mucosal lymphoid infiltrate identifiable in many of the mucosal biopsy fragments co-existing with lymphoepithelial lesions extending beyond the mucosa into muscularis mucosae and submucosa and associated with cytological atypia [44, 70]. Wotherspoon et al had tabulated important histological features to relate to likelihood of MALT lymphoma [69].

These low-grade lymphomas exhibit a tendency to spread to certain sites like Waldeyer's rings having 5 year survival rate of 94%. Presence of 5–10% of scattered immature lymphoid cells does not alter disease behaviour [71]. Co-existence of MALT lymphoma and DLBCL should not be reported only as high-grade MALT lymphoma but as DLBCL with the presence of MALT lymphoma [67, 71]. There may be focal collection of sheets of centrocyte-like cells often with residual germinal centre and lymphoepithelial lesions. Occasionally also the tumour cells may have signet ring cell appearance [72]. The adjoining to the nodular abnormal mucosa may show varied morphology like epithelial erosions and ulcerations, and chronic gastritis with or without metaplasia. Chronic gastritis can be patchy or diffuse, usually associate with atrophy either of the antrum or the body mucosa, variable grades and types of inflammatory cell infiltration, foveolar hyperplasia and metaplastic epithelium. There can be variable grades of regenerating epithelium and dysplasia. Presence of *H. pylori* should be documented in the biopsies sampled from the non-tumorous, non-ulcerated and non-metaplastic adjoining mucosa. Lymphoid follicles in the lamina propria is invariably present, and may sometimes be a prominent feature qualifying for the diagnosis of follicular gastritis in the adjoining mucosa [44, 68, 70].

Immunohistological features. Malignant lymphomas are primarily classified based on routine H&E stain sections and histological typing with the help of immunohistochemistry staining using specific markers [71]. They are classified based on presence of abnormal genes demonstrable with FISH, various types of PCRs and clonality analysis documented by translocation and gene rearrangement [72, 73]. Marginal zone lymphoma (MZL), a low-grade B cell, lacks specific marker, diagnosis is based on cell morphology and the growth pattern [73]. Hallmark of extra-nodal MZL of MALT type is lymphoepithelial lesions, with no specific immunomarker still so far [73–75] (Fig. 17.1a–h). In nodal MZL, cells proliferate around reactive follicles; splenic MZL cells surround and replace splenic white pulp germinal centres [76, 77]. MALT lymphoma cells express similar immunophenotype to native marginal zone B cells, i.e. CD20+, CD79a+, Bcl2+, IgD2-, IgM+>IgA+>IgG+, CD5-, CD10-, CD23-, Bcl6-, Cyclin D1-, CD43+/-, CD11c+/- [41, 44, 74, 78]. Evaluation of the phenotype is a necessity to establish lineage of the atypical proliferating lymphoid cells and immunoglobulin light chain restriction. Presence of diffuse CD20+ cells +/- CD3+ cells between gastric glands +/- reactive follicles is highly suggestive of lymphoma [74, 77]. Light chain restriction will exclude reactive lymphoid or plasma cells. CD21 and CD10 identify follicular dendritic cell network highlighting the unrecognizable lymphoid follicles. Positive IgD demonstrates follicular mantle zones. Cytokeratin helps to identify the remnant of the epithelial cells in lymphoepithelial lesion. Half of MALT lymphoma cells co-express CD43 and CD20+. Other close differential diagnosis for a low-grade MALToma can be excluded by demonstrating negativity for IgD, CD5, CD10, Bcl6 and cyclin D, rarely MALToma cell may be positive for CD5 or IgD [76, 77]. Ki67 index is usually low in this group of lymphoma but the intervening reactive follicles may have high index [68]. Immunoglobulin superfamily receptor translocation-associated 1 (IRTA1) was identified in myeloma cell line and has been observed to be expressed in MALTOMA [78, 79]. IRTA1 protein has 5 surface receptors involved in humeral immune responses, cellular communication and cell migration. IRTA1 is expressed by marginal zone B cells; IRTA2 by centrocytes, marginal zone B cells and immunoblast, IRTA3 by germinal centre cells, intra-epithelial and interfollicular regions, IRTA4 and IRTA5 by cells in mantle zone [73, 78, 79]. Myeloid cell nuclear differentiation antigen (MNDA) present in leukaemic cell line is a useful marker for normal marginal zone and nodal marginal zone lymphoma cells [80]. MNDA gives an intense nuclear signal in neutrophils, also primary lymphoid follicles a weak nuclear staining. MNDA can be used in differentiating low-grade follicular lymphomas from marginal zone lymphomas [81, 82]. MALT lymphoma may be differentiated from mantle cell lymphoma by the negative staining for cyclinD1, SOX11 and CD5 and from follicular lymphoma by a positive staining by the follicular lymphoma cells for CD10/BCL6 and BCL2 [55, 83–86].

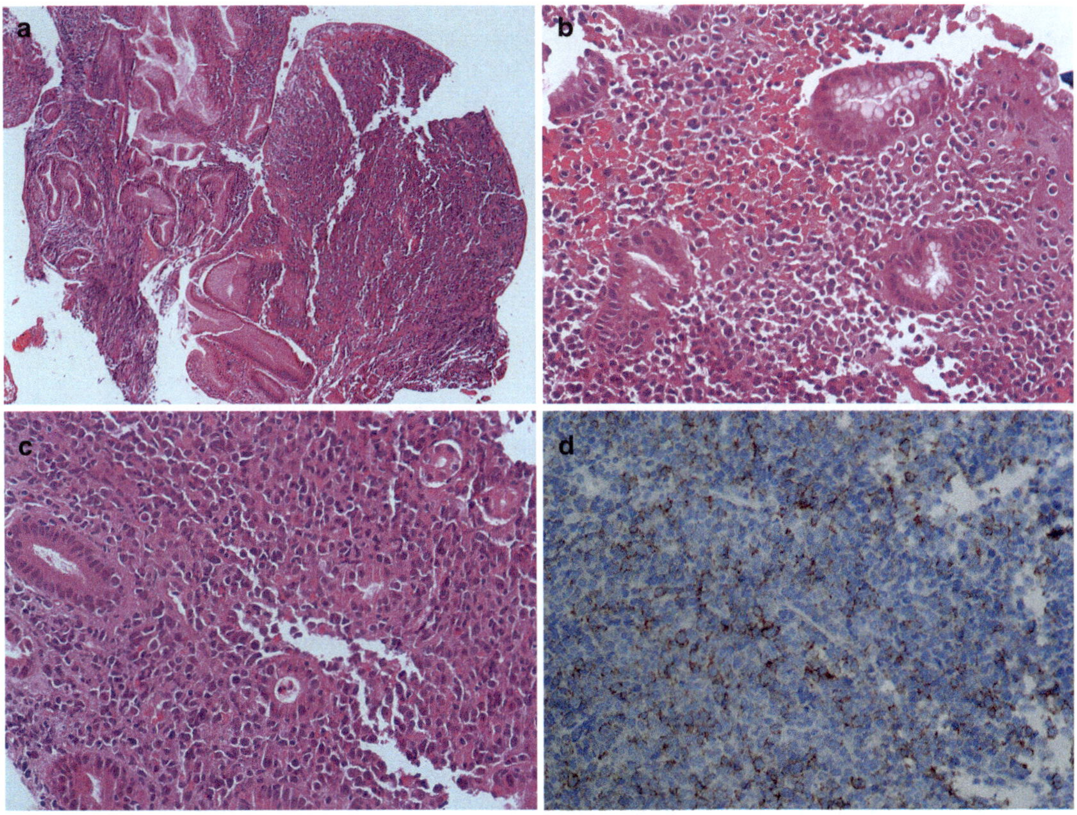

Fig. 17.1 Photomicrographs of a biopsy of MALTOMA. (**a**, **b**) Low- and high-power pictures of HE stained section to show histological changes of chronic gastritis with lamina propria infiltration by monomorphic population of cells. (**c**) High-power picture to show the plasmacytoid cells with destruction of the glands along with scattered eosinophils (HE, ×350). (**d**, **e**) Photomicrographs of immunostained sections using CD138 and CD20, respectively, showing only a few positively stained scattered cells (PAP, ×350). (**f**) Photomicrograph of an immunostained section using cytokeratin to highlight loss of glands (PAP, ×350). (**g**, **h**) Photomicrographs to show almost all the cells are stained positive for kappa light chain and negative for lambda light chain (PAP, ×350)

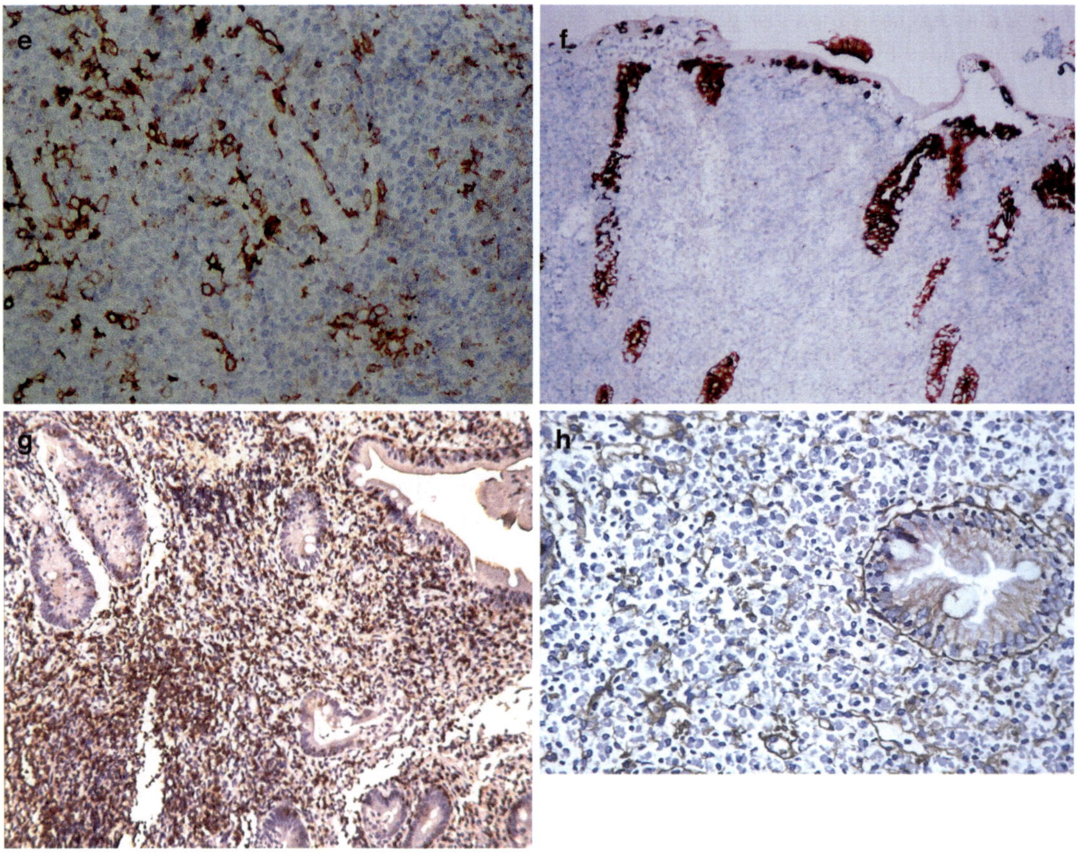

Fig. 17.1 (continued)

Differential Diagnosis. While considering a diagnosis of MALToma, the following differentials must be kept in mind: (a) long-standing chronic inflammatory lesions—these lesions do not produce lymphoepithelial lesions. (b) splenic marginal zone lymphoma involving the gastric mucosa. (c) mantle cell lymphoma which will be positive for CD5. (d) follicular lymphoma—a B cell neoplasm that expresses CD10 and exhibits t(14;18) rearrangements involving BCL2 gene. (e) DLBCL and MALToma are B cell neoplasms and pure DLBCL has more rapid growth with poor prognosis. This differential is possible on morphology only with tumour cells of DLBCL having large cell size and large nuclei.

Diffuse large B cell lymphoma. It constitutes about 60% of gastric lymphomas, seen in middle-aged and elderly individuals with predominance [87, 88] (Fig. 17.2a–f). High-grade gastric lymphoma has lower complete remission rate and shorter survival [89]. bcl-6 located on chromosome 3q27 is frequently involved in majority of extra-nodal DLBCL. bcl-6 promoter region can be altered due to translocations, hypermutations or deregulation that results in bcl-6 overexpression, and predicts better prognosis [90]. Histomorphology of primary gastric DLBCL and DLBCL (MALT) is similar to nodal variant. The tumour cells are in sheets with high proliferative index. Majority of the cells resemble centroblasts or immunoblasts, occasionally appearing anaplastic with marked anisonucleosis. All cells express one or more of B cell markers like CD19, CD20, CD79a, PAX5 or surface or cytoplasmic immunoglobulins [91, 92]. A possibility of high-grade lymphoma arising from a low-grade tumour can be excluded with the help of appropriate immunomarkers. In

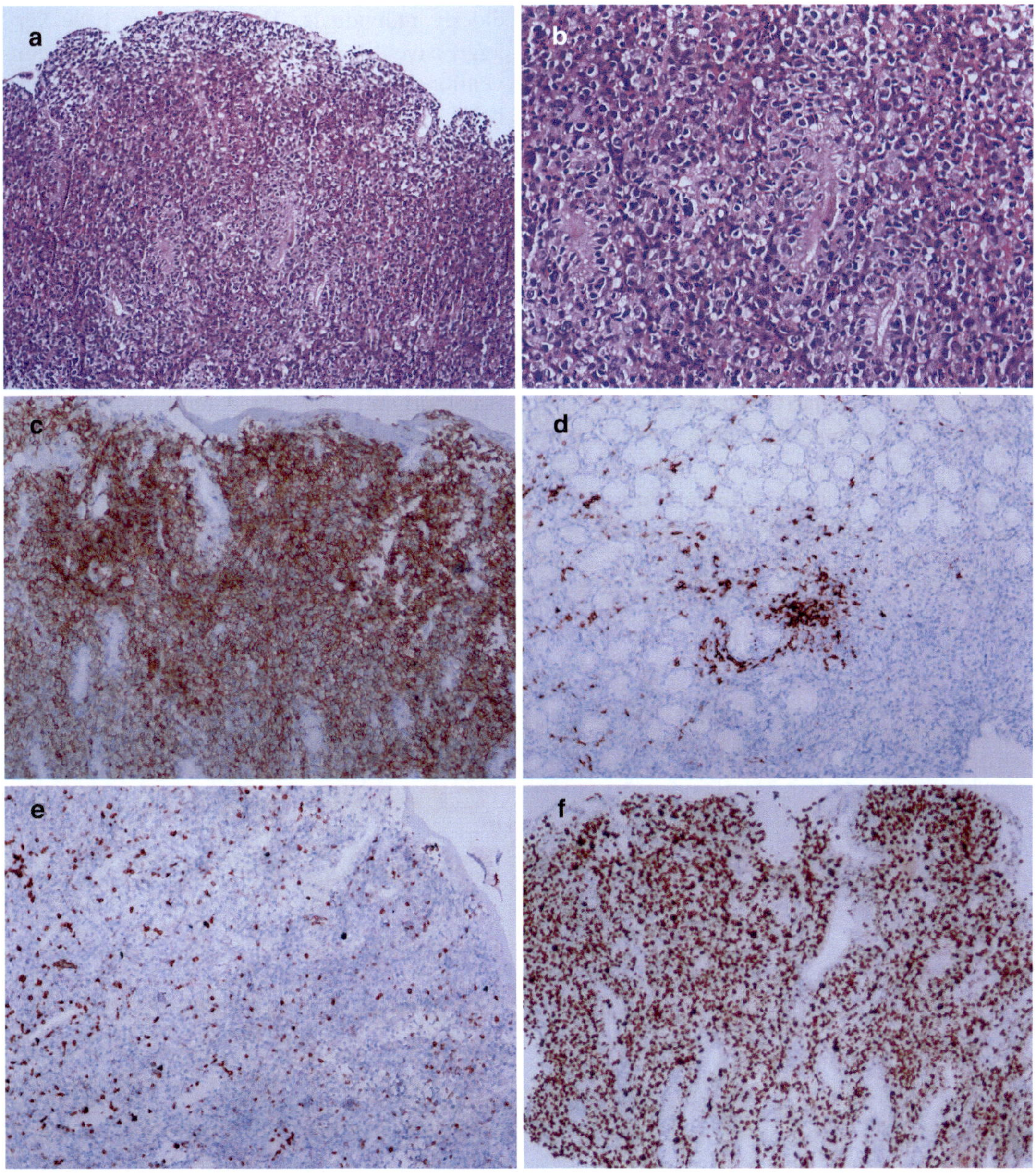

Fig. 17.2 Panel of photomicrographs showing features of a high-grade lymphoma in (**a**) and (**b**) pictures; (**c**–**f**) photomicrographs of immunostaining using CD45, CD20, CD3 and Ki-67, respectively showing CD 45 positivity and high proliferative index (PAP, ×350)

a grossly anaplastic looking tumour in an endoscopic biopsy, a differential diagnosis of other tumours like a poorly differentiated gastric carcinoma or any high-grade mesenchymal tumour may be considered. All these important differential diagnoses can be excluded by carrying out immunohistochemistry. Though it may not be absolute, but pure form of DLBCL arises de-novo with minimal changes of chronic gastritis in the adjoining gastric mucosa. In poorly differentiated gastric cancer of a high-grade lymphoma arising from a low-grade MALT lymphoma, the surrounding non-tumorous gastric mucosa will be showing changes of chronic gastritis, with variable grades of atrophy, metaplasia and/or dysplasia. Sometimes, even *H. pylori* may be demonstrable. Varying grades of lymphoepithelial lesion may also be observed in varying subtypes of DLBCL (Fig. 17.3a–g). GCB DLBCLs are more often positive for CD10, GCET1 and LMO2, and the ABC type expresses strongly IRF4 (MUM1) and FOXp1 [93]. A strong bcl-6 positivity with weak or negative MUM1 favours a GCB subtype. EBV associated primary gastric DLBCLs have been described in non-immunocompromised individuals. These tumours tend to show variable degree of plasmablastic differentiation. These cases can be seen both in young adults and elderly individuals. These tumours have very aggressive disease course compared to the conventional primary gastric DLBCL [94–96]. bcl-6 expression is present in germinal centre B cell (GCB) irrespective of genetic aberration and non-GCB lymphoma expressing bcl-6 is due to deregulation of the gene with no survival benefit [92]. CD10 expression is useful in identifying GC B-like DLBCL. B cell lymphomas expressing bcl-6 are follicular and Burkitt lymphoma. CD10 (a traditional marker for GC B cell) with bcl-6 can identify tumours of GC B-cell origin [1, 97, 98]. A bcl-6 positive staining requires awareness that it may also be expressed by non-GC B cell and T cell lineages. In contrary to bcl-6, bcl-2 is expressed significantly low in primary gastric DLBCL; however,

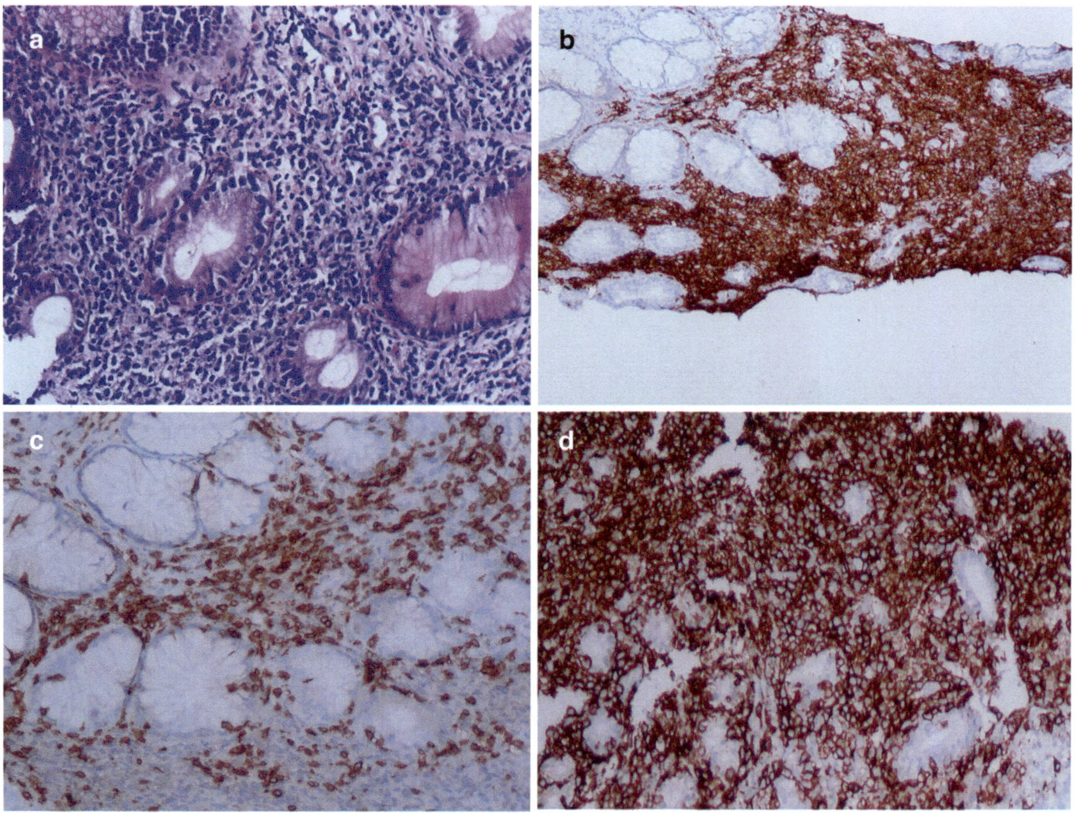

Fig. 17.3 Panel of another gastric lymphoma. (**a**) Photomicrograph of HE stained section to show immature lymphoid cell infiltration in between the gastric glands (HE, ×350). (**b**, **d**) Photomicrographs of immunostained sections of CD20, CD3 and CD30, where all the markers showed positively stained cells, almost all the cells were positive for CD30 (PAP, ×350). (**e**, **g**) Photomicrographs of BCL6, BCL2 and MUM1 immunostained sections showing BCL6 positivity and negative staining for BCL2 and MUM1 (PAP, ×350)

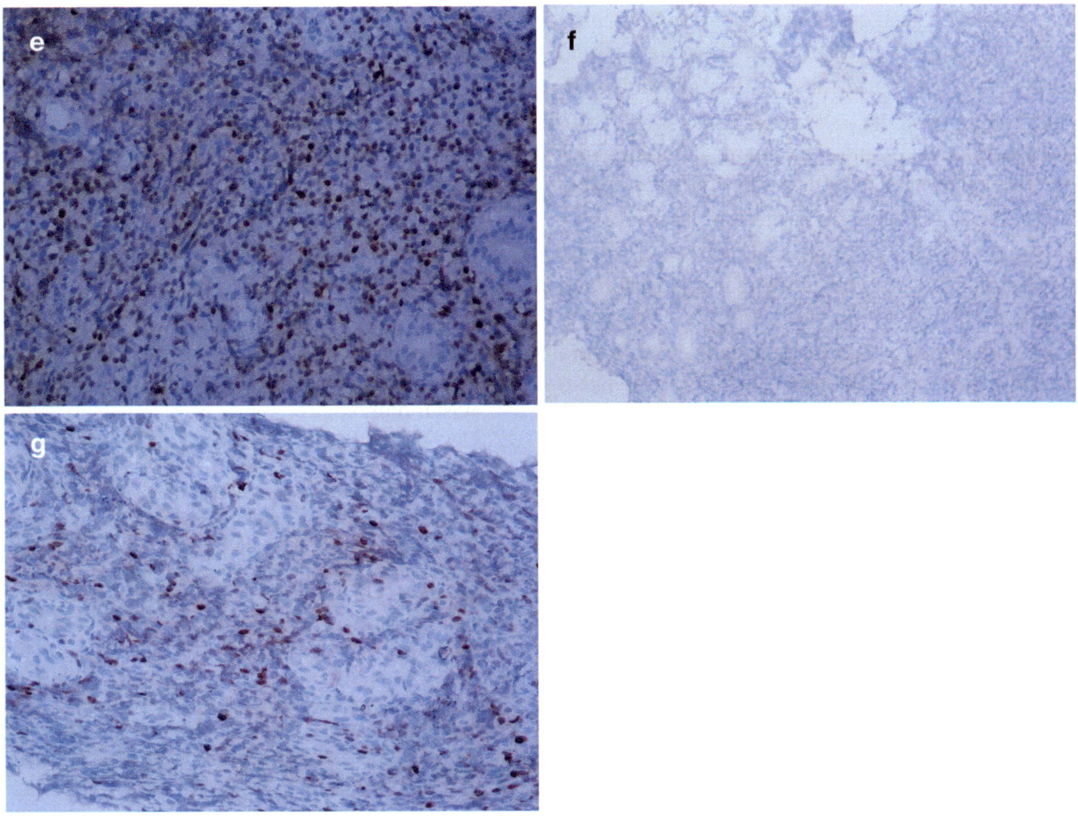

Fig. 17.3 (continued)

p53 protein expression does not differ between gastric and other extra-nodal lymphomas [99–102].

Burkitt's lymphoma (BL). BL is considered as a nodal lymphoma but extra-nodal involvement is present in more than 80% of the cases. Extra-nodal BL can be seen in many organs including gastrointestinal tract. In more than 60% of the cases, the overall survival is below 5 months [103–105]. Primary sporadic BL of the stomach is mostly a secondary spread from a retroperitoneal BL [104]. The cases diagnosed are due to clinical symptoms related to upper GI including haematemesis and perforation. Gastric BL has been observed in association with *H. Pylori* associated chronic gastritis [106, 107]. Other documented aetiological factors are EBV and HIV, environmental factors and a genetically disposed individual with germline mutations in ATM, BLM and SH2D1 [108–114]. EBV associated BL is seen in 25 to 40% of patients co-existing with immunodeficiency, and EBV has been documented in 20 to 30% of sporadic BL. BL is characterized by a de-regulated MYC gene by translocating to one of Ig gene loci at band 8q24 IGH locus located in chromosome 14q32, t(8:14) (q24:q32) and it is also associated but less frequently with translocation to IGK light chain locus on 2p12 or IGL light locus on 22q11 [112–114]. Exact roles of these translocating genes in disease pathogenesis are not well understood. Inhibitor of DNA binding (ID) protein 3(ID3) mutation has been documented in one third of BL cases [115]. ID3 mutation results in increased cell proliferation due to activation of the genes responsible for cell cycle and MYC as a human oncogene was first discovered in Burkitt lymphoma [115]. Still there is minimal understanding of other genes that collaborate with MYC deregulation in BL [115–118]. Macroscopic appearance—during endoscopic examination, there is no characteristic feature described for

BL; however, BL tumours are usually large mucosal protruding mass, soft, tan, fleshy and necrotic tumour infiltrating the gastric wall. Histologically: the characteristic cells are arranged diffusely and the tumour cells intermediate-sized lymphoid cells having monomorphic nuclei along with small visible multiple nucleoli. Cytoplasm is scanty with pale pink in colour. Mitotic activity is brisk with many degenerated apoptotic bodies [119, 120]. Tumour cells show positive staining for mature B cell antigens and follicle centre B cells such as CD10 and bcl-6 with 100% Ki67 proliferative index [120]. Half of the tumour cells show translocation of C-myc break-apart probe in FISH [116–118]. Gastric Bl is an aggressive tumour having an overall survival rate in low and high stage diseases 90% and 60% to 80%, respectively [119]. Differential diagnosis of BL is DLBCL having much pleomorphic and larger cell morphology [119]. BL tumour cells show positive staining for CD10, CD19, CD20, Ki67/MIB1 (almost 100%), CD22, CD33 (myeloid antigen), CD43, CD79a, BCL6, surface IgM and nuclear staining with new c-MYC antibody. Negative stains for CD5, CD23, TdT and BCL2 (positive in 20%) [119, 120].

References

1. Juárez-Salcedo LM, Sokol L, Chavez JC, et al. Primary gastric lymphoma, epidemiology, clinical diagnosis, and treatment. Cancer Control. 2018;25:1–12.
2. Groves F, Linet M, Travis L, et al. Cancer surveillance series: non-Hodgkin's lymphoma incidence by histologic subtype in the united states from 1978 through 1995. J Natl Cancer Inst. 2000;92:1240–51.
3. Chiu B, Weisenburger D. An update of the epidemiology of non-Hodgkin's lymphoma. Clin Lymphoma. 2003;4:161–8.
4. Ghimire P, Wu GY, Zhu L. Primary gastrointestinal lymphoma. World J Gastroenterol. 2011;17:697–707.
5. Al-Akwaa AM, Siddiqui N, Al-Mofleh IA. Primary gastric lymphoma. World J Gastroenterol. 2004;10:5–11.
6. Shimm DS, Dosoretz DE, Anderson T, et al. Primary gastric lymphoma. An analysis with emphasis on prognostic factors and radiation therapy. Cancer. 1983;52:2044–8.
7. Cogliatti S, Schmid U, Schumacher U, et al. Primary B-cell gastric lymphoma: a clinicopathological study of 145 patients. Gastroenterology. 1991;101:1159–70.
8. Herrmann R, Panahon AM, Barcos MP, et al. Gastrointestinal involvement in non-Hodgkin's lymphoma. Cancer. 1980;46:215–22.
9. Ruskoné-Fourmestraux A, Fischbach W, EGILS group, et al. EGILS consensus report. Gastric extranodal marginal zone B-cell lymphoma of MALT. Gut. 2011;60:747–58.
10. Jaffe ES, Harris NL, Stein H, et al. Classification of lymphoid neoplasms: the microscope as a tool for disease discovery. Blood. 2008;112:4384–99.
11. Swerdlow SH, Campo E, Harris NL, et al. The World Health Organization classification of tumours of haematopoietic and lymphoid tissues. Lyon, France: WHO; 2008.
12. Doglioni C, Ponzoni M, Ferreri AJ, et al. Gruppo Italiano Patologi Apparato Digerente (GIPAD); Societ `a Italiana di Anatomia Patologica e Citopatologia Diagnostica/International Academy of Pathology, Italian division (SIAPEC/IAP). Gastric lymphoma: the histology report. Dig Liver Dis. 2011;43:S310–8.
13. Kuo SH, Chen LT, Wu MS, et al. Differential response to H. pylori eradication therapy of coexisting diffuse large B-cell lymphoma and MALT lymphoma of stomach-significance of tumour cell clonality and BCL10 expression. J Pathol. 2007;211:296–304.
14. Jaffe ES, Harris NL, Stein H, et al. World Health Organization classification of tumours. Pathology and genetics of tumours of haematopoietic and lymphoid tissues. Lyon, France: IARC Press; 2001.
15. Zucca E, Dreyling M. ESMO guidelines working group. Gastric marginal zone lymphoma of MALT type: ESMO clinical practice guidelines for diagnosis, treatment and follow-up. Ann Oncol. 2010;21:v175–6.
16. Chen LT, Lin JT, Tai JJ, et al. Long-term results of anti-Helicobacter pylori therapy in early-stage gastric high-grade transformed MALT lymphoma. J Natl Cancer Inst. 2005;97:1345–53.
17. Nakamura S, Matsumoto T, Suekane H, et al. Predictive value of endoscopic ultrasonography for regression of gastric low grade and high grade MALT lymphomas after eradication of Helicobacter pylori. Gut. 2001;48:454–60.
18. Morgner A, Miehlke S, Fischbach W, et al. Complete remission of primary high-grade B-cell gastric lymphoma after cure of Helicobacter pylori infection. J Clin Oncol. 2001;19:2041–8.
19. Mitsuhashi K, Yamashita K, Goto A, et al. Gastric diffuse large B-cell lymphoma cured with Helicobacter pylori eradication regardless of whether it contains features of MALT lymphoma or not. Intern Med. 2014;53:695–8.
20. Engels EA. Infectious agents as causes of non-Hodgkin lymphoma. Cancer Epidemiol Biomarkers Prev. 2007;16:401–4.
21. Lecuit M, Abachin E, Martin A, et al. Immunoproliferative small intestinal disease asso-

ciated with Campylobacter jejuni. N Engl J Med. 2004;350:239–48.
22. Juarez-Salcedo LM, Sokol L, Chavez JC, et al. Primary gastric lymphoma, epidemiology, clinical diagnosis and treatment. Cancer Control. 2018;25:1–12.
23. Ferrucci PF, Zucca E. Primary gastric lymphoma pathogenesis and treatment: what has changed over the past 10 years? Br J Haematol. 2007;136:521–38.
24. Medina-Franco H, Germes SS, et al. Prognostic factors in primary gastric lymphoma. Ann Surg Oncol. 2007;14:2239–45.
25. Parsonnet J, Hansen S, Rodriguez L, et al. Helicobacter pylori infection and gastric lymphoma. N Engl J Med. 1994;330:1267–71.
26. Taal BG, Burgers JM. Primary non-Hodgkin's lymphoma of the stomach: endoscopic diagnosis and the role of surgery. Scand J Gastroenterol Suppl. 1991;188:33–7.
27. Uotani T, Graham DY. Diagnosis of Helicobacter pylori using the rapid urease test. Ann Transl Med. 2015;3:9.
28. Brown JA, Carson BW, Gascoyne RD, et al. Low grade gastric MALT Lymphoma: radiographic findings. Clin Radiol. 2000;55:384–9.
29. Chou CK, Sheu RS, Yang CW, et al. Abdominal pseudotumors and simulated lymphadenopathy in MRI: differential features with the use of retrograde air insufflation. Abdom Imaging. 1994;19:503–6.
30. Püspök A, Raderer M, Chott A, et al. Endoscopic ultrasound in the follow up and response assessment of patients with primary gastric lymphoma. Gut. 2002;51:691–4.
31. Radan L, Fischer D, Bar-Shalom R, et al. FDG avidity and PET/CT patterns in primary gastric lymphoma. Eur J Nucl Med Mol Imaging. 2008;35:1424–30.
32. Wu J, Zhu H, Li K, et al. 18F-fluorodeoxyglucose positron emission tomography/computed tomography findings of gastric lymphoma: comparisons with gastric cancer. Oncol Lett. 2014;8:1757–64.
33. Rizvi MA, Evens AM, Tallman MS, et al. T-cell non-Hodgkin lymphoma. Blood. 2006;107:1255–64.
34. Doglioni C, Ponzoni M, Ferreri AJ, et al. Gastric lymphoma: the histology report. Dig Liver Dis. 2011;43:S310–8.
35. Farinha P, Gascoyne RD. Molecular pathogenesis of mucosa-associated lymphoid tissue lymphoma. J Clin Oncol. 2005;23(26):6370–8.
36. Zucca E, Bertoni F, Vannata B, et al. Emerging role of infectious etiologies in the pathogenesis of marginal zone B-cell lymphomas. Clin Cancer Res: Off J Am Assoc Cancer Res. 2014;20:5207–16.
37. Isaacson PG. Pathogenesis and early lesions in extranodal lymphoma. Toxicol Lett. 1993;67:231–41.
38. Schreuder MI, van den Brand M, Hebeda KM, et al. Novel developments in the pathogenesis and diagnosis of extranodal marginal zone lymphoma. J Hematopathol. 2017;10:91–107.
39. Zucca E, Roggero E, Pileri S. B-cell lymphoma of MALT type: a review with special emphasis on diagnostic and management problems of low-grade gastric tumours. Br J Haematol. 1998;100:3–14.
40. Isaacson P, Muller-Hermelink H, Piris M, et al. Extranodal marginal zone B-cell lymphoma of mucosa-associated lymphoid tissue (MALT lymphoma). In: Jaffe ES, Harris NL, Stein H, Vardiman JW, editors. Pathology and genetics of tumours of haematopoietic and lymphoid tissues. World Health Organization classification of tumours. Lyon, France: IARC Press; 2001. p. 157–60.
41. de Leval L, Jaffe E. Lymphoma classification. Cancer. 2020;26:176–85.
42. Ponzoni M, Ferreri AJ, Pruneri G, et al. Prognostic value of bcl-6, CD10 and CD38 immunoreactivity in stage I-II gastric lymphomas: identification of a subset of CD10þ large B-cell lymphomas with a favourable outcome. Int J Cancer. 2003;106:288–91.
43. Zelenetz AD, Gordon LI, Wierda WG, et al. Non-Hodgkin's lymphomas, version 4.2014. J Natl Compr Canc Netw. 2014;12:1282–303.
44. Bacon CM, Du MQ, Dogan A. Mucosa-associated lymphoid tissue (MALT) lymphoma: a practical guide for pathologists. J Clin Pathol. 2007;60:361–72.
45. Nakamura S, Sugiyama T, Matsumoto T, et al. JAPAN GAST Study Group. Long-term clinical outcome of gastric MALT lymphoma after eradication of Helicobacter pylori: a multicentre cohort follow-up study of 420 patients in Japan. Gut. 2012;61:507–13.
46. Zullo A, Hassan C, Ridola L, et al. Gastric MALT lymphoma: old and new insights. Ann Gastroenterol. 2014;27:27–33.
47. Greiner A, Knorr C, Qin Y, et al. Low-grade B cell lymphomas of mucosa-associated lymphoid tissue (MALT-type) require CD40-mediated signalling and Th2-type cytokines for in vitro growth and differentiation. Am J Pathol. 1997;150:1583–93.
48. Craig VJ, Arnold I, Gerke C, et al. Gastric MALT lymphoma B cells express polyreactive, somatically mutated immunoglobulins. Blood. 2010;115:581–91.
49. Novak U, Basso K, Pasqualucci L, et al. Genomic analysis of non-splenic marginal zone lymphomas (MZL) indicates similarities between nodal and extranodal MZL and supports their derivation from memory B-cells. Br J Haematol. 2011;155:362–5.
50. Ruland J, Duncan GS, Elia A, et al. Bcl10 is a positive regulator of antigen receptor-induced activation of NF-kappa B and neural tube closure. Cell. 2001;104:33–42.
51. Bertoni F, Zucca E. Delving deeper into MALT lymphoma biology. J Clin Invest. 2006;116:22–6.
52. Zhang Q, Siebert R, Yan M, et al. Inactivating mutations and overexpression of BCL10, a caspase recruitment domain containing gene, in MALT lymphoma with t(1;14)(p22;q32). Nat Genet. 1999;22:63–8.
53. Willis TG, Jadayel DM, Du MQ, et al. Bcl10 is involved in t(1;14)(p22;q32) of MALT B cell lym-

phoma and mutated in multiple tumor types. Cell. 1999;96:35–45.
54. Yeh KH, Kuo SH, Chen LT, et al. Nuclear expression of BCL10 or nuclear factor kappa B helps predict Helicobacter pylori-independent status of low-grade gastric mucosa-associated lymphoid tissue lymphomas with or without t(11;18)(q21;q21). Blood. 2005;106:1037–41.
55. Raderer M, Kiesewetter B, Ferreri A. Clinicopathologic characteristics and treatment of marginal zone lymphoma of mucosa associated lymphoid tissue (MALT lymphoma). CA Cancer J Clin. 2016;66:153–71.
56. Foster LH, Portell CA. The role of infectious agents, antibiotics, and antiviral therapy in the treatment of extra-nodal marginal zone lymphoma and other low-grade lymphomas. Curr Treat Options Oncol. 2015;16:28.
57. Thieblemont C, Cascione L, Conconi A, et al. A MALT lymphoma prognostic index. Blood. 2017;130:1409–17.
58. Cogliatti SB, Griesser H, Peng H, et al. Significantly different BCL-2 expression profiles in gastric and nongastric primary extranodal high-grade B-cell Lymphomas. J Pathol. 2000;192:470–8.
59. Horn H, Ziepert M, Becher C, et al. MYC status in concert with BCL2 and BCL6 expression predicts outcome in diffuse large B-cell lymphoma. Blood. 2013;121:2253–63.
60. Swerdlow SH. Diagnosis of 'double hit' diffuse large B-cell lymphoma and B-cell lymphoma, unclassifiable, with features intermediate between DLBCL and Burkitt lymphoma: when and how, FISH versus IHC. Haematology Am Soc Haematol Educ Program. 2014;2014:90–9.
61. He M, Chen K, Li S, et al. Clinical significance of "double-hit" and "double-protein" expression in primary gastric B-cell lymphomas. J Cancer. 2016;7:1215–25.
62. The International Non-Hodgkin's Lymphoma Prognostic Factors Project. A Predictive Model for Aggressive Non-Hodgkin's Lymphoma. NEJM. 1993;329:987–94.
63. Terada T. Histopathological study using computer database of 10 000 consecutive gastric specimens: benign conditions. Gastroenterol Rep (Oxf). 2015;3:238–42.
64. Isaacson P, Wright DH. Malignant lymphoma of mucosa-associated lymphoid tissue. A distinctive type of B-cell lymphoma. Cancer. 1983;52:1410–6.
65. Spencer J, Finn T, Isaacson PG. Human Peyer's patches: an immunohistochemical study. Gut. 1986;27:405–10.
66. Spencer J, Finn T, Pulford KAF, et al. The human gut contains a novel population of B-lymphocytes which resemble marginal zone cells. Clin Exp Immunol. 1985;62:607–10.
67. Swerdlow SH, Campo E, Pileri SA, et al. The 2016 revision of the World Health Organization classification of lymphoid neoplasms; clinical trials & observations. Blood. 2016;127:2375–90.
68. Zukerberg LR, Ferry JA, Southern JF, et al. Lymphoid infiltrates of the stomach. Evaluation of histologic criteria for the diagnosis of low-grade gastric lymphoma on endoscopic biopsy specimens. Am J Surg Pathol. 1990;14:1087–99.
69. Wotherspoon AC, Doglioni C, Diss TC, et al. Regression of primary low-grade B-cell gastric lymphoma of mucosa-associated lymphoid tissue type after eradication of Helicobacter pylori. Lancet. 1993;342:575–7.
70. Arista-Nasr J, Herrera-Goepfert R, Lazos-Ochoa M, et al. Histologic changes of the gastric mucosa associated with primary gastric lymphoma in endoscopic biopsy specimens. Arch Pathol Lab Med. 2000;124:1628–31.
71. Ferreri AJ, Freschi M, Dell'Oro S, et al. Prognostic significance of the histopathologic recognition of low- and high-grade components in stage I-II B-cell gastric lymphomas. Am J Surg Pathol. 2001;25:95–102.
72. Swerdlow SH, Campo E, Harris NL, et al. World Health Organization classification of tumours of haematopoietic and lymphoid tissues. Lyon, France: IARC Press; 2008.
73. Ikeda J, Kohara M, Tsuruta Y, et al. Immunohistochemical analysis of the novel marginal zone B-cell marker IRTA1 in malignant lymphoma. Hum Pathol. 2017;59:70–9.
74. Isaacson PG, Chott A, Nakamura S, et al. Extranodal marginal zone lymphoma of mucosa-associated lymphoid tissue (MALT lymphoma). In: Swerdlow SH, Campo E, Harris NL, et al., editors. World Health Organization classification of tumours of haematopoietic and lymphoid tissues. Geneva: IARC Press; 2008. p. 214–7.
75. De Leval L. Lymphoid tumours of the stomach. In: Shepherd NA, Warren BF, Williams GT, et al., editors. Morson and Dawson's gastrointestinal pathology. 5th ed. Wiley-Blackwell Publication; 2012. p. 241–69.
76. Ballesteros E, Osborne BM, Matsushima AY. CD5+ low-grade marginal zone B cell lymphomas with localized presentation. Am J Surg Pathol. 1998;22:201–7.
77. Mullangi S, Lekkala MR. Mucosa-associated lymphoma tissue. In: StatPearls [Internet]. Treasure Island, FL: StatPearls Publishing; 2021.
78. Falini B, Agostinelli C, Bigerna B, et al. IRTA1 is selectively expressed in nodal and extranodal marginal zone lymphomas. Histopathology. 2012;61:930–41.
79. Bob R, Falini B, Marafioti T, et al. Nodal reactive and neoplastic proliferation of monocytoid and marginal zone B cells: an immunoarchitectural and molecular study highlighting the relevance of IRTA1 and T-bet as positive markers. Histopathology. 2013;63:482–98.

80. Kanellis G, Roncador G, Arribas A, et al. Identification of MNDA as a new marker for nodal marginal zone lymphoma. Leukemia. 2009;23:1847–57.
81. Manohar V, Peerani R, Tan B, et al. Myeloid Cell Nuclear Differentiation Antigen (MNDA) positivity in primary follicles: potential pitfall in the differential diagnosis with marginal zone lymphoma. Appl Immunohistochem Mol Morphol. 2020;28:384–8.
82. Metcalf RA, Monabati A, Vyas M, et al. Myeloid cell nuclear differentiation antigen is expressed in a subset of marginal zone lymphomas and is useful in the differential diagnosis with follicular lymphoma. Hum Pathol. 2014;45:1730–6.
83. Rattotti S, Croci G, Ferretti VV, et al. Mantle cell lymphoma mimicking Mucosa-Associated Lymphoid Tissue (MALT) lymphomas: a pathological characterization (on behalf of the "Fondazione Italiana Linfomi (FIL) – postgraduate master course"). Blood. 2017;130:4049.
84. Narurkar R, Alkayem M, Liu D. SOX11 is a biomarker for cyclin D1-negative mantle cell lymphoma. Biomark Res. 2016;4:6–8.
85. Kojima M, Nakamura S, Murase T, et al. Follicular colonization of nodal marginal-zone B-cell lymphoma resembling follicular lymphoma: report of 6 cases. Int J Surg Pathol. 2005;13:73–8.
86. Naresh KN. Nodal marginal zone B-cell lymphoma with prominent follicular colonization – difficulties in diagnosis: a study of 15 cases. Histopathology. 2008;52:331–9.
87. Harris NL, Jaffe ES, Stein H, et al. A revised European-American classification of lymphoid neoplasm: a proposal from the International Lymphoma Study Group. Blood. 1994;84:1361–92.
88. Harris NL, Jaffe EX, Diebold J, et al. The World Health Organization classification of neoplastic diseases of the haematopoietic and lymphoid tissues: report of the clinical advisory committee meeting, Airlie House, Virginia, November 1997. Histopathology. 2000;36:69–87.
89. Koch P, del Valle F, Berdel WE, et al. German Multicenter Study Group. Primary gastrointestinal non-Hodgkin's lymphoma: I. Anatomic and histologic distribution, clinical features, and survival data of 371 patients registered in the German Multicenter Study GIT NHL 01/92. J Clin Oncol. 2001;19:3861–73.
90. Offit K, Lococo F, Louie DC, et al. Rearrangement of the bcl-6 gene as prognostic marker in diffuse large cell lymphoma. N Engl J Med. 1994;331:74–80.
91. Li S, Young KH, Medeiros LJ. Diffuse large B-cell lymphoma. Pathology. 2018;50:74–87.
92. Rosenwald A, Wright G, Wing C, et al. The use of molecular profiling to predict survival after chemotherapy for diffuse large-B-cell lymphoma. N Engl J Med. 2002;346:1937–347.
93. Guo Y, Takeuchi I, Karnan S, et al. Array-comparative genomic hybridization profiling of immunohistochemical subgroups of diffuse large B-cell lymphoma shows distinct genomic alterations. Cancer Sci. 2014;105:481–9.
94. Hu M, Trevino J, Yang L, et al. Primary gastric EBV-positive diffuse large B cell lymphoma (DLBCL) of the elderly with plasmablastic differentiation. In Vivo. 2018;32:413–7.
95. Castillo JJ, Beltran BE, Miranda RN, et al. EBV-positive diffuse large B-cell lymphoma of the elderly: 2016 update on diagnosis, risk-stratification, and management. Am J Hematol. 2016;91:529–37.
96. Lu TX, Liang JH, Miao Y, et al. Epstein-Barr virus positive diffuse large B-cell lymphoma predict poor outcome, regardless of the age. Sci Rep. 2015;5:12168.
97. Huang JA, Sanger WG, Greiner TC, et al. The t(14;18) defines a unique subset of diffuse large B-cell lymphoma with a germinal center B-cell expression profile. Blood. 2002;99:2286–90.
98. Flenghi L, Ye BH, Fizzotti M, et al. A specific monoclonal antibody (PG-B6) detects expression of the Bcl-6 protein in germinal center B cells. Am J Pathol. 1995;147:405–11.
99. Ree HJ, Kadin ME, Kikuchi M, et al. Bcl-6 expression in reactive follicular hyperplasia, follicular lymphoma, and angioimmunoblastic T-cell lymphoma with hyperplastic germinal centers: heterogeneity of intrafollicular T-cells and their altered distribution in the pathogenesis of angioimmunoblastic T-cell lymphoma. Hum Pathol. 1999;30:403–11.
100. Ree HJ, Yang WI, Kim CW, et al. Coexpression of Bcl-6 and CD10 in diffuse large B-cell lymphomas: significance of Bcl-6 expression patterns in identifying germinal center B-cell lymphoma. Hum Pathol. 2001;32:954–62.
101. Ree HJ. Bcl-6 expression in primary mediastinal large cell lymphoma [letter]. Am J Surg Pathol. 2002;26:1087–92.
102. Yonezumi M, Suzuki R, Suzuki H, et al. Detection of AP12-MALT1 chimaeric gene in extranodal and nodal marginal zone B-cell lymphoma by reverse transcription polymerase chain reaction (PCR) and genomic long and accurate PCR analyses. Br J Haematol. 2001;115:588–94.
103. Jang SJ, Yoon DH, Kim S, et al. A unique pattern of extra-nodal involvement in Korean adults with sporadic Burkitt lymphoma: a single center experience. Ann Hematol. 2012;91:1917–22.
104. Kesik V, Safali M, Citak EC, et al. Primary gastric Burkitt lymphoma: a rare cause of intraabdominal mass in childhood. Pediatr Surg Int. 2010;26:927–9.
105. Mitra S, Mehta A, Sk G, et al. Primary gastric Burkitt's lymphoma. Rare Tumours. 2014;6:5300.
106. Grewal SS, Hunt JP, O'Connor SC, et al. Helicobacter pylori associated gastric Burkitt lymphoma. Pediatr Blood Cancer. 2008;50:888–90.
107. Baumgaertner I, Copie-Bergman C, Levy M, et al. Complete remission of gastric Burkitt's lymphoma after eradication of Helicobacter pylori. World J Gastroenterol. 2009;15:5746–50.

108. De Falco G, Antonicelli G, Onnis A, et al. Role of EBV in microRNA dysregulation in Burkitt lymphoma. Semin Cancer Biol. 2009;19:401–6.
109. Van den Bosch CA. Is endemic Burkitt's lymphoma an alliance between three infections and a tumour promoter? Lancet Oncol. 2004;5:738–46.
110. Knowles DM. Etiology and pathogenesis of AIDS-related non-Hodgkin's lymphoma. Hematol Oncol Clin North Am. 2003;17:785–820.
111. Neri A, Barriga F, Knowles DM, et al. Different regions of the immunoglobulin heavy-chain locus are involved in chromosomal translocations in distinct pathogenetic forms of Burkitt lymphoma. Proc Natl Acad Sci U S A. 1988;85:2748–52.
112. Amato T, Abate F, Piccaluga P, et al. Clonality analysis of immunoglobulin gene rearrangement by next-generation sequencing in endemic Burkitt lymphoma suggests antigen drive activation of BCR as opposed to sporadic Burkitt lymphoma. Am J Clin Pathol. 2016;145:116–27.
113. Dalla-Favera R, Martinotti S, Gallo RC, et al. Translocation and rearrangements of the c-myc oncogene locus in human undifferentiated B-cell lymphomas. Science. 1983;219(4587):963–7.
114. Barth TF, Muller S, Pawlita M, et al. Homogeneous immunophenotype and paucity of secondary genomic aberrations are distinctive features of endemic but not of sporadic Burkitt's lymphoma and diffuse large B-cell lymphoma with MYC rearrangement. J Pathol. 2004;203:940–5.
115. Richter J, Schlesner M, Hoffmann S, et al. Recurrent mutation of the ID3 gene in Burkitt lymphoma identified by integrated genome, exome and transcriptome sequencing. Nat Genet. 2012;44:1316–20.
116. Rodig SJ, Vergilio JA, Shahsafaei A, et al. Characteristic expression patterns of TCL1, CD38, and CD44 identify aggressive lymphomas harbouring a MYC translocation. Am J Surg Pathol. 2008;32:113–22.
117. Ruzinovo MB, Caron T, Rodig SJ. Altered subcellular localization of c-Myc protein identifies aggressive B-cell lymphomas harboring a c-MYC translocation. Am J Surg Pathol. 2010;34:882–91.
118. Casares S, Rodríguez JM, Martin A, et al. Rearrangements of c-myc and c-abl genes in tumour cells in Burkitt's lymphoma. J Clin Pathol. 1993;46:778–9.
119. Steven H, Swerdlow EC, Harris NL, et al. WHO classification of tumours of haematopoietic and lymphoid tissues. Lyon: IARC; 2008.
120. Ruzinova MB, Caron T, Rodig SJ. Altered subcellular localization of c-Myc protein identifies aggressive B-cell lymphomas harbouring a c-MYC translocation. Am J Surg Pathol. 2010;34:882–91.

18 Lymphocytic and Other Autoimmune-Related Gastritis

Lymphocytic gastritis (LG), first described by Haot et al. in 1988, is characterized histopathologically by lymphocytosis of surface and foveolar epithelium with increased chronic inflammation in the lamina propria [1] (Fig. 18.1a and b). Lymphocytic gastritis is an uncommon chronic gastritis: the prevalence has been reported to be 0.83% of upper endoscopic examinations and 1.7–4.5% of chronic active gastritis [2, 3]. LG has been reported in patients with celiac disease (prevalence of 36–45%) [4–6], *Helicobacter pylori* (HP) gastritis (13%) [7] and gastropathies with inconsistent histopathological-endoscopic correlation. These include varioliform gastritis, which has distinctive endoscopic findings of large folds in the fundus and erosive mucosal bulging in the fundus and antrum with biopsy findings of LG (74–82%) [8–10] and hypertrophic lymphocytic gastritis [11–14] with Menetrier's-like protein losing gastropathy, sometimes associated with HP infection [14–16]. Some patients with LG are asymptomatic.

Collagenous gastroenteritides refers to a spectrum of diseases which include collagenous gastritis (CG), collagenous sprue and collagenous colitis. These conditions are relatively uncommon and are characterized by excess amount of subepithelial collagen deposition associated with varying degrees of mucosal lymphocytosis [17–19] (Fig. 18.2a–c). The underlying aetiology of these conditions remains unclear. Clinical manifestations are usually related to the site of involvement of the gastrointestinal tract. Compared to collagenous colitis, collagenous gastritis and collagenous enteritis are rarer [20]. CG was described for the first time by Colletti and Trainer (1989) in a 15-year-old patient who presented with recurrent abdominal pain and gastrointestinal bleeding [21]. CG can have two forms of clinical presentations, i.e. in paediatric patients usually present with abdominal pain and anaemia and adult patients present with chronic watery diarrhoea with diffuse collagenous involvement of the gastrointestinal tract [22].

These are rarer forms of gastritis. With increasing awareness, these conditions have been histologically diagnosed increasingly. Normally gastric mucosa is very innocuous looking with no or minimal mononuclear cells in lamina propria, seldom any intra-epithelial lymphocytes (IEL). Whenever there is an increase in IEL, it requires attention in order to exclude the possibility of an underlying systemic autoimmune disorder or an isolated autoimmune gastritis. Besides the clinical history, exclusion of any infective agents like *H. pylori* requires to be excluded first. In such a situation, it is essential to examine the status of the basement membrane, for any thickening. Basement membrane in gastric and foregut biopsies normally is almost imperceptible, just a few microns thick. Whenever there is a visibly thick basement membrane measuring 5 or more microns, a diagnosis of collagenous gastritis can be considered. This may be an isolated condition

K. Vaiphei, *Interpretation of Endoscopic Biopsy - Gastritis, Gastropathies and Beyond*,
https://doi.org/10.1007/978-981-16-6026-9_18

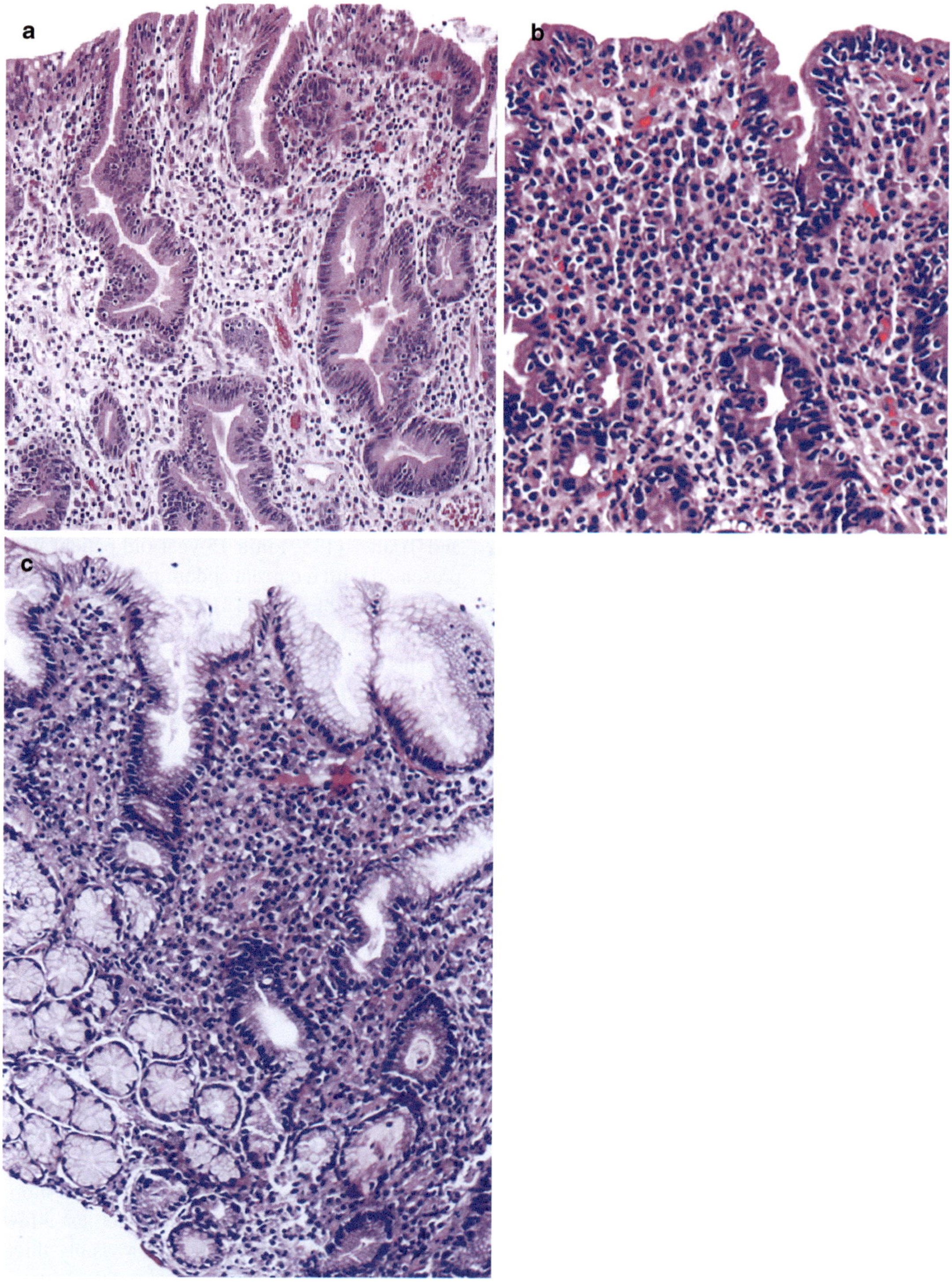

Fig. 18.1 Photomicrographs of a gastric biopsy showing (**a**)—features of chronic gastritis as indicated by foveolar hyperplasia and heavy mononuclear cell infiltration of lamina propria. Also to be noted is the disproportionate increase in the number of intraepithelial lymphocytes (HE, ×150); (**b**)—another closer view of the biopsy to show the heavier infiltration of the epithelial cells by lymphocytes along with an increase in mononuclear cells in the lamina propria (HE, ×300); (**c**)—this particular picture has been added to compare the number of intra-epithelial lymphocytes in spite the heavy mucosal inflammation and also to be noted is the normal basement membrane along the surface lining epithelium (HE, ×300)

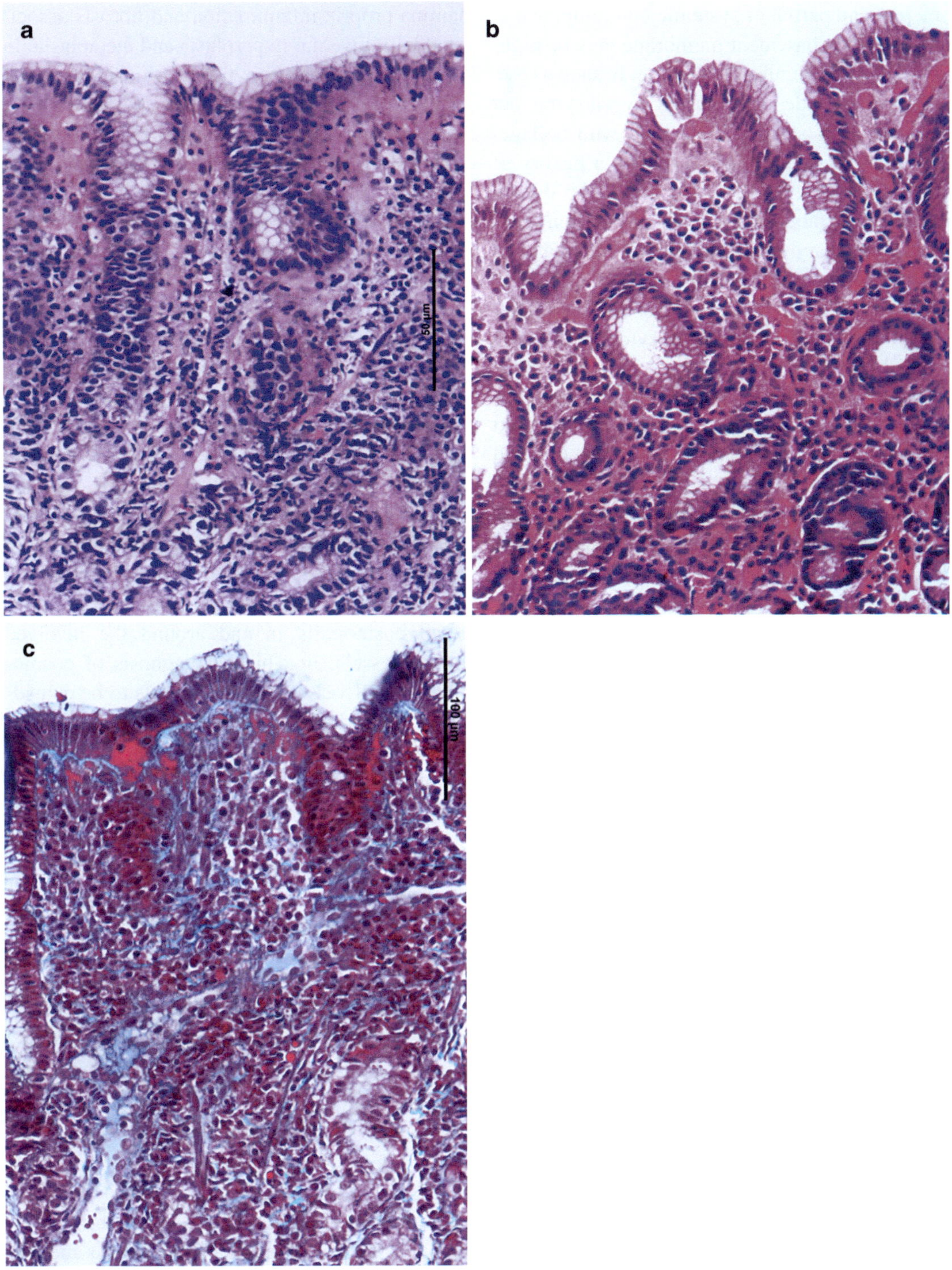

Fig. 18.2 Panel of photomicrographs showing (**a**) quite significantly inflamed gastric mucosa with fluffy looking eosinophilic material along the basement membrane of surface epithelium. To be noted is the not-increased number of intra-epithelial lymphocytes (HE, ×250); (**b**) Another photomicrograph of gastric biopsy with milder mucosal inflammation to show thicken basement membrane along the surface lining, sparing the foveolar epithelium (HE, ×250); (**c**) Photomicrograph to highlight the thicken basement membrane better in connective tissue staining (Masson's trichrome, ×300)

or a part and partial of systemic autoimmune disorder. A thick basement membrane may be highlighted better by collagen staining. In such a case, one may exclude amyloidosis by carrying out histochemistry staining. A patient with collagenous gastritis usually presents with a history of upper GI bleed. The bleed tends to be due to recurrent surface injury and the presence of dilated capillary channels within the collagen band. Lamina propria inflammation with relatively well preserve gastric glands. On higher power, intra-epithelial lymphocytosis is visibly prominent, which may involve surface as well as the glandular lining epithelial cells. Lamina propria inflammatory cells are dominantly composed of lymphocytes and plasma cells, maybe with scattered eosinophils and neutrophils. There may be lymphoid aggregate formation. This condition is rare and more frequently seen in females. Treatment is non-specific and symptomatic in an isolated condition, otherwise, in systemic autoimmune disorders, it may be treated as the spectrum of the primary disorder. It is very rare in paediatric age group and is relatively benign condition and these children may come with the complaints of non-specific abdominal pain [17, 19, 20, 22].

In children who are suffering from gluten sensitivity may have features of lymphocytic gastritis and in such a setting the intra-epithelial lymphocytes in stomach have been observed to be increased to a similar number to that observed in a duodenal biopsy. If one comes across a gastric antral biopsy with heavy lymphocytosis, Celiac disease needs to be excluded, after having excluded other common aetiologies. Presence of dyspepsia and other serological markers for celiac disease do not show any significant relationship with gastric lymphocytosis. Apart from Celiac disease, another condition, which may be more frequently observed with gastric lymphocytosis is *H. pylori* gastritis [23–27]. The latter is a body and pyloric antrum dominant lesion. Rarely lymphocytic gastritis may give endoscopic appearances of varioliform gastritis. In longstanding autoimmune gastritis or lymphocytic gastritis, there may be development of atrophic gastritis with loss of specialized gastric glands, lamina propria inflammation and fibrosis associated with foveolar hyperplasia and metaplasia. In any form of lymphocytic gastritis in an adult female where there is dominant body and fundic mucosa involvement, a possibility autoimmune gastritis or gastritis associated with megaloblastic anaemia needs to be excluded. In such a setting, small vessels in the deeper area of lamina propria and the capillaries and venules located in between the smooth muscle fibres may show mononuclear cell aggregate in and around swollen endothelial cells. If one is lucky enough, these thin wall small-sized blood vessels may have extravasated red blood cells and perivascular oedema. Small vessel vasculitis in an endoscopic biopsy is identified only by careful examination of the capillaries and venules mainly on the deeper portion of the lamina propria by tracing them out and need to be differentiated from muco-depleted crypts. More frequently than not, along with the lymphocytes, there may be scattered eosinophils in and around the involved blood vessels, in which a diagnosis of eosinophilic small vessel vasculitis needs to be considered. The finding of these few subtle but important features will be enough to document the presence of small vessel vasculitis in gastric biopsy. This may be seen in any age groups including children who usually present with unexplained pain abdomen, sometimes with evidence of upper GI bleed. If a part of submucosa is included in such biopsy, it may also show similar changes in the larger arterioles and veins. In such a situation, it is also important to study the status of basement membrane along the surface lining. Basement membrane in the foregut mucosa is almost imperceptible normally, quite different from that of hindgut mucosa. Lining epithelium is seen just attached to the underlying fine basement membrane. Hence, any obviously visible basement membrane without paying attention to the thickness, may be considered as significantly thick, and a diagnosis of collagenous gastritis may be entertained. If the thick basement membrane is well developed, there be many entrapped vasculature, some of them may be gaping explaining the clinical presentation of upper GI bleed. This condition is usually seen in young or middle-aged females presenting with upper GI bleed. Endoscopic examination tends to be non-specific, may be focal areas of erosions or mucosal haemorrhages. Majority may not have any other extra-intestinal manifestation. In any of these conditions, *H. pylori* infection and other associated changes need to look for and commented on appropriately. Any of these conditions are not mutually exclusive.

Systemic vasculitis disorder associated with immunoglobulin A most frequently presents with gastrointestinal involvement. To name some of the common ones—Henoch-Schönlein purpura, ANCA-associated vasculitis, polyarteritis nodosa and Behçet's disease [28]. In one-third of these conditions have GI involvement [29, 30]. Clinical manifestations due to GI vasculitides are the result of ischaemia of the affected organ and main presenting symptoms are—abdominal pain, nausea, vomiting, diarrhoea which may be associated with frank or occult blood [31]. In an endoscopic biopsy, it is the capillaries and venules, and in deep biopsy occasionally a portion of the submucosa may be included in the biopsy. The changes in the mucosa tends to be enhanced focally and the enhanced inflammation may be traced along the blood vessel. The involved vessel will have swollen endothelial cells and the inflammatory cells may be neutrophils, lymphocytes and plasma cells, and occasionally eosinophil-rich infiltrate (Fig. 18.3a–d). Useful clue that I have

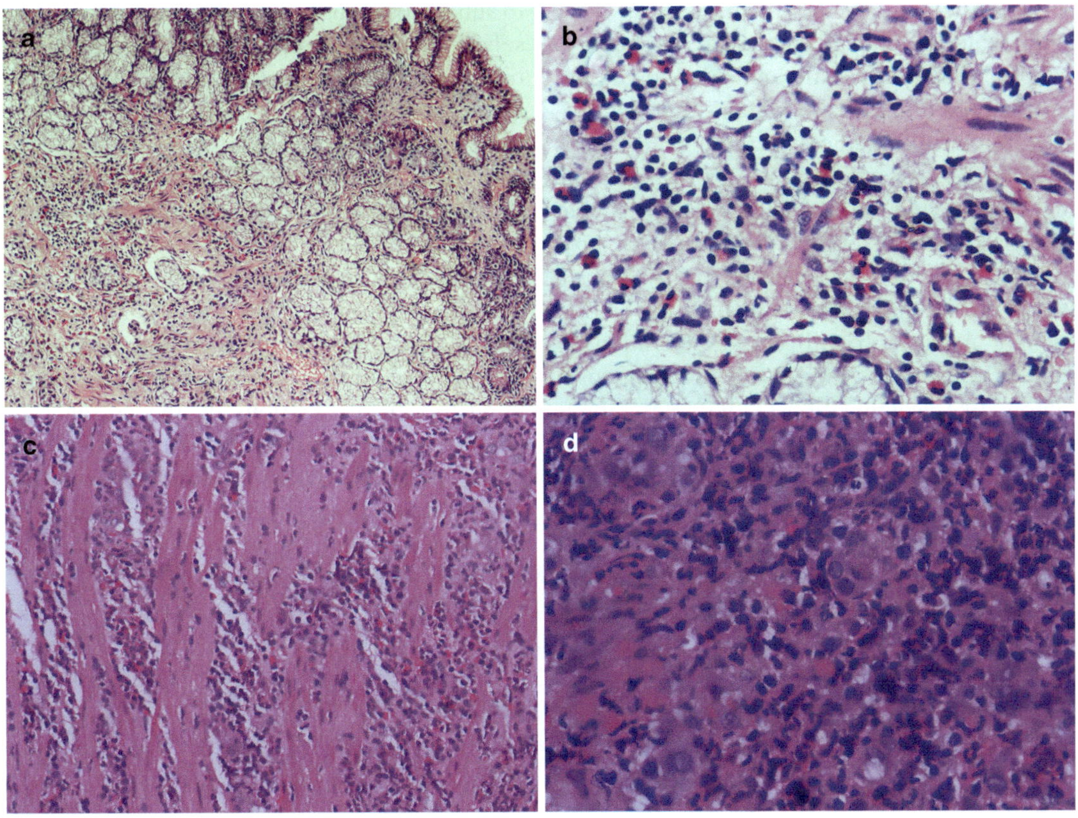

Fig. 18.3 Panel of photomicrographs of vasculitides. (**a**) Highlight a low-power view of antral biopsy highlighting grossly expanded and busy submucosa with splaying of muscularis mucosae. Patchy replacement fibrosis of lamina propria is also present (HE, ×100). (**b**) The same biopsy on a higher power show multiple small vessels with endothelial swelling and infiltration by lymphocytes mixed with eosinophils (HE, ×350). (**c**) Photomicrograph of another biopsy show hypertrophied and splayed muscularis mucosae intersected by conglomerates of eosinophil-rich inflammatory cells with prominence of small vasculatures (HE, ×300). (**d**) High-power photomicrograph of another biopsy show swollen endothelial cells occluding the lumen along with heavy inflammatory cell infiltration including many neutrophils (HE, ×500)

observed in routine practice is unexplained aggregation of inflammatory cells around small vessels with swollen endothelial cells on between smooth muscle bundles in muscularis mucosae layer. These focally enhanced inflammatory lesions may be associated with patchy fibrosis depending on disease duration. Tissue infarction in vasculitides is unusual, if present, the possibility of larger vessel vasculitis needs to be considered.

Amyloidosis refers to morphological features encompassing heterogeneous spectrum of underlying aetiologies and wide varieties of clinical presentations. It is diagnosed by identifying deposits of amorphous extracellular pale eosinophilic material [32]. Amyloidosis may be genetic or acquired. Localized gastric amyloidosis is a rare disorder [33]. The clinical manifestations of localized gastric amyloidosis are often uncharacteristic and subclinical, and patient may present with weight loss, dyspepsia refractory to medical therapy or GI bleeding. With respect to stomach, endoscopic features include mucosal erythema, friable mucosal with erosion or ulcers, mucosal protrusions and thickened folds. AA amyloidosis was more associated with diffuse deposition causing mucosal friability and ulceration or there may be mucosal bulge due to submucosal tumour like accumulation of the extracellular material [34, 35]. Imaging studies and endoscopy are helpful in localising the lesion but determining a definite clinical diagnosis is almost impossible [33–35]. Differential diagnosis for a localized gastric amyloidosis includes stromal tumours, gastric cancer including of both epithelial and lymphoid malignant tumours and a healing gastric ulcer. Amyloidosis has been observed to be the commonest type in gastrointestinal tract in about 10%–70% and AL type has been reported in a fewer number of cases [36]. Under the microscope, there is abundant the pale pink substance deposited in mucosal lamina propria in and around and also within the wall of arterioles, freely in the lamina propria in between the gastric glands. The adjoining gastric mucosa tends to show florid changes of chronic gastritis rich in plasma cells. Deposits may also extend and intersect in between smooth muscle fibres of muscularis mucosae extending to submucosa, mainly in and around blood vessels (Fig. 18.4a–c). Congo red staining gives a beautiful bright orangie congophilia. Before the era of immunohistochemistry typing of the primary (light chain or AL type) (Fig. 18.4d–h) and secondary amyloid was done with their sensitivity to potassium permanganate pretreatment. It was confirmed to be a secondary type if it is sensitive as indicated loss of congophilia and birefringence, whereas light-chain amyloid (AL) will be resistant. All these post-treatment sections can be confirmed by examining the treated sections by the presence or absence of birefringence while examining under polarized light microscopy with the observation of apple-green birefringence by the amyloid protein.

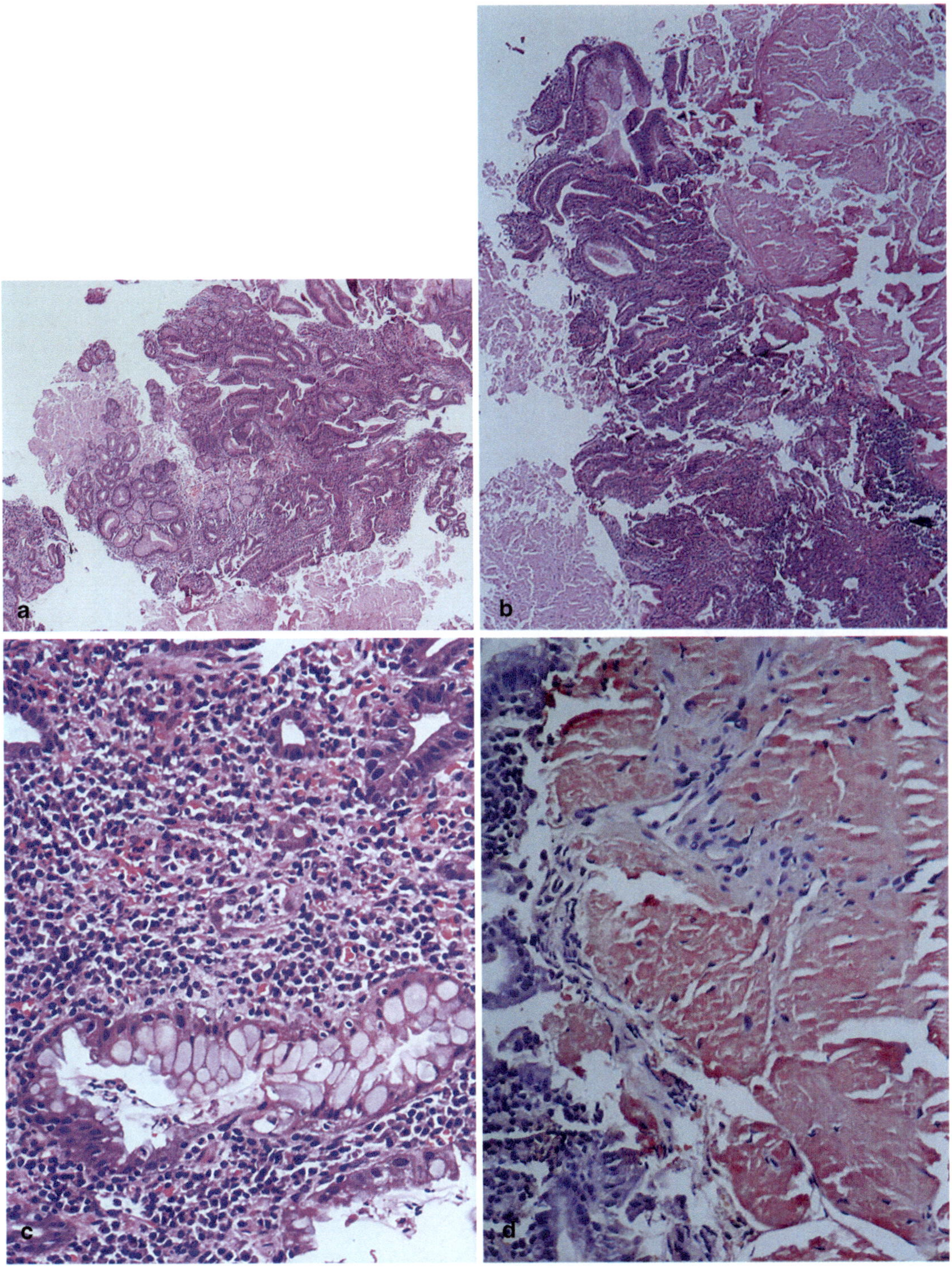

Fig. 18.4 Photomicrographs showing panels of HE stained section. (**a**) Low-power view show the presence of the pale pink amorphous material in lamina propria (JE, ×100). (**b**) Higher power view to show the character of the pink material better and histology of adjoining mucosa to be heavily infiltrated by inflammatory cells with cystic dilatation of the glands and foveolar hyperplasia (HE, ×200). (**c**) To show the dominant cell population in lamina propria infiltrate is plasma cells (HE, ×300). (**d**) and (**e**) Photomicrographs of Congo red stain section show the congophilia of the amorphous material. In (**e**) the material is also seen within an arteriole (HE, ×250). (**f**)–(**h**) Panel of photomicrographs of immunohistochemistry staining, (**f**) show the positive staining for SAA, (**g**) for lambda light chain and (**h**) negative staining for kappa light chain (PAP, ×300)

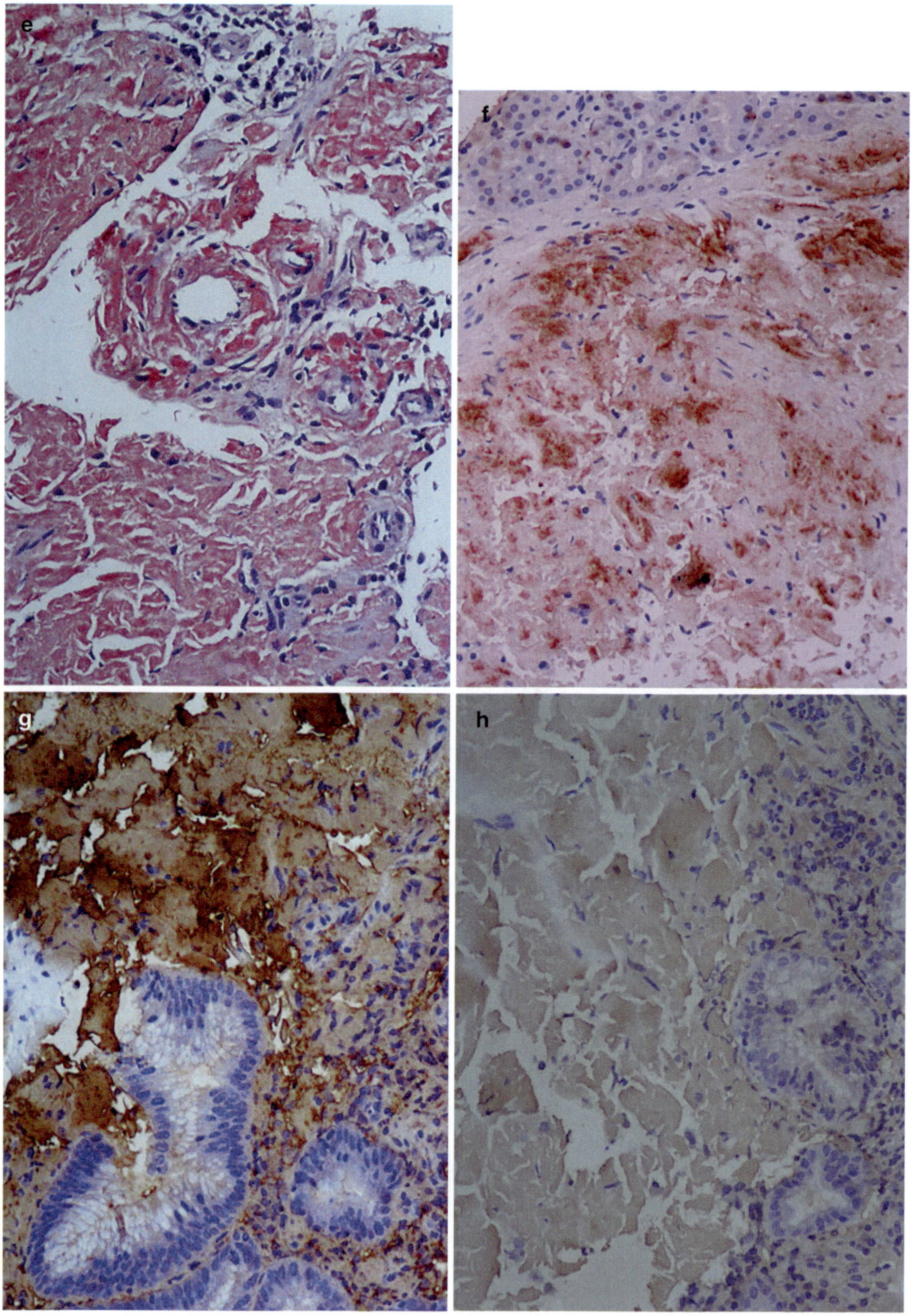

Fig. 18.4 (continued)

References

1. Haot J, Hamichi L, Wallez L, et al. Lymphocytic gastritis: a newly described entity: a retrospective endoscopic and histological study. Gut. 1988;29:1258–64.
2. Dixon MF, Wyatt JI, Burke DA, et al. Lymphocytic gastritis-relationship to Campylobacter pylori infection. J Pathol. 1988;154:125–32.
3. Jaskiewicz K, Price SK, Zak J, et al. Lymphocytic gastritis in nodular dyspepsia. Dig Dis Sci. 1991;36:1079–83.
4. Giacomo CD, Gianatti A, Negrini R, et al. Lymphocytic gastritis: a positive relationship with celiac disease. J Pediatr. 1994;124:57–62.
5. Wolber R, Owen D, DelBuono L, et al. Lymphocytic gastritis in patients with celiac sprue or spruelike intestinal disease. Gastroenterology. 1990;98:310–5.
6. Tsung-The W, Stanley H. Lymphocytic gastritis: association with etiology and topology. Am J Surg Pathol. 1999;23:153–8.
7. Niemela S, Karttunen T, Kerola T, et al. Ten year follow up study of lymphocytic gastritis: further evidence on Helicobacter pylori as a cause of lymphocytic gastritis and corpus gastritis. J Clin Pathol. 1995;48:1111–6.
8. Haot J, Berger F, Andre C, et al. Lymphocytic gastritis versus varioliform gastritis. A historical series revisited. J Pathol. 1989;158:19–22.
9. Haot J, Jouret A, Willette M, Gossuin A, et al. Lymphocytic gastritis-prospective study of this relationship with varioliform gastritis. Gut. 1990;31:282–5.
10. Lambert R, Andre C, Moulinier B, et al. Diffuse varioliform gastritis. Digestion. 1978;17:159–67.
11. Crampton JR, Hunter JO, Neale G, et al. Chronic lymphocytic gastritis and protein losing gastropathy. Gut. 1989;30:71–4.
12. Haot J, Bogomoletz WV, Jouret A, et al. Menetrier's disease with lymphocytic gastritis: an unusual association with possible pathogenic implications. Hum Pathol. 1991;22:379–86.
13. Wolber RA, Owen DA, Anderson FH, et al. Lymphocytic gastritis and giant gastric folds associated with gastrointestinal protein loss. Mod Pathol. 1991;4:13–5.
14. Wolfsen HC, Carpenter HA, Talley NJ. Menetrier's disease: a form of hypertrophic gastropathy or gastritis. Gastroenterology. 1993;104:1310–9.
15. Bayerdorffer E, Ritter MM, Hatz R, et al. Healing of protein losing hypertrophic gastropathy by eradication of Helicobacter pylori-is Helicobacter pylori a pathogenic factor in Menetrier's disease? Gut. 1995;35:701–4.
16. Groisamn GM, George J, Berman D, et al. Resolution of protein-losing hypertrophic lymphocytic gastritis with therapeutic eradication of Helicobacter pylori. Am J Gastroenterol. 1994;89:1548–51.
17. Brain O, Rajaguru C, Warren B, et al. Collagenous gastritis: reports and systematic review. Eur J Gastroenterol Hepatol. 2009;21:1419–24.
18. Nielsen OH, Riis LB, Danese S, et al. Proximal collagenous gastroenteritides: clinical management. A systematic review. Ann Med. 2014;46:311–7.
19. Rustagi T, Rai M, Scholes JV. Collagenous gastroduodenitis. J Clin Gastroenterol. 2011;45:794–9.
20. Gopal P, McKenna BJ. The collagenous gastroenteritides: similarities and differences. Arch Pathol Lab Med. 2010;134:1485–9.
21. Colletti RB, Trainer TD. Collagenous gastritis. Gastroenterology. 1989;97:1552–5.
22. Lagorce-Pages C, Fabiani B, Bouvier R, et al. Collagenous gastritis. Am J Surg Pathol. 2001;25:1174–9.
23. Müller H, Rappel S, Volkholz H, et al. Die lymphozytäre Gastritis—eine seltene Erkrankung der Magenschleimhaut. Pathologe. 2001;22:56–61.
24. Feeley KM, Heneghan MA, Stevens FM, et al. Lymphocytic gastritis and coeliac disease: evidence of a positive association. J Clin Pathol. 1998;51:207–10.
25. Tsai HF, Hsu PN. Interplay between Helicobacter pylori and immune cells in immune pathogenesis of gastric inflammation and mucosal pathology. Cell Mol Immunol. 2010;7:255–9.
26. Vakiani E, Yantiss R. Lymphocytic gastritis: clinicopathologic features, etiologic associations, and pathogenesis. Pathol Case Rev. 2008;13:167–71.
27. Puderecki M, Wronecki L, Cięszczyk K, et al. Lymphocytic gastritis. Pol J Pathol. 2019;70:155–61.
28. Hatemi I, Hatemi G, Çelik AF. Systemic vasculitis and the gut. Curr Opin Rheumatol. 2017;29:33–8.
29. Scott DG, Bacon PA, Elliott PJ, et al. Systemic vasculitis in a district general hospital 1972–1980: clinical and laboratory features, classification and prognosis of 80 cases. Q J Med. 1982;51:292–311.
30. Lopez LR, Schocket AL, Stanford RE, et al. Gastrointestinal involvement in leukocytoclastic vasculitis and polyarteritis nodosa. J Rheumatol. 1980;7:677–84.
31. Hatemia I, Hatemib G, Celika AF. Systemic vasculitis and the gut. Curr Opin Rheumatol. 2016;29:33–8. https://doi.org/10.1097/BOR.0000000000000344.
32. Sipe JD, Benson MD, Buxbaum JN, et al. Nomenclature 2014: amyloid fibril proteins and clinical classification of the amyloidosis. Amyloid. 2014;21:221–4.
33. Ebert EC, Nagar M. Gastrointestinal manifestations of amyloidosis. Am J Gastroenterol. 2008;103:776–87.
34. Ding Y, Li Y, Sun L. A rare case of asymptomatic primary gastric localized amyloidosis. Clin Gastroenterol Hepatol. 2019;17:A41–2.
35. Liu XM, Di LJ, Zhu JX, et al. Localized primary gastric amyloidosis: three case reports. World J Clin Cases. 2020;8:4667–75.
36. Petre S, Shah IA, Gilani N. Review article: gastrointestinal amyloidosis—clinical features, diagnosis and therapy. Aliment Pharmacol Ther. 2008;27:1006–16.

Uncommon Types of Gastritis and Gastropathies Including Anti-parietal Cell, GVHD, Reactive and Granulomatous Gastritis

19

19.1 Anti-parietal Cell Antibody Related Autoimmune Gastritis

It is an immune-mediated persistent inflammatory disorder affecting the gastric body and fundus. There is persistent destruction of the parietal cells present by autoantibody against the parietal cell producing mucosal atrophy resulting in reduction in acid and intrinsic factor production. Parietal cell plays important role in maintenance of acid medium in the stomach through H+/K+ ATPase and proton pump supported by G cells located in gastric antrum producing gastrin [1]. Gastrin production is regulated by the low Ph in antrum. A few scattered enterochromaffin-like (ECL) cells located in oxyntic mucosa assist in maintenance of acid medium by secreting histamine. Mucosal atrophy is the result of loss or destruction of parietal cells by lymphocytes, also affecting the chief cells which normally secretes pepsinogen and gastric lipase. In this conventional autoimmune gastritis (AIG), gastric mucosa is infiltrated by CD4-positive T cells targeting parietal and chief cells resulting in their destruction. The resulting mucosal atrophy gives rise to a state of achlorhydria prompting G cells activation and hypergastrinemia. Atrophic gastritis is the end result of chronic long-standing mucosal inflammation and destruction of specialized glands and AIG is one such important condition and any other condition that may result in mucosal inflammation and destruction of the specialized glands will result in morphologically similar mucosal histology. One such non-AIG associated condition is *H. pylori*-associated gastritis. Mucosal changes in AIG selectively involves corpus and fundus as the autoantibody is targeting parietal cells Gastritis due to other underlying aetiology like *H. pylori*, stress or drug-induced, the involvement may be pyloric antral dominant or multifocal in distribution including the body and fundus regions of the stomach (Fig. 19.1a–g). Long-standing destruction of the parietal cells by ongoing chronic inflammation leads ultimately to mucosal atrophy producing high gastric pH and loss of intrinsic factor resulting in pernicious anaemia. In 1909, achylia gastrica was identified as the underlying aetiology for iron deficiency anaemia by Faber [2]. It is pertinent to differentiate between primary lymphocytic autoimmune gastritis from AIG associated with B12 deficiency. The first condition is not restricted to body, antrum may also be involved by the lymphocytic inflammation and the affected individual does not present with megaloblastic anaemia. On the other hand, the second condition is selectively seen in middle-aged females presenting with refractile megaloblastic anaemia, selective involvement of the body and fundus sparing the antrum, along with a positive serology for anti-parietal cell antibody; a certain number of patients having involvement of antrum may also have a positive serology for anti-parietal cell antibody [3, 4].

K. Vaiphei, *Interpretation of Endoscopic Biopsy - Gastritis, Gastropathies and Beyond*,
https://doi.org/10.1007/978-981-16-6026-9_19

Hence, the most sensitive marker for AIG is serology testing for anti-parietal cell antibodies, which may be positive in 90% of patients. And more than half of these patients may be positive for antibodies against intrinsic factor and H^+/K^+ ATPase [5]. Intrinsic factor antibody is considered diagnostic for pernicious anaemia, but does not show correlation with histological extent of gastric mucosa disease and clinical manifestation. Serology may be positive for the antibody years before the clinical symptom. Anti-H^+/K^+ ATPase antibody is non-specific, as it is also positive in an individual with long-standing *H. pylori* gastritis. Hence, the role of *H. pylori* in AIG is still unclear. Serum gastrin and pepsinogen levels help in predicting the severity of the AIG per se. *H. pylori* gastritis with mucosal atrophy positive autoantibodies may resemble AIG clinically and pathologically. Besides about 80% of AIG individuals harbour antibodies to *H. pylori* though gastric mucosal biopsies failed to demonstrate colonization by the organism [5, 6].

In AIG, it is essential to have biopsies from antrum and body, and in a classic AIG case, antral mucosa will be of normal morphology with inflamed body and fundus mucosa. In a biopsy with early-stage morphological changes, there will be a diffuse basal predominant mucosal inflammation, dominantly comprising of CD4+ T cells intermixed with scatter plasma cell, eosino-

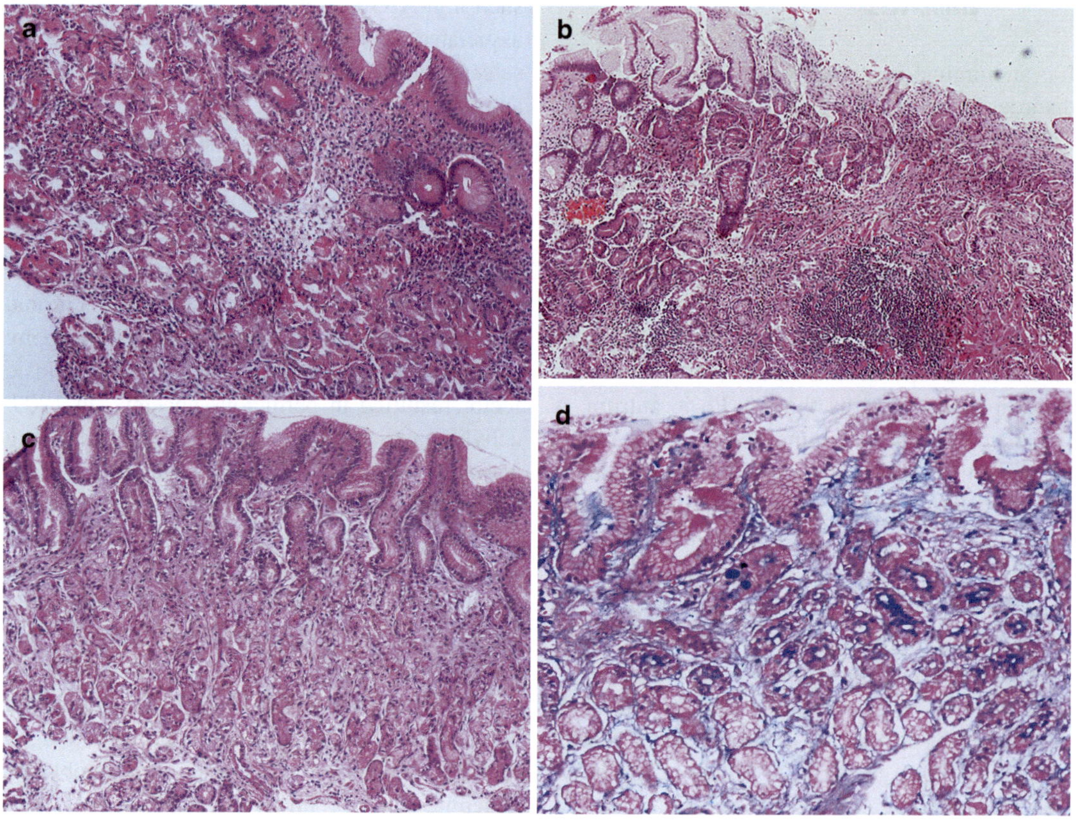

Fig. 19.1 (**a**)–(**c**) Highlights different stages of atrophic gastritis from early patchy destruction of parietal cells by lymphocytes to almost near-total destruction and pylori metaplasia and moderately heavy mononuclear cell infiltration to almost total loss of specialized gastric glands and replacement fibrosis (H#, ×350). (**d**) and (**e**) Photomicrographs of alcian blue PAS stain sections to show scattered alcian blue positive metaplastic cells in the background of atrophic changes and grossly hyperplastic foveolae with metaplastic epithelium (AB-PAS, ×350). (**f**) and (**g**) Photomicrographs of immunohistochemistry stain sections using gastrin and chromogranin A primary antibodies respectively and showing many gastrin-positive cells along the deeper portion of the atrophic mucosa and very few scattered chromogranin A-positive cells (PAP, ×350)

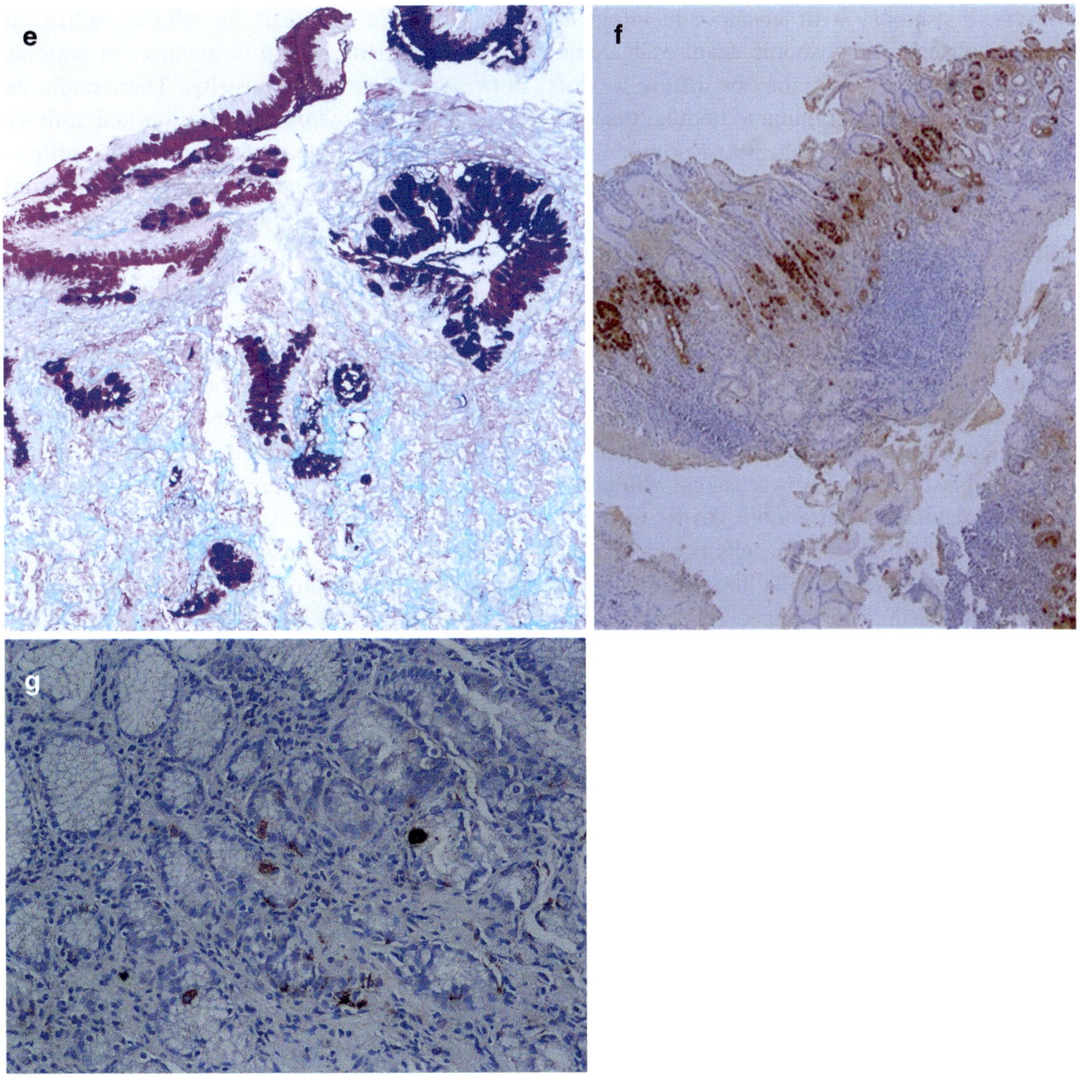

Fig. 19.1 (continued)

phil and occasional mast cell. There will be lymphocytic infiltration of glands with active epithelial/parietal cell destruction. Metaplastic epithelial cells may be identifiable in a biopsy carried out in early-stage disease. Metaplastic cells are like mucous cells/glands, pseudo-pyloric metaplasia and pancreatic acinar cells. There may be florid proliferation of immature neck cells. Atrophic changes indicated by loss of parietal cells which may be with metaplastic epithelial cells may be of variable extend. Sometimes, the residual parietal cells may undergo hypertrophy as a response to increased gastrin production resulting in nodular mucosa in the endoscopic examination. In an advanced disease, the body and fundus mucosa show almost to total loss of specialized cells with diffuse lamina propria lymphoplasmacytic infiltration, with sometimes appreciable metaplastic epithelium. Later stage of the disease, ECL cells start proliferating and the biopsy from the pyloric antrum shows gastrin secreting cell hyperplasia. Biopsy in late-stage disease, the mucosa becomes thin with variable degree of fibrosis of the lamina propria and reduction in lymphoplasmacytic cells. The proliferating ECL cells are best identified by immunomarkers. In a biopsy with advanced histological mucosal changes, endoscopic features become more heterogenous, there may be diffuse loss of mucosal fold pattern, granular to nodular mucosa ranging from a few millimetres to 1 or more cms in size, which are sessile but rarely pedunculated. Multiple site biopsies are required in such mucosa in order to identify areas of dysplasia, intestinal metaplasia and, type and extend of ECL cells proliferation. ECL cell proliferation requires classification according to the pattern and distributions, which can be simple, linear and nodular proliferation. ECL cells in HE stained section appear small cells with a moderate amount of clear cytoplasm, nuclei appear round with compact chromatin. In any random gastric atrophy, best way of identifying ECL cells is by utilizing IHC for neuroendocrine cells like chromogranin A, synaptophysin, neuron-specific enolase and gastrin. Any one or more may be positive, KI-67 IHC will help to interpret extent of the cellular proliferation of the cells of interest as the proliferative zone of native gastric mucosa may exhibit many positive nuclei [7–9].

Biopsies from the polypoidal lesions will frequently show hyperplastic polyp in the background of atrophic gastritis and these polyps tend to be multiply mimicking a polyposis. Hence, multiple site biopsy including biopsy from non-polypoidal mucosa to establish changes in the background gastric mucosa. Besides immunohistochemistry, it is all advisable to have alcian blue periodic acid Schiff stained section in gastric biopsies and this will help to highlight all the gastric mucous cells containing partially or totally metaplastic mucin. Many of the cells may contain purplish mucin indicating partially or incompletely modified acid mucin, especially in the ones with micro-vesicular changes. And further, this will also help to identified unsuspected invasive carcinomas in the lamina propria, as these cells may be innocuous vacuolated cells. Varying degree of lamina propria fibrosis tends to be present. These fibrotic areas may give alcian blue positivity due to associated stromal degenerative changes. Ideally, biopsies should be received in labelled separate vials [7–9].

Differential diagnosis for AIG is multifocal strophic gastritis, which in majority of patients is *H. pylori*-associated gastritis. There could be evidence of *H. pylori* colonization and activity in form of focal mucosal neutrophilic infiltration in the background of atrophic gastritis and hyperplastic pseudopolyps. These changes may be observed both in corpus biopsy also in pyloric antral biopsy. Frequently, neutrophil infiltration may be result of associated mucosal erosions and ulcerations, which may be identifiable. In a developing country like ours with frequent occurrence of *H. pylori*-associated gastritis, possibility of superadded infection remains high. If biopsy interpretation from different areas of the stomach is being used as the gold standard, one may miss AIG. Hence, serology study for the autoimmune markers should be made a routine essential in addition to the other clinical and haematological parameters. Multifocal atrophic gastritis is not rare amongst the population where gastric carcinoma is endemic [7–9]. All histological changes are similar in all atrophic gastritis irrespective of the underlying aetiology.

19.2 Focally Enhanced Gastritis

It is one specific condition that has been described and mentioned in many textbooks as the gastric manifestation of inflammatory bowel disease (IBD). As the term suggests, there are focal aggregates of mixed inflammatory cells. The inflammatory cells aggregate more towards the gastric pits and the glands. Amongst the paediatric population, this condition has been documented more frequently in Crohn's disease (CD) than in ulcerative colitis (UC) patients [10–14]. A wide range of incidences of upper GI involvement have been reported, the reported frequency varied from 5% to 70% amongst all IBD cases. Similar to paediatric group, gastric involvement has been documented in more numbers of CD patients both in endoscopic as well as histological examinations, although gastric mucosa looked normal frequently [15, 16]. Light microscopic features are similar between the two conditions except for the presence of compact epithelioid cell granuloma in CD not associated with a ruptured crypt (cryptolytic granuloma). And the termed focally enhanced gastritis (FEG) was described by Oberhuber et al. as a specific condition for CD though subsequently similar features were observed in UC patients and also other non-IBD patients [16–18]. Endoscopic features may show mild erythema, erosions, granular and nodular mucosa involving antrum and body. All the changes that have been described may be observed with an underlying infective aetiology as well.

The histological features of FEG are characterized by a focal pit or gland inflammation with epithelial cell injury. The inflammatory cells are dominantly consisting of lymphocytes and macrophages, often with scattered plasma cells, eosinophils and/a few neutrophils. A distinctive feature is the relatively normal looking background gastric mucosa, otherwise similar morphological features may be observed in many other types of gastritis (Fig. 19.2a and b). Several studies have reported FEG in 43 to 76% of CD and 20% of UC patients [15–18]. Hence, it is considered to be a characteristic feature for IBD in general, though it is a non-specific feature. FEG is reportedly more frequently observed in IBD children.

19.3 Graft Versus Host Disease

It is a clinical condition observed in allogenic haematopoietic stem cell transplant patients. Gastrointestinal tract (GIT) is one more frequently involved system, both upper and lower GITs are involved. It is an immunologic disorder in which functionally competent donor T lymphocytes interact with the epithelial cells of the recipient [19]. An increasing trend of Graft Versus Host Disease (GVHD) has been observed in spite of advancement in immunosuppressive therapy. Radiology of the affected organ plays important role in the initial step of diagnosing early phase of GVHD, follow-up and surveillance of GVHD. Frequently affected organs are skin, gastrointestinal system and hepatobiliary systems. Radiological features in GIT are bowel wall thickening with mucosal enhancement, oedema of the mesentery and engorged blood vessels. These features are non-specific but with a known history of HSCT, GVHD may be considered [20]. The morphological changes of GVHD are patchy, hence multiple tissue biopsy from multiple sites is necessary to document the morphological evidence. Biopsies from upper and lower GI are usually sampled. The time of presentation is variable and common presenting symptoms are nausea, vomiting and diarrhoea,

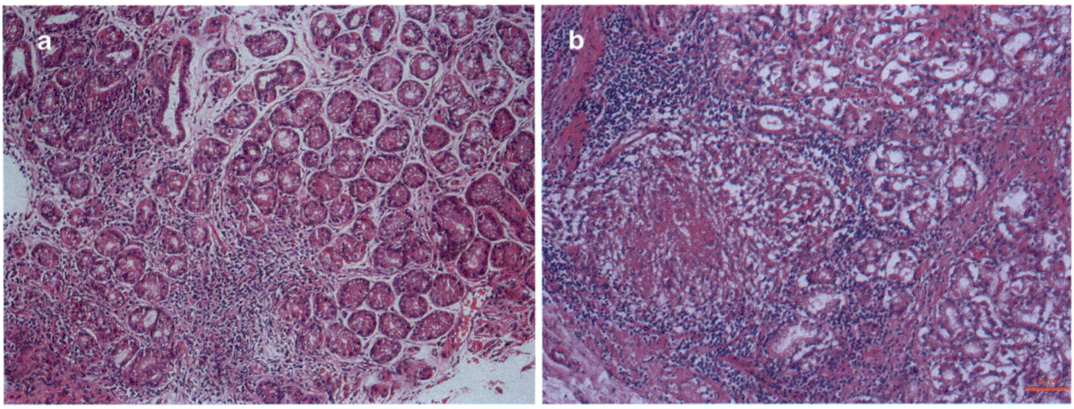

Fig. 19.2 (**a**) Photomicrograph showing focally enhanced mucosal inflammation where aggregates of mononuclear cells are seen in one particular focus in the lamina propria with destruction of the glands and relatively less inflamed mucosa in the adjoining area (HE, ×250). (**b**) Photomicrograph showing an inflamed body mucosa with a focus of compact epithelioid cell granuloma surrounded by lymphomononuclear cells (HE, ×250)

more severe ones may also have GI bleed and protein losing enteropathy. Endoscopic evaluation may show normal mucosa, mild erythema, erosions, friable, loss of normal mucosal folds and deep ulcers. This is one condition where there may be a gross disparity between endoscopic features and histological findings. The diagnosis of GVHD is established only with the existence of a specific history [21, 22]. Similar clinical and pathological features, though maybe of lesser intensity, can also be seen following transfusion of unirradiated blood.

Though, there are no validated histopathological criteria for GVHD, most common feature observed in a biopsy form GIT is the presence of crypt/foveolae epithelial cell apoptosis, affecting the regenerative zone. The affected cells may show either cytoplasmic vacuolization or condensation indicated as dense eosinophilia containing clumped hyperchromatic or karyorrhectic nuclei, which requires differentiation from a cell in mitosis (Fig. 19.3a and b). This can be done easily from the character of the cytoplasm [23–26]. Identification of small individual cell apoptosis in gastric biopsies may be quite challenging and the help of specific immunomarkers for apoptotic body may be incorporated in reporting [27, 28]. In addition, other histological features include glandular dilatation, crypt cast or debris within the glands, denudation of surface lining epithelium, mucodepletion, degenerative changes of the glandular lining epithelial cells, glandular fragmentation, disappearance or loss of glands. Epithelial cells showing regeneration may also be observed side by side. Prominence of the mucosal and submucosal blood vessels, mixed inflammatory cell infiltration of lamina propria including many eosinophils and occasionally neutrophils. Morphological changes in mucosa will depend on the severity of the disease and may be patchy [21–25].

The exact pathophysiology of chronic GVHD is not well understood but is believed to be an immune dysregulation resulting in continuous inflammatory process results in stimulation of fibroblasts resulting in fibrosis and chronic GVHD patient histologically exhibits prominent fibrosis of mucosa, submucosa and serosa. Mucosa tends to show disorganized crypt architecture though with mild inflammation, Paneth cell metaplasia and prominent hyalinosis of mucosal and submucosal blood vessels. Morphological changes of chronic GVHD may coexist frequently with acute changes. Documented incidence of chronic GVHD differs widely from centre to centre ranging between 30 and 65% following HSCT, and also depends on the regime the patient is receiving. Acute GVHD is usually seen within the first 10–40 days and for diagnosing acute GVHD, maximum cut-off number of days is the first 100 days. After 100 days, there can be persistent, recurrent or late-onset acute GVHD. The time schedule for the diagnosis of a chronic GVHD is >100 days. Skin tends to be the first organ to be involved followed by GIT and liver. GI and liver manifestations without skin involvement happen rarely. Majority of acute GVHD is frequently followed by the process of chronic GVHD. Chronic GVHD may develop insidiously with no pre-existing acute GVHD. Incidence of both acute and chronic GVHDs are more frequently observed following unrelated transplant recipients and these patients tend to have chronic events more than an acute event. Though a chronic GVHD is typically diagnosed after 100 days of transplantation, it may occur any time before 100 days as well [28–32].

Histological features may help to differentiate between acute and chronic forms of GVHD, there is a grey zone between the two that has been referred to as overlap syndrome. National Institutes of Health recognizes two main categories of GVHD, each with two subcategories, based on clinical manifestations [28–30]. An acute GVHD can have varieties of clinical presentations, i.e. classic, persistent, recurrent or a late onset after day 100. Similarly, a chronic maybe classic or an overlap clinical features for both acute and chronic conditions. GVHD has been classified into acute for those cases presenting with characteristic skin, GIT and liver involvement regardless of the time factor. And for the diagnosis of chronic GVHD, presence of at least one distinctive clinical manifestation and confirmed histologically or any other relevant test in the same or another organ [28–30].

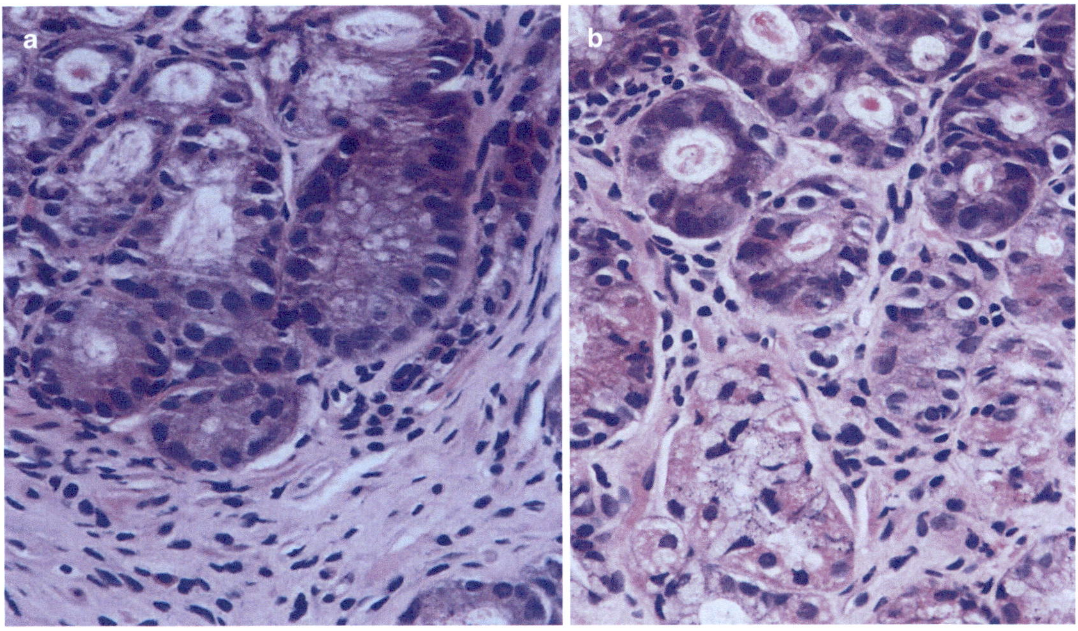

Fig. 19.3 (**a**) and (**b**) Both photomicrographs show gastric mucosa of antral and body origin respectively on high power. Deeper portion of the mucosa in both the biopsies shows replacement fibrosis. The gastric glands show apoptotic bodies and vacuolization of the gastric glands indicating acute and chronic graft versus host disease (HE, ×500)

The first histological feature one looks for the diagnosis of acute GVHD is apoptotic body. There is no validated optimum number of apoptotic bodies. It is, however, good to remember that an apoptotic body is seldom normally observed structure in a crypt or in gastric mucosa. Besides, any diseased organ tends to show a spectrum of morphological changes and not just one particular feature. Presence of one or few more apoptotic and pre-apoptotic bodies in one biopsy piece may be considered adequate for the diagnosis of acute GVHD in the right clinical setting. The best way to practice in clinical material is to study ribbon sections examining the biopsy at multiple levels. There are just a few other conditions that may produce similar morphological changes in an endoscopic biopsy like drugs, otherwise, the histological features diagnostic for GVHD though not specific. Hence diagnosis of GVHD is a clinicopathological entity. No definite serological marker is still so far been established. There are many reports studying the possible roles of key inflammatory factors like IL-2, TNFα, TGFβ, IL-7 and IL-15 as the possible markers for acute GVHD but all were found to be non-specific [21, 23, 30, 31]. Apoptosis of regenerating epithelial cell is considered as the hallmark of acute GVHD and correlation have been observed between serum levels of cytokeratin18 fragments (CK18F) and total CK18 correlated with acute hepato-intestinal GVHD [26, 27]. There are studies reporting lower frequency of infused naïve CD8+ T cells to be associated with reduced risk for GVHD and bone marrow graft with CD4:CD8 $\geq$1.16 to be associated with increased risk of severe GVHD [31, 32].

Symptom of GVHD is believed to developed by about 15 days post-transplant, some studied reporting it to occur within a few days following stem cell transplant. However, histological features that may be consistent with GVHD could be seen by about three weeks post-transplant. It is important to be knowledgeable about the plausible effects of conditioning chemotherapy and total body irradiation on the intestinal mucosa, which may produce similar histological changes in GI mucosa. GVHD of autologous stem cell transplantation seems to be due to failure of self-tolerance where chemotherapy regimens diminish regulatory T-cells allowing development of GVHD. A biopsy carried out <21 days of post-transplantation shows less CD8, FoxP3 and CD4 cells in lamina propria [32].

National Health Institute consensus guidelines (2015) recommends examination of 8 to 20 serial sections of the mucosal biopsy. A 4 tier grading system is in use which was described by Lerner later modified by Sale [28] is given below appropriately modified for gastric biopsy. Grade I refers to individual cell apoptosis with a rare apoptotic body involving a deeper region of foveolae with sparse or no lymphocyte. Grade II—more number exhibiting apoptosis, almost extending along the length of foveolae with luminal necrotic cell debris along with lymphocytes, neutrophils and eosinophils. Grade III—destruction of many foveolae in continuity resulting in lack of epithelial cells in the mucosa. Grade IV—mucosal loss along with surface epithelial cell loss and loss of foveolae. Histological features and the gradings may not correlate with clinical course and treatment received. The consensus acknowledges high-grade (III–IV) lesions relevant for treatment decision and grade IV lesion as an independent parameter for lack of response to treatment and worse outcome [19, 28–30]. Certain categories for biopsy reporting in a patient suspected to be a case of GVHD (NIH guidelines), i.e. not GVHD, possible GVHD and likely GVHD [19, 28–30]. The possible category refers to when a few features are identified but viral infection or adverse drug reaction cannot be excluded. For a likely category refers to unequivocal features for the diagnosis, i.e. minimal histological changes are present with no explainable alternative condition, or a biopsy carried out long enough after chemotherapy or radiotherapy, or along with positive serology for cytomegalovirus but no morphological evidence within apoptotic cells. Some clinically relevant differential diagnoses for mucosal biopsies in the case of GVHD are effects of chemotherapeutic agents, mycophenolate mofetil, non-steroidal anti-inflammatory drugs, proton pump inhibitor, bowel preparation and viral infection. Similar to colonic mucosa, gastric mucosa may also show metaplastic epithelium, basal plasmacytosis, collection of epithelioid histiocytes and rarely pseudo-membrane formation, all with negative for microorganisms and viruses [29, 30].

19.4 Drugs and Chemical-Related Gastritis or Reactive Gastropathy

William Beaumont in 1833 documented an association between bile in stomach with gastric mucosal damage [33]. Morphological features observed in such gastric mucosa were described much later in the 1960s and 1970s, were referred to as post-operative gastritis with malignant potential [34–40]. In the 1980s, these mucosal changes were referred to as bile reflux gastritis [41, 42]. Similar histological features were described with regular intake of NSAIDs and the term of chemical gastritis was recommended [43, 44]. The term reactive gastropathy has been interchangeably used with chemical gastropathy or chemical gastritis or gastritis of C type which are the effects of bile, alcohol, drugs, haematinic supplements like iron, instrumentation, radiation and prolapsed antral mucosa or may be idiopathic with no known exposure to any particular chemical compound. Gastric mucosa in these conditions shows minimal inflammation [45]. Gastritis refers to inflammation of gastric mucosa and often refers to any clinical condition associated with upper gastrointestinal symptoms. Gastropathy, on the other hand, refers to nonspecific microscopic features of stomach mucosa with minimal or no inflammatory cell infiltration. Both conditions may be asymptomatic or may have similar clinical presentation. Clinical symptoms in drugs or chemical-related gastritis or reactive gastropathy will be like any other gastritis patient and will present with definite temporal relationship with causative agent. Diagnosis is established based on characteristic histological feature, which can be seen in any part of the gastric mucosa, more frequently in antral mucosa [44, 46–48]. This may be related to more frequently examined mucosa that happens to be of antral origin and alternatively antral mucosa gets exposed to the irritant content longer duration due to its strategic physiological position. Endoscopic features are non-specific and the mucosa may appear normal, erythematous, congested, oedematous or erosive. In bile reflux-associated reactive changes, mucosa may be bile stained in the endoscopic examination, which possibly sometimes may also be visible histologically. Depending on the underlying etiology or associated condition, there may be crystals of different colors, shapes and sizes along the surface of the gastric lining mucosal epithelium and foveolae, identifying these structures appropriately may help in diagnosing the causative agent. Histological changes may be observed after four to five weeks of intake of the irritating agent. It is characterized by hyperplastic foveolar cells along with grossly tortuous giving a cock screw appearance along with glandular dilatation. Lamina propria tends to show minimal or mild inflammatory cells which dominantly are chronic inflammatory cells (Fig. 19.4a and b). These changes may be associated with regenerative activity observed at the foveolar neck cells where there may be nucleomegaly and nuclear hyperchromasia with occasional mitosis. There may be scattered eosinophils and neutrophils invading the gastric epithelial cells and also in lamina propria. These changes dominantly involve pyloric antrum, however, any portion of the stomach may show similar features. Overall mucosal thickness may be increased due to associated characteristic changes observed in the glands and foveolae. These mucosal changes are associated with

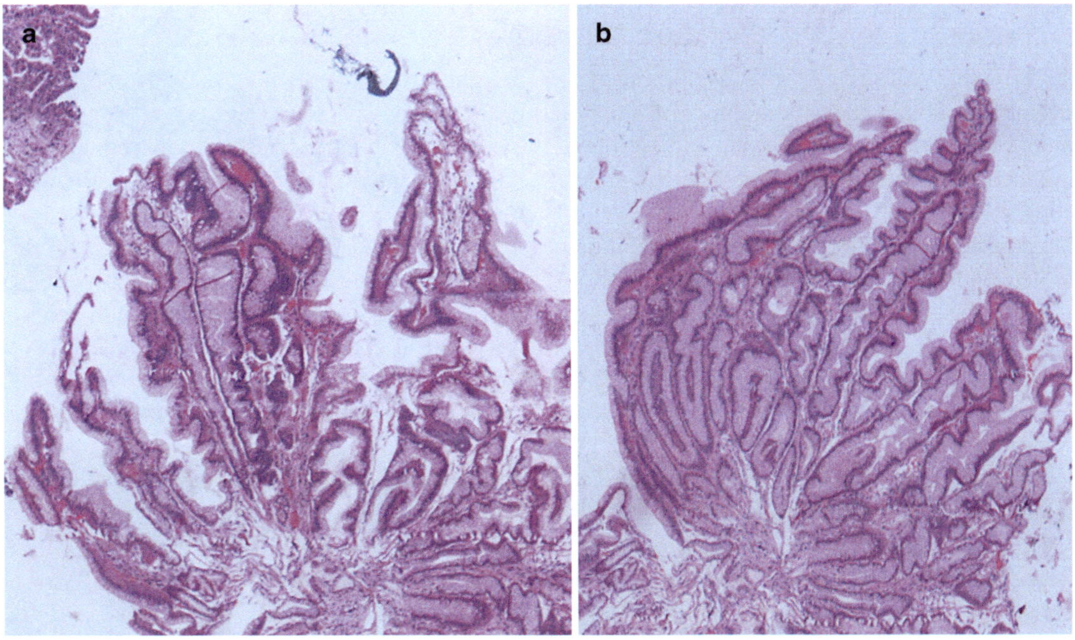

Fig. 19.4 (**a**) and (**b**) Both the photomicrographs show elongated and cock screw-like gastric foveolae with total loss of the gastric glands which are the characteristic appearances observed in long-standing reactive gastropathy of any aetiology (HE, ×150). (**c**) Higher power photomicrograph in similar condition showing in addition to the foveolar epithelial changes, lamina propria included is showing oedema and strands of smooth muscle (HE, ×250). (**d**)–(**f**) Photomicrographs of gastric biopsy to show mucosal injury related to intake of haematinics (iron-based tonics). In (**d**), there is an erosion of the surface lining epithelium along with disorganization of the glands lined by irritated epithelium and lamina propria early collagenization. Overlying the surface are clusters of fluffy eosinophilic materials (HE, ×300). (**e**) Another photomicrograph shows necrotic gastric mucosa along with golden brown pigment on the ulcer and within the necrotic gastric glands (HE, ×300). (**f**) Photomicrograph highlights presence of perl's positive pigments corresponding to those seen as golden brown in (**e**) (Perls, ×300)

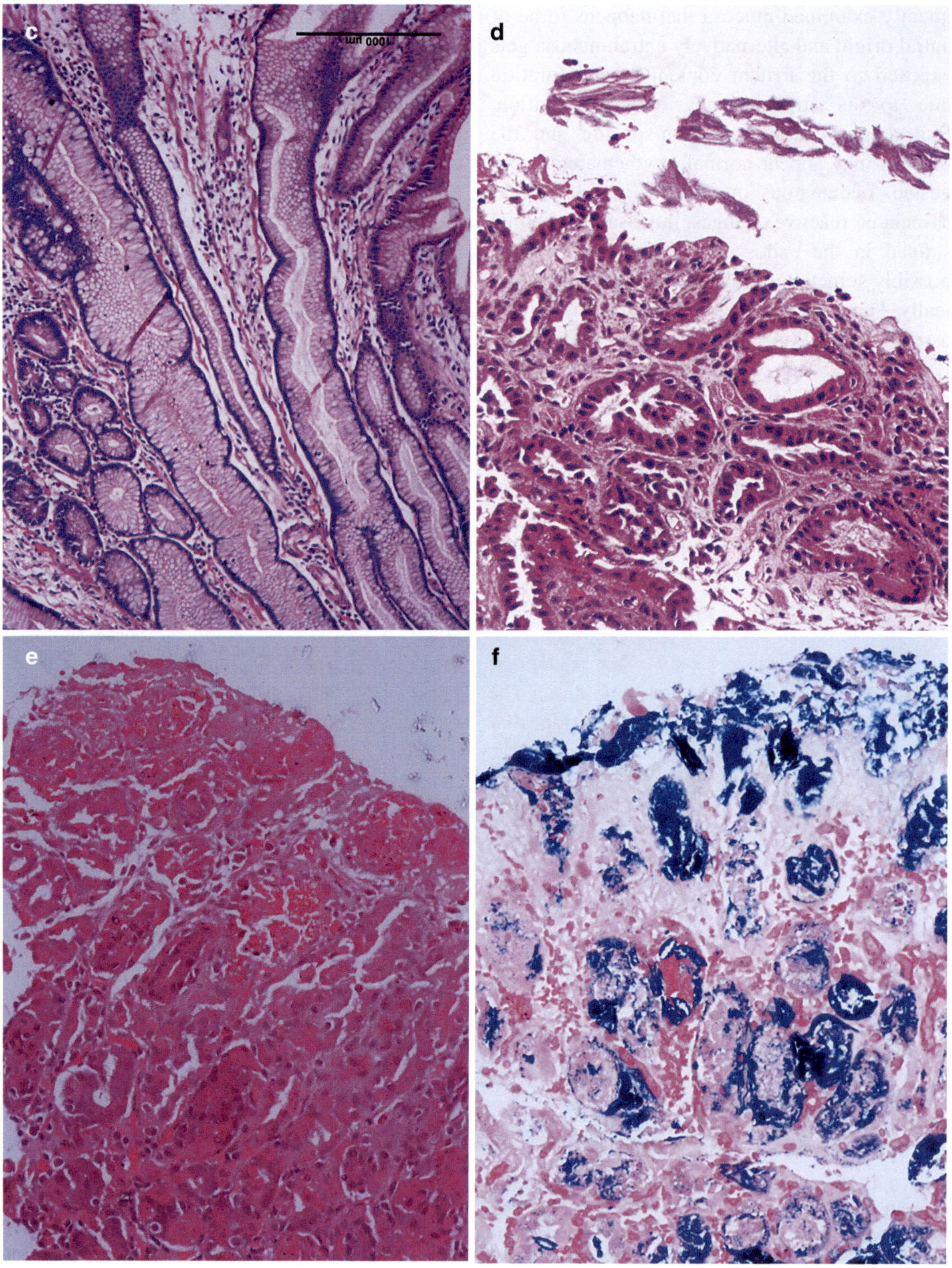

Fig. 19.4 (continued)

hyperplasia accompanied by splaying and extension of the muscularis mucosae into lamina propria. In biopsy taken from the body, parietal cells are usually well preserved or reduced with replacement fibrosis. Lamina propria may show oedema, vascular congestion along with few scattered ectatic thin-walled mucosal vessels (Fig. 19.4c). Lamina propria in addition may also show an excess of loose stromal components or patchy fibrosis and superficial epithelial erosion [44, 46–50]. Following ingestion of iron supplements, there can be variable grades of mucosal erosion, fibrosis, changes of mucosal atrophy and inflammation depending on the duration of exposure associated with the mucosal injury. Deposition of iron pigment along the eroded surface and sometimes entrapped within healed mucosa may be demonstrable (Fig. 19.4d–f).

It gives immense pleasure to learn the history of describing a particular condition. According to the report by Bensley in 1959, the damaging effect of bile in gastric mucosa was first documented by William Beaumont (1833) in his decade-long observation of Alexis St. Martin's permanent open gastric fistula [33]. Effects of bile and duodenopancreatic juice in reflux conditions following partial gastrectomy were referred to as post-operative gastritis [34–36, 50]. In the series of publications on gastric mucosal changes in reflux diseases, the term bile reflux gastritis was proposed and used as a distinct clinicopathological entity [50, 51]. A broader term of chemical gastritis was recommended by Updated Sydney System as similar mucosal changes were also associated in patients who were on regular NSAIDs [43]. Since then, many histopathologists have used interchangeably the term reactive gastropathy, although in significant number of patients, the clinical symptoms and the morphological changes observed in the gastric mucosa remain unexplained and associated with gradual increase with increasing age of the individuals [42–44]. Genta had described morphological features of reactive gastropathy as gastric mucosa showing combinations of foveolar hyperplasia, surface epithelial regeneration, lamina propria oedema and/or hyperaemia, erosions and splaying of muscularis mucosae [44]. Malguilnik et al. observed morphological changes in oesophagus and duodenum in association with reactive gastropathy in high percentages. Though the study has not specified the aetiology of the reactive gastropathy, i.e. any history of intake of any irritant or idiopathic variant [50].

19.5 Granulomatous Gastritis

Granulomas in gastric mucosa is a rarely observed condition and it is believed to be due to a low pH of gastric content, making unsuitable for an organism to survive [52]. Granulomatous Gastritis (GG) refers to a broad spectrum of histopathologic features ranging from vague ill-defined collections of mucosal and or submucosal epithelioid histiocytes intermixed with other inflammatory cells to well-formed epithelioid cell granulomas, multinucleated giant cells and lymphoplasmacytic cells. Usually, gastric granuloma tends to be small and compact, areas of necrosis may be an occasional feature (Fig. 19.5a–c). These granulomas are distributed in a background of heavy dense mucosal inflammation along with lymphoid aggregates [52–56]. Estimated incidence varies between 0.27 and 0.35% amongst all gastric biopsies and a large series reported only 56 cases out of 15,947 biopsies/resections [52, 53, 56]. There may be associated mucosal ulceration and patchy mucosal fibrosis. Changes in mucosal atrophy may also be present indicating that majority of the granulomatous gastritis patients undergo endoscopic examination accompanied by biopsy much later in the course of the disease. This indicates that granulomatous gastritis is a chronic slowly progressing inflammatory condition. However, this statement requires verification and will depend on the associated condition, i.e. either an isolated primary gastric disorder or gastric involvement as a part and partial of systemic disseminated

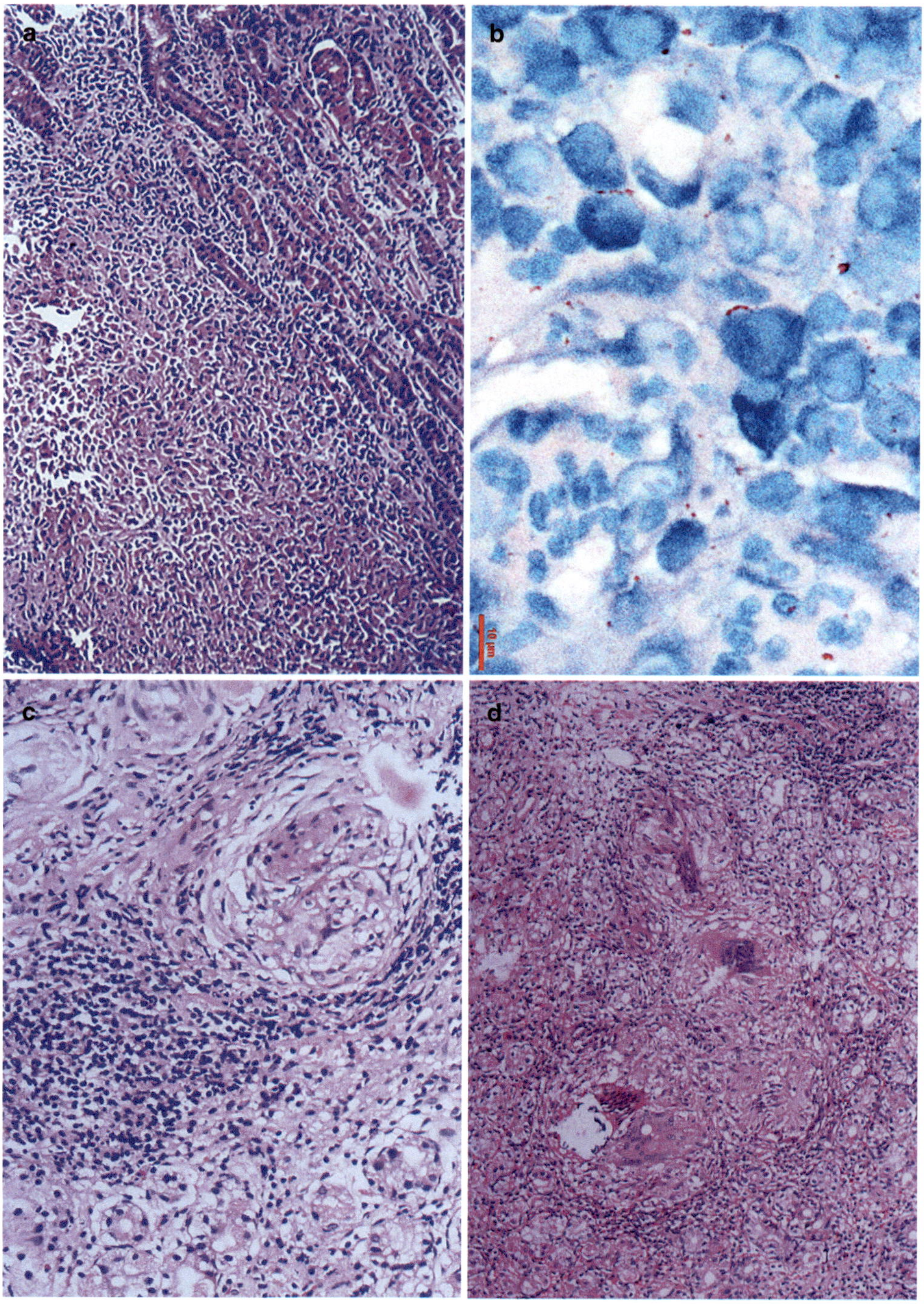

Fig. 19.5 (**a**) Medium power view of gastric biopsy showing heavily inflamed gastric mucosa with epithelioid cells granuloma in the lamina propria (HE, ×300). (**b**) Oil immersion view of the same biopsy to show the presence of a few scatter beaded appearing acid-fast bacilli (Z N stain, ×1000). (**c**) Another medium power photomicrograph showing a compact epithelioid cell granuloma surrounded by lymphomononuclear cells and fibrous tissue (HE, ×400). (**d**) A photomicrograph of a gastric biopsy showing multiple epithelioid cell granulomas with heavy lamina propria inflammation. Many Langhan, as well as foreign body type multinucleated giant cells, are seen within the granulomas. These giant cells are seen to have many vacuoles and negative shadows which did not stain with PAS (HE, ×150)

disorder. GG may be infective, non-infective or idiopathic [54, 56]. Shapiro et al. documented the commonest aetiology being Crohn's disease followed by foreign body reaction, malignant conditions and sarcoidosis [54]. They further stated that determining underlying aetiology may often be difficult in significant number of GG cases and are frequently given the label of idiopathic GG. Infecting agents may be identifiable in many of the biopsy specimens; underlying aetiology is likely to vary according to geographical location of the patient and its ethnic origin. Majority of GG diagnosed in developed countries are non-infective type, whereas in developing countries it is likely to be infective aetiology [56, 57]. The usual common infective conditions to be considered are tuberculosis, atypical mycobacterial infection, syphilis, Whipple's disease, actinomycosis, nocardia, a variety of fungal infections including cryptococcosis as well as anisakidosis, taeniasis and infestations with other parasitic worms and schistosomes [56, 57]. *H. pylori* has been associated with granulomatous gastritis and those patients responded to *H. pylori* eradication [58–60]. Amongst the subtypes of leprosy, tuberculoid leprosy is one condition where granulomatous reaction is a characteristic feature. However, still so far there is no report or record of tuberculoid leprosy in the world literature and also based on personnel communication with dermatologists; rarely there has been incidence of histoid leprosy involving the stomach. Any organism or bacteria which is known to result in granulomatous inflammation in other body areas may produce a similar lesion in the stomach. Whenever one comes across any granulomatous gastritis, all the possibilities are to be considered and exclude one by one. Criteria for the diagnosis of a particular condition is never 100 percent airtight. When dealing with a single case, percentages, frequencies and incidences are never applicable, the particular case requires to be analyzed and studied in isolation. In endoscopic biopsy, obliquely cut isolated or small cluster of smooth muscle or myofibroblasts in lamina propria scared area may appear like collections of epithelioid histiocytes, in such situation if these cells are accompanied by multinucleated giant cell, it can simplify the diagnosis. Alternatively, one may use immunohistochemistry to differentiate between smooth muscle or myofibroblast from a histiocyte.

Non-infectious granulomatous gastritis is rarer than infectious GG. However, the following conditions require discussion so that morphologists are aware of the rare conditions and should be able to differentiate one from another [60]. Crohn's disease (CD) is rare, however, this is the most common condition of granulomatous gastritis observed in developed countries (Fig. 19.5d). Other rare non-infectious causes of GG include tumorous conditions (adenocarcinoma and MALT lymphoma), vasculitides, eosinophilic granulomatosis, polyangiitis, drugs like cocaine, carbimazole and interferon, xanthogranulomatous gastritis, foreign body reactions to stomach contents within an ulcer repair zone or to surgical material (suture granuloma), crystalline drugs (antacids containing magnesium, aluminium and silicon), reaction to endogenous materials (mucin, lipid or crystalline material), Langerhans cell histiocytosis (more common in children) and chronic granulomatous disease (more common in childhood and adolescence) [61–70]. Clinically apparent gastritis is seen in 2 to 7 percent of CD patients, microscopic involvement may be seen in up to 75 percent of patients in a normal appearing mucosa endoscopically [60]. Very characteristically, the mucosa, like in other sites of intestine, is described as focally enhanced inflammation where there are focal aggregates of inflammatory cells comprising of lymphocytes, macrophages, plasma cells and scattered neutrophils and eosinophils. Gastric mucosa usually show chronic gastritis, maybe with activity and variable extend of lamina propria fibrosis or there may be features of lymphocytic gastritis. CD involves antrum more frequently than the body or fundus. There can be associated infection by *H. pylori*, cryptosporidium or virus(es) as these patients are usually on steroid therapy. An isolated gastric involvement is almost unknown and gastric involvement in CD tends to be a part of the multicentric disease process and pick-up rate of gastric involvement may be increased proportionately with increasing number of tissue samples available for microscopic examination. Granulomas may be located in any portion of the lamina propria, not necessarily on the deeper portion only. These granulomas are compact and noncaseating, may be small and compact, but presence of a larger size granuloma will not exclude a possibility of CD. Characteristic fistulising ulcer is not usually documented in stomach but the inflammation may be more prominent on the deeper aspect of the mucosa with a relatively preserved surface epithelium. Necrosis is a rare phenomenon and if present appears more of eosinophilic hyaline or fibrinoid. This is one condition where one may also have coexisting small vessel lymphocytic vasculitis. A few scattered eosinophils and neutrophils shall not deter you from considering the possibility of CD. It is good to remember at this point that many of these patients' problems might have lasted months together where they have been treated with various types of medicines. Many of the medicines are associated with tissue eosinophilia. *In children*, CD tends involve the stomach more frequently compared to an adult counterpart and gastric manifestation, sometimes along with duodenal involvement, may be the presenting symptomatology [53–55].

Other rare variants of GG: Common variable immunodeficiency (CVID) is one condition where there can be granulomatous inflammation anywhere along the whole length of gastrointestinal tract [71]. These granulomas are noncaseating and tend to be small, discrete, maybe with Langhans as well as foreign body types of giant cells along with variable amount of lymphoplasmacytic infiltration in mucosa; there may be chronic or atrophic gastritis. Such diagnosis will only be established with the history of a documented CVID, otherwise, the histological features in a mucosal biopsy will not specific. In gastric neoplastic conditions of carcinomas, lymphomas and stromal tumours and vice versa, there may be coexisting granulomatous inflammation in the adjoining mucosa, which may result in misdiagnosis depending upon the site of sampling in endoscopic biopsy [72–75]. Many of the vasculitis conditions may also affect the stomach rarely as a primary isolated focus or as a part and partial of systemic vasculitic disorders. In such a setting, the mucosa may show variable appearances on endoscopic examinations ranging from erythema, oedema, erosions and ulcers. In an endoscopic biopsy, capillaries and venules will be identifiable in the lamina propria and in between small bundles of smooth muscles of muscularis propria. The involves vessels may show perivascular oedema, endothelial swelling and infiltration by inflammatory cells, which tend to be mainly mononuclear cells. The granulomas will be present in and around these vascular structures and may be compact or necrotising, which may be intermixed with eosinophils. The necrotic tissue tends to show eosinophilic appearance, quite distinctly different from the pale eosinophilic character of caseous necrosis. Main vasculitides that may be considered are granulomatosis with polyangiitis and eosinophilic granulomatosis with polyangiitis. The granulomas in eosinophilic polyangiitis are small discrete present in and around the involved blood vessels (both arteries and veins) [62–65]. This kind of granuloma requires to be differentiated from tuberculosis with the help of clinical profiles and other laboratory investigations, as an active tubercular granuloma is known to be associated with vasculitis [60]. Apart from certain bacteria like *Streptococcus* spp. and *Staphylococcus aureas*, there are viruses like herpes simplex, varicella zoster, hepatitis C and Human immunodeficiency viruses, which may produce granulomatous inflammation. Hence the importance of clinical profiles remains very strong in order to differentiate these many conditions and also examining the biopsy for any unsuspected findings remain critical to identify these unusual and rare conditions in a given gastric biopsy. Herpes group of viruses produces intense fibrinoid necrosis of the infected tissue. Other conditions are (1) drugs like cocaine, carbimazole, interferon, antacids or silicon; (2) xanthogranulomatous gastritis, (3) foreign body reactions to stomach contents within an ulcer repair zone or surgical material like gauze pieces, dressing or suture materials; (4) reaction to endogenous materials like mucin, lipid or crystalline material; (5) Langerhans cell histiocytosis usually in paediatric age group and (6) chronic granulomatous diseases. The granulomas may be seen anywhere and usually in vasculitis, the involved vessels are more at the deeper area of the mucosa, extending across the muscularis mucosae and a bit of involved submucosa comes along with the mucosal fragment, where one may be able to find arterioles with the characteristic changes. The crystals which may be observed in biopsy tend to be towards the upper half of the mucosa, sometimes entrapping within the foveolae with epithelial destruction and mucin entrapment. Inflammatory cell infiltrate is variable and mixed type, sometimes lymphoid cell population will be prominent with lymphoid follicle formation. Variable degrees of changes in the adjoining mucosa, which sometimes, like in Crohn's disease, maybe strikingly exhibiting focal enhanced inflammation. Langerhan's histiocytosis is a challenge to establish the diagnosis and as there are no obvious characteristic features that may stand out in casual examination of the biopsy. If the mucosal infiltrate appear to be relatively sparing the epithelial cells but aggregating in between in lamina propria, and the cells also contain larger histiocytes with atypical irregular and hyperchromic nuclei, a possibility of LCH may be considered in the differential diagnosis. The granulomas in this setting will be loose and composed of epithelioid histiocytes rather than the classic compact epithelioid cells. Immunohistochemistry by selecting the right primary antibodies will help to clinch the diagnosis [66, 67].

Sarcoidosis-stomach is the most commonly affected site in the gastrointestinal tract (GIT). Gastric granulomas are usually incidental findings in systemic sarcoidosis. Subclinical GIT involvement in sarcoidosis is known, while a symptomatic granulomatous gastritis has been reported in less than 1 percent of the patients [61]. The clinical presentation will depend on the site of involvement of the stomach. The gastric mucosa may show nodular and thicken gastric mucosal folds, erosion, ulcers or polypoidal lesion obstructing gastric outlet. Infiltrative and hyperplastic mucosa may mimic Ménétrier's disease or linitis plastica [68, 69].

Idiopathic granulomatous gastritis. In up to one-fourth of the patients, the underlying cause for granulomatous gastritis may not be identifiable and this group of patients is labelled as idiopathic granulomatous gastritis. The clinical importance of these patients is that the granulomas are considered to be idiopathic and its existence as a distinctive condition is uncertain, and the granulomatous response may be a non-specific inflammatory reaction to an unclassified unknown agent and over the years some of these patients may develop either Crohn's disease or sarcoidosis. Clinical and endoscopic findings are similar to other types where definitely associated conditions or underlying aetiology are identifiable. Histological features including the location of the granulomas, adjoining mucosal changes, all will be similar to non-infective subgroups with no specific findings. Hence, it may be advisable to give a descriptive terminology of granulomatous gastritis of uncertain aetiology.

The following paragraph highlights some of the important points to be noted while reporting a case of granulomatous gastritis:

1. Clinical history should include a history of residence in or travel to areas endemic for certain infectious diseases.
2. High-risk behaviour (e.g. cocaine and syphilis).
3. Medications (e.g. antacids).
4. Pulmonary or systemic symptoms like evidence of lower gastrointestinal symptoms.
5. Careful endoscopic inspection of stomach with mapping of biopsy and noting the presence of any suture site or material.
6. Examination of HE stained sections examining the granuloma for its character, number, location, any identifiable structures and inflammatory background of the surrounding gastric mucosa.
7. Depending upon the findings on HE, further special stains are to be ordered appropriately.
8. If there are negative unstained or negatively stained areas or visible materials polarized microscopy is to be performed to look for birefringent material.
9. Certain immunohistochemistry is to be carried out based on HE features.

References

1. Toh BH, Sentry JW, Alderuccio F. The causative H+/K+ ATPase antigen in the pathogenesis of autoimmune gastritis. Immunol Today. 2000;21:348–54.
2. Faber K. Achylia gastrica mit Anamie. Med Klin. 1909;5:1310–25.
3. Cabrera de León A, Almeida González D, Almeida AA, et al. Factors associated with parietal cell autoantibodies in the general population. Immunol Lett. 2012;147:63–6.
4. Toh BH, Chan J, Kyaw T, Alderuccio F. Cutting edge issues in autoimmune gastritis. Clin Rev Allergy Immunol. 2012;42:269–78.
5. Lenti MV, Rugge M, Lahner E, et al. Autoimmune gastritis. Nat Rev Dis Primers. 2020;6:56.
6. El-Zimaity H, Riddell R. Stomach and proximal duodenum: inflammatory and miscellaneous disorders. In: Riddell R, Jain D, editors. Lewin, Weinstein, and Riddell's gastrointestinal pathology and its clinical implications. Philadelphia, PA: Wolters Kluwer; 2014. p. 635–43.
7. Hall SN, Appelman HD. Autoimmune gastritis. Arch Pathol Lab Med. 2019;143:1327–31.
8. Minalyan A, Benhammou JN, Artashesyan A, et al. Autoimmune atrophic gastritis: current perspectives. Clin Exp Gastroenterol. 2017;10:19–27.
9. Neumann WL, Coss E, Rugge M, et al. Autoimmune atrophic gastritis—pathogenesis, pathology and management. Nat Rev Gastroenterol Hepatol. 2013;10:529–41.
10. Abdullah BA, Gupta SK, Croffie JM, et al. The role of esophagogastroduodenoscopy in the initial evaluation of childhood inflammatory bowel disease: a 7-year study. J Pediatr Gastroenterol Nutr. 2002;35:636–40.
11. Burke KE, Boumitri C, Ananthakrishnan AN. Modifiable environmental factors in inflammatory bowel disease. Curr Gastroenterol Rep. 2017;19:21.
12. McHugh JB, Gopal P, Greenson JK. The clinical significance of focally enhanced gastritis in children. Am J Surg Pathol. 2013;37:295–9.
13. Kundhal PS, Stormon MO, Zachos M, et al. Gastric antral biopsy in the differentiation of pediatric colitides. Am J Gastroenterol. 2003;98:557–61.
14. Putra J, Ornvold K. Focally enhanced gastritis in children with inflammatory bowel disease: a clinicopathological correlation. Correspondence. 2017;49:808–10.
15. Meining A, Bayerdörffer E, Bästlein E, et al. Focal inflammatory infiltrations in gastric biopsy specimens are suggestive of Crohn's disease. Scand J Gastroenterol. 1997;32:813–8.
16. Oberhuber G, Püspök A, Oesterreicher C, et al. Focally enhanced gastritis: a frequent type of gastritis in patients with Crohn's disease. Gastroenterology. 1997;112:698–706.
17. Parente F, Cucino C, Bollani S, et al. Focal gastric inflammatory infiltrates in inflammatory bowel disease: prevalence, immunohistochemical characteristics, and diagnostic role. Am J Gastroenterol. 2000;95:705–11.
18. Xin W, Greenson JK. The clinical significance of focally enhanced gastritis. Am J Surg Pathol. 2004;28:1347–51.
19. Westerhoff M, Lamps L. Mucosal biopsy after bone marrow transplantation. Surg Pathol Clin. 2017;10:909–30.
20. Lubner MG, Menias CO, Agrons M, et al. Imaging of abdominal and pelvic manifestations of graft-versus-host disease after hematopoietic stem cell transplant. Am J Roentgenol. 2017;209:33–45.
21. Salomao M, Dorritie K, Mapara MY, et al. Histopathology of graft-vs-host disease of gastrointestinal tract and liver: an update. Am J Clin Pathol. 2016;145:591–603.
22. Brodoefel H, Bethge W, Vogel M, et al. Early and late-onset acute GvHD following hematopoietic cell transplantation: CT features of gastrointestinal involvement with clinical and pathological correlation. Eur J Radiol. 2010;73:594–600.
23. Washington K, Jagasia M. Pathology of graft-versus-host disease in the gastrointestinal tract. Hum Pathol. 2009;40:909–17.
24. Malard F, Mohty M. New insight for the diagnosis of gastrointestinal acute graft-versus-host disease. Mediators Inflammation. 2014;2014:701013.
25. Spencer GD, Shulman HM, Myerson D, et al. Diffuse intestinal ulceration after marrow transplantation: a clinicopathologic study of 13 patients. Hum Pathol. 1986;17:621–33.
26. Sauer S, Radujkovic A, Hegenbart U, et al. Cytokeratin (CK)-18 and CK18 fragments as sensitive and specific biomarkers of acute hepato-intestinal GVHD: results of a prospective observational study. Blood. 2015;126:3083.
27. Sauer S, Hüsing J, Hajda J, et al. A prospective study on serum cytokeratin (CK)-18 and CK18 fragments as biomarkers of acute hepato-intestinal GVHD. Leukemia. 2018;32:2685–92.
28. Shulman HM, Cardona DM, Greenson JK, et al. NIH consensus development project on criteria for clinical trials in chronic graft-versus-host disease: II. The 2014 Pathology Working Group Report. Biol Blood Marrow Transplant. 2015;21:589–603.
29. Jagasia MH, Greinix HT, Arora M, et al. National Institutes of Health consensus development project on criteria for clinical trials in chronic graft-versus-host disease: I. The 2014 Diagnosis and Staging Working Group Report. Biol Blood Marrow Transplant. 2015;21:389–401.
30. Lee SJ, Wolff D, Kitko C, et al. Measuring therapeutic response in chronic graft-versus-host disease. National Institutes of Health consensus development project on criteria for clinical trials in chronic graft-versus-host disease: IV. The 2014 Response Criteria Working Group Report. Biol Blood Marrow Transplant. 2015;21:984–99.

31. Peled JU, Hanash AM, Jenq RR. Role of the intestinal mucosa in acute gastrointestinal GVHD. Hematol Am Soc Hematol Educ Prog. 2016;2016:119–27.
32. Hartley CP, Carrillo-Polanco LF, Rowan DJ, et al. Colonic graft-vs.-host disease in autologous versus allogeneic transplant patients: earlier onset, more apoptosis, and lack of regulatory T-cell attenuation. Mod Pathol. 2018;31:1619–26.
33. Bensley EH. Alexis St Martin. Can Med Assoc J. 1959;80:907–9.
34. Cotton PB, Rosenberg MT, Axon AT, et al. Diagnostic yield of fibre-optic endoscopy in the operated stomach. Br J Surg. 1973;60:629–32.
35. Krentz K. Gastroscopic and aspiration biopsy findings on the operated stomach. Dtsch Med Wochenschr. 1964;89:664–71.
36. Lechner HJ, Anton D. The histology of gastric mucosa in B II-stomach. Z Gastroenterol. 1979;17:674–9.
37. Mosimann F, Sorgi M, Wolverson RL, et al. Bile reflux after duodenal ulcer surgery. A study of 114 asymptomatic and symptomatic patients. Scand J Gastroenterol Suppl. 1984;92:224–6.
38. Langhans P, Bues M, Bunte H. Morphological changes in the operated stomach under the influence of duodenogastric reflux. Clinical follow-up over 20 years. Scand J Gastroenterol Suppl. 1984;92:145–8.
39. Langhans P, Heger RA, Stegemann B. The cancer risk in the stomach subjected to nonresecting procedures. An experimental long-term study. Aliment Pharmacol Ther. 2012;36:736–43.
40. Offerhaus GJ, Stadt J, Huibregtse K, et al. Endoscopic screening for malignancy in the gastric remnant: the clinical significance of dysplasia in gastric mucosa. J Clin Pathol. 1984;37:748–54.
41. Dewar P, Dixon MF, Johnston D. Bile reflux and degree of gastritis in patients with gastric ulcer: before and after operation. J Surg Res. 1984;37:277–84.
42. Dixon MF, O'Connor HJ, Axon AT, et al. Reflux gastritis: distinct histopathological entity? J Clin Pathol. 1986;39:524–30.
43. Dixon MF, Genta RM, Yardley JH. Classification and grading of gastritis. The updated Sydney System. International Workshop on the histopathology of gastritis, Houston 1994. Am J Surg Pathol. 1994;20:1161–81.
44. Genta RM. Differential diagnosis of reactive gastropathy. Semin Diagn Pathol. 2005;22:273–83.
45. Wyatt JI, Dixon MF. Chronic gastritis—a pathogenesis approach. J Pathol. 1988;40:113–24.
46. De Nardi F, Riddell RH. Reactive (chemical) gastropathy and gastritis. In: Graham DY, Genta RM, Dixon MF, editors. Gastritis. Philadelphia, PA: Lippincott Williams & Wilkins; 1999. p. 125–47.
47. Owen D. Gastritis and carditis. Mod Pathol. 2003;16:325–41.
48. Srivastava A. Pathology of non-infective gastritis. Histopathology. 2007;50:15–29.
49. Ramos S, del Pilar M, Baquero M, et al. Reactive gastropathy: frequency in endoscopic biopsies evaluated at the Universidad Nacional de Colombia. Rev Colomb Gastroenterol. 2011;26:253–60.
50. Maguilnik WL, Neumann A, Sonnenberg R, et al. Reactive gastropathy is associated with inflammatory conditions throughout the gastrointestinal tract. Aliment Pharmacol Ther. 2012;36:736–43.
51. Nakos A, Kouklakis G, Pitiakoudis M, et al. The histological and immunohistochemical aspects of bile reflux in patients with gastroesophageal reflux disease. Gastroenterol Res Pract. 2011;2011:905872. https://doi.org/10.1155/2011/905872.
52. Raja J, Meriam S, Meriam N, et al. Granulomatous gastritis: a clinicopathologic analysis of 39 biopsy cases. J Spleen Liver Res. 2018;1:10–5.
53. Ectors NL, Dixon MF, Geboes KJ, et al. Granulomatous gastritis: a morphological and diagnostic approach. Histopathology. 1993;23:55–61.
54. Shapiro JL, Goldblum JR, Petras RE. A clinicopathologic study of 42 patients with granulomatous gastritis. Is there really an "idiopathic" granulomatous gastritis? Am J Surg Pathol. 1996;20:462–70.
55. Maeng L, Lee A, Choi K, et al. Granulomatous gastritis: a clinicopathologic analysis of 18 biopsy cases. Am J Surg Pathol. 2004;28:941–5.
56. Genta RM. Granulomatous gastritis. In: Graham DY, Genta RM, Dixon MF, editors. Gastritis. Philadelphia, PA: Lippincott Williams & Wilkins; 1999.
57. Amarnath S, Deeb L, Philipose J, et al. A comprehensive review of infectious granulomatous diseases of the gastrointestinal tract. Gastroenterol Res Pract. 2021;2021:8167149. https://doi.org/10.1155/2021/8167149.
58. Miyamoto M, Yoshihara K, Haruma M, et al. isolated granulomatous gastritis: successfully treated by H pylori eradication: a possible association between gastritis granulomatous and Helicobacter pylori. J Gastroenterol. 2003;38:371–5.
59. Dor-Ben D, Landa E, Delgado S. Granulomatous gastritis and H pylori Infection. Isr Med Assoc J. 2013;15:385–6.
60. Lauwers GY. Gastritis: beyond Helicobacter pylori. Int J Surg Pathol. 2010;18:28S.
61. Vahid B, Spodik M, Braun KN, et al. Sarcoidosis of gastrointestinal tract: a rare disease. Dig Dis Sci. 2007;52:3316.
62. Masiak A, Zdrojewski Ł, Zdrojewski Z, et al. Gastrointestinal tract involvement in granulomatosis with polyangiitis. Przegl Gastroenterol. 2016;11:270–5.
63. Zheng Z, Ding J, Li X, et al. Gastric presentation (vasculitis) mimics a gastric cancer as initial symptom in granulomatosis with polyangiitis: a case report and review of the literature. Rheumatol Int. 2015;35:1925–9.
64. Temmesfeld-Wollbrueck B, Heinrichs C, Szalay A, et al. Granulomatous gastritis in Wegener's disease: differentiation from Crohn's disease supported by a positive test for antineutrophil antibodies. Gut. 1997;40:550–3.

65. Liang WY, Lauwers GY. Granulomatous gastritis. In: Carneiro F, Chaves P, Ensari A, editors. Pathology of the gastrointestinal tract. Encyclopedia of pathology. Cham: Springer; 2017. https://doi.org/10.1007/978-3-319-40560-5_1614.
66. Yan F, Zhou Q, Gao Y, et al. Isolated Langerhans cell histiocytosis of the stomach: a case report and literature review. Int J Clin Exp Pathol. 2018;11:5962–8.
67. Lee SJ, Hwang CS, Huh GY, et al. Gastric Langerhans cell histiocytosis: case report and review of the literature. J Pathol Transl Med. 2015;49:421–3.
68. Leeds JS, McAlindon ME, Lorenz E, et al. Gastric sarcoidosis mimicking irritable bowel syndrome—cause not association? World J Gastroenterol. 2006;12:4754–6.
69. Bhattarai B, Mandal A, Lamichhane J, et al. A symptomatic gastric sarcoidosis and asymptomatic pulmonary sarcoidosis: a rare manifestation. J Community Hosp Intern Med Perspect. 2019;9:440–2.
70. Sameh S, Mohamed Salah H, Mohamed G, et al. Gastric sarcoidosis: rare revealing feature of systemic sarcoidosis. Arab J Gastroenterol. 2020;21:62–4.
71. Uzzan M, Ko H, Mehandru S, et al. Gastrointestinal disorders associated with common variable immune deficiency (CVID) and chronic granulomatous disease (CGD). Curr Gastroenterol Rep. 2016;18:17–29.
72. Bigotti G, Coli A, Magistrelli P, De Ninno M, Antonacci V, Crucitti A, Federico F, Antinori A, Massi G. Gastric adenocarcinoma associated with granulomatous gastritis. Case report and review of the literature. Tumori. 2002;88(2):163–6.
73. El Demellawy D, Otero C, Radhi J. Primary gastric lymphoma with florid granulomatous reaction. J Gastrointest Liver Dis. 2009;18(1):99–101.
74. Barros MHM, Leite E, Chabay P, et al. Diagnosing lymphoma in a setting with a high burden of infection: a pediatric case of Epstein-Barr virus-associated aggressive B-cell lymphoma with t(8,14) (q23;q32) and extensive necrosis mimicking tuberculosis. Rev Soc Bras Med Trop. 2015;48:108–11.
75. Niitsu H, Tanabe K, Tokumoto N, et al. Idiopathic granulomatous gastritis resembling a gastrointestinal stromal tumor. Case Rep Gastroenterol. 2012;6:502–9.

Gastric Polyps: Gastritis cystica profunda, Hyperplastic Gastropathies, Ménétrier's Disease, Zollinger-Ellison (ZE) Syndrome

20

Gastric polyp is a rarely encountered disorder in routine practice and do not have any specific clinical presentation. It is detected incidentally during the process of upper GI endoscopy. It may be a benign or malignant lesion (Fig. 20.1a–d). It may be defined as a localized proliferative lesion, usually of epithelial cells in origin or occasionally may be of mesenchymal cells, sessile or pedunculated, producing luminal protrusion due to the elevated property of the lesion, which may be a non-neoplastic or neoplastic in type. Gastric polyps are detected during routine upper GI endoscopic examination in up to 6% of the cases and incidentally may be detected in <1% of autopsy cases [1]. In a retrospective analysis by Viudez et al. in 41,253 gastroscopies, 2% were found to have gastric polyps, mean age being 65.6 years, 62% were women, 54% had multiple polyps and 83% of the polyps were less than 1 cm in size. Most frequent site was fundus and the most common histological type was hyperplastic in 43% followed by fundic gland in 38% of the cases [2]. Hypothetically these polyps are believed to be formed due to focal hyperproliferative response of the mucosa response to irritants and inflammation [3]. Foveolar epithelium are believed to be cells that respond first and involved in the process resulting in hipping up of the epithelium producing the polyp. The commonest aetiology for the mucosal injury being *H. pylori*-associated chronic gastritis. Other important causes are chemicals, drugs, bile reflux, gastroesophageal reflux disease and autoimmune gastritis. Though rare, there may be focus on dysplasia. During the time of endoscopy, thorough examination and description of the gastric mucosa is advisable including the area where there is no polyp and biopsy of the non-polypoidal surrounding mucosa. Grossly the polyp may be just polypoidal mucosal lesion to well define polyp with or without a stalk, and may have smooth velvety to granular to villiform surface, which may be associated with surface erosion or ulcer. Standard technique of grossing and blocking to be followed embedding the whole tissue including the resection plane. On microscopy, classic low-power view of hyperplastic polyp will give a look at varying dilated spaces which will represent dilated and hyperplastic glands and foveolae, which may be prominent finger-like or villiform processes, and loss of the normal architecture. There may be extension of the smooth muscle fibres in between the dilated glands intermixed with a variable amount of collagen. The mucous type of epithelial cells will show varying degrees of hyperplasia, may be globoid or rarely with goblet cell metaplasia. To characterize the type of cells, a simple alcian blue periodic acid Schiff stain is more than adequate, which may give you three types of mucin, i.e. the conventional magenta colour neutral mucin, blue colour acid or sialomucin and intermediate purplish colour mucin indicating the presence of incomplete mucin, which tend to be exhibited by

K. Vaiphei, *Interpretation of Endoscopic Biopsy - Gastritis, Gastropathies and Beyond*,
https://doi.org/10.1007/978-981-16-6026-9_20

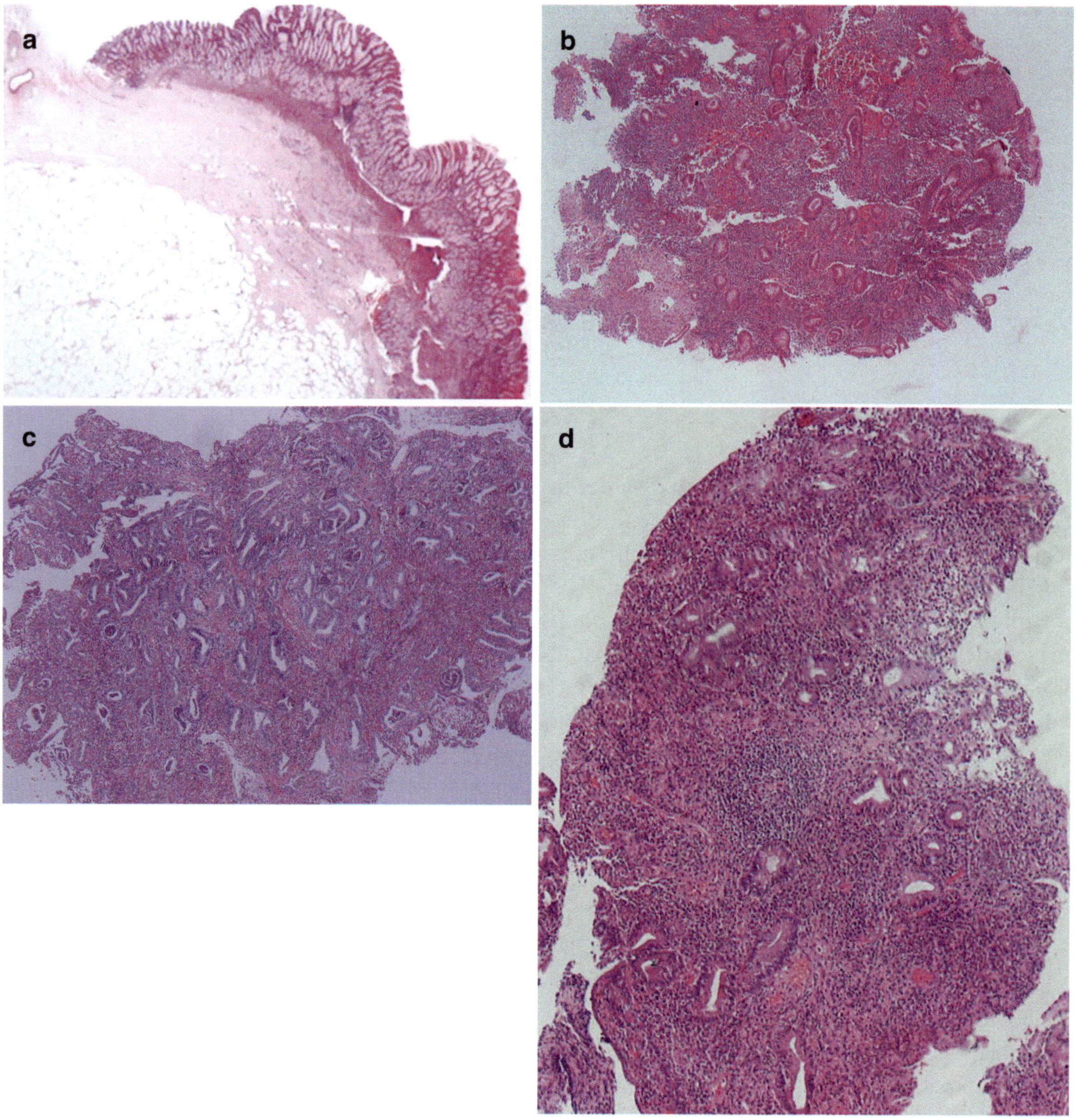

Fig. 20.1 (**a** to **c**) The three photomicrographs are of different polypoidal growth in stomach. (**a**) Low power view of a lipoma covered by antral mucosa (HE, x50). (**b**) Another low power view of an endoscopic biopsy, one fragment shows hyperplastic and inflamed gastric mucosa, and the second fragment shows a polypoidal structure with gross expansion of lamina propria by monomorphic population of lymphomatous cells (HE, x150). (**c**) Another low power view of an endoscopic biopsy from a polypoidal gastric mucosal lesion with ulceration showing collections of atypical dysplastic glands (HE, x150). (**d**) Another endoscopic biopsy to show an inflammatory pseudo-polyp composed of inflammatory granulation tissue entrapping scatter benign gastric glands (HE, x150)

globoid cell. Hence, this stain, i.e. a combination of alcian blue with PAS in the same section ay be carried out in every gastric biopsy, which will help to identify many of the cells with incomplete metaplastic change by the mucin type. Lamina propria may show oedema with acute and chronic inflammatory cells including scattered eosinophils and occasional lymphoid follicles, and vascular congestion. Sometimes in a larger polyp, the blood vessels may have a thick wall but are of venous type and will not qualify for any vascular malformation. Inflammatory cells may be located more towards the superficial portion of the polyp, and if erosions and ulcers are present, the surface may show neutrophilic exudate with or without granulation tissue formation. Very occasionally, these polyps may show near-total replacement by inflammatory granulation tissue along with few hyperplastic glands, lined by mucodepleted epithelial cells due to associated inflammation. This can be a tricky situation where presence of dysplastic epithelium or adenoma needs to be excluded. Step serial section study or examination of the remaining mucosal fragments may be much help. The polyp may also be seen at gastro-oesophageal junction, sometimes in association with pink mucosa at lower end of oesophagus and this group of polyps may show focal areas of intestinal metaplasia. Regenerative epithelial cells may be prominent and require to be differentiated from true dysplastic epithelium, in these foci there may also be brisk mitosis. In cases where there is dysplastic epithelium with complex glandular architecture including a cribriform pattern of the epithelial cells, it is an essential requisite to examine multiple-step serial sections to exclude an invasive tumour that may be limited to lamina propria. The non-polypoidal mucosa should be examined and look for *H. pylori* [4–8].

20.1 Gastritis cystica profunda

It is a rare benign condition benign and the polypoidal mucosa comprising multiple cystically dilated hyperplastic gastric glands extending into the submucosa. The mucosal changes were described in 1947 [9]. The term gastritis cystica profunda (GCP) was coined two decades later and the cystically dilated gastric type of glands present in submucosa was considered to be reactive and postsurgical [10]. There is no unified diagnostic criterion, pathological examination of the resected specimen remains gold standard for the diagnosis. In endoscopy and naked eye examinations may show a localized lesion or more diffuse mucosal fold thickening involving the whole stomach including the fundic mucosa. Morphological light microscopic features include abnormal mucosa infiltrating deep into submucosa. The abnormal mucosa is comprising of many benign cystically dilated gastric glands along with connective tissue hyperplasia including smooth muscles of muscularis mucosae origin and variable grades of inflammatory cells dominantly chronic inflammatory cells, which may be intermixed with acute and scattered eosinophils. With the advancement in endoscopic ultrasound, GCP has been diagnosed in the hands of experienced radiologists with the typical imaging features of the lesion originating from gastric basal mucosa extending gradually to submucosa in association with thickening of gastric wall, often in some patients, there may be irregular hypoechoic area in muscularis propria with abnormal overlying mucosa [11] (Fig. 20.2a–e). The three EUS features described are—anechoic, heterogeneous and increased mucosal thickness, and hypoechoic with cystic spaces. GCP may develop following any form of intervention resulting in mucosal defects like mucosal biopsy, polypectomy, chronic ischaemia and inflammation though it has also been reported in patients with no history of any previous intervention [12]. Radiology differential diagnoses are stromal tumour, Ménétrier's disease, inverted hyperplastic polyp and any other polyps [12–15]. Endoscopic examination usually reveals a smooth surface mucosa, localized bulge or grossly thicken mucosal folds that may extend variably involving a variable number of mucosal folds. Overlying mucosa is usually normal looking or shiny, or maybe erosions and ulcers. Presenting symptoms may be upper GI bleed, abdominal pain, anorexia, nausea, dyspepsia or may be asymptomatic. In the majority of patients, site of previous gastric-related surgery may be visible. GCP has been observed in elderly individuals and mostly in males. Differential diagnosis based on radiological features and endoscopic findings will be one of gastric mucosal nodular lesion which will include benign mucosal polyps to malignant polypoidal lesions to submucosal benign and malignant tumours including mesenchymal tumours. In almost all cases, first and foremost, the patient will be subjected to an endoscopic biopsy. In a given biopsy, there will be gross disorganization of the glandular architecture, cystically dilated glands, foveolar

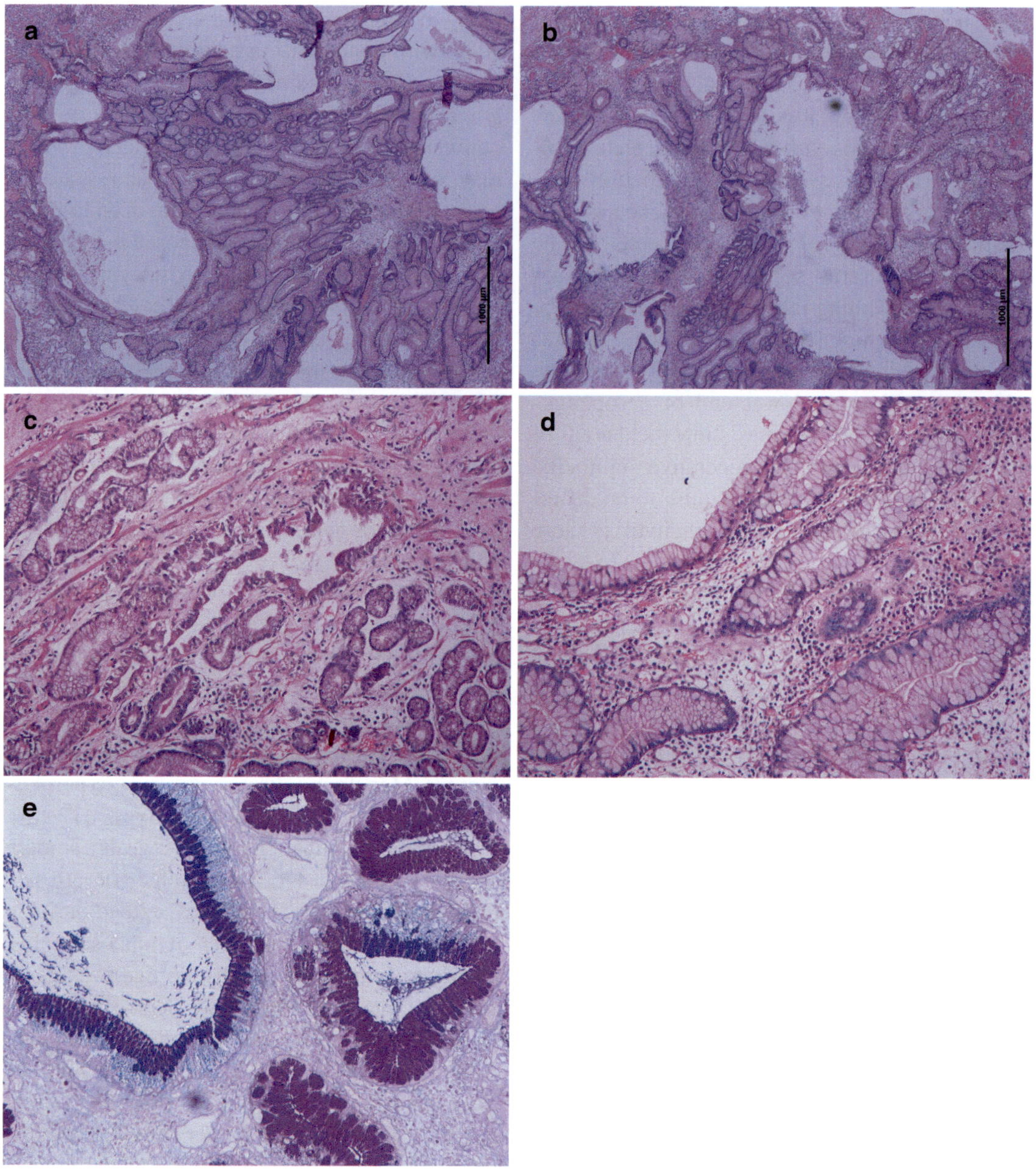

Fig. 20.2 (**a**) Low-power photomicrograph of the gastric polyp showing grossly disorganized gastric mucosal architecture as indicated by multiple cystically dilated glands (HE, x50). (**b**) Another area of the same polyp where the surface lining epithelium is visible on one aspect and deeper area contains a few residual specialized gastric glands. There is an increase in lamina propria stromal component (HE, x150). (**c**) The deeper portion of the polyp showing smooth muscle fibre strands in between the glands (HE, x200). (**d**) High-power photomicrograph to show hyperplastic lining epithelial cells (HE, x300). (**e**) A photomicrograph to show the metaplastic epithelium in special stain (AB-PAS, x300)

hyperplasia and lamina propria fibrosis, variable amount inflammatory cells, which may range from acute to chronic inflammatory cells including lymphoid aggregation. Lamina propria will show variable degrees of fibrosis and splaying of the smooth muscle. The surface lining may be denuded or ulcerated and covered by inflammatory cell exudate, maybe with granulation tissue formation. Some of the epithelial cells may show features of regeneration, metaplasia including goblet cell. The true picture will be visible in the resected specimen where there will be discontinuation of the hypertrophied and splayed muscularis mucosae entrapping the disorganized gastric glands showing hyperplastic elongated and dilated foveolae. These abnormal shaped sizes glands are seen to be displaced towards the deep submucosa across the muscularis mucosae. In an operated specimen, there may be evidence of previous surgery in the form of large areas of hyalinization and presence of foreign body or suture granulomas. These changes may also involve the muscularis propria entrapping the abnormal shaped and sized gastric glands. On closure examination, the displaced epithelial cells will fail to exhibit atypia to suggest any evidence of malignancy or atypia, though there may be some degree of muco-depletion in the inflamed mucosa or regenerating epithelium. Rarely, GCP may show giant mucosal folds, a submucosally located mass or as a single polyp. The cases where features of GCP were described were all operated cases in relates to stomach. As the condition has been well recognized as a separate entity, there are many more cases that have been reported with no history of any kind of surgery in the past [16–18].

20.2 Hyperplastic Gastropathies

It is a premalignant disorder of stomach characterized by overgrowth of gastric mucosa associated with hypoalbuminemia due to albumin loss by gastric mucosa. The abnormalities include characteristic giant mucosa folds with excessive mucus secretion with hypochlorhydria. It was Menetrier who had described this condition 94 years ago and it still carries his name [19]. This eponym has been associated with various different terminologies [20]. Similar looking mucosal changes may be an observation feature for some of the malignant disorders of stomach and this grossly thick abnormal mucosal fold has been described characteristically in primary HG (PHG). It was first introduced by Ming by classifying into 3 types: (i) mucous cell hyperplasia, (ii) gastric glandular cell hyperplasia and (iii) mixed type where both mucous cells and glandular cells undergo hyperplasia [21]. Menetrier's disease (MD) is one such condition with thick mucosal fold and its features correspond to Ming's first type. MD has four distinct features comprising of increased mucosal fold thickness, low or near normal gastric acid secretion, increased gastric protein loss and characteristic histological changes in the mucosa [22]. Histological features include elongated and grossly distorted and coiled foveolae associated with loss of parietal and chief cells, pseudopyloric metaplasia, cystic dilatation of glands, splayed and hyperplastic smooth muscle and displaced epithelium into submucosa (Fig. 20.3a–c). Grossly the thicken mucosal fold height may range up to 3 to 4 cm affecting fundus and body sparing antrum. However, the whole stomach may be involved in certain cases. Symptoms are similar to any other gastritis and peptic ulcer disease including weight loss, bleeding and pedal oedema. Investigations are similar to any other dyspeptic conditions. Although decreased gastric acid production is a frequent association, serum gastrin levels remain relatively normal [23, 24]. Diagnosis of this condition rests on histological examination of a full-thickness gastric mucosa, routine conventional endoscopic biopsy provides a sample that is too shallow. MD is known to have increased risk for gastric cancer [25]. A similar kind of condition is known in children who present with self-limiting protein-losing gastropathy with an allergic background or frequently in association with cytomegalovirus infection, and paediatric MD appears to be unrelated to adult type [24]. The credit for endoscopic diagnosis of thicken hypertrophic gastric mucosal fold should go to the pioneer work of Rudolf Schindler, the first person to have described histological features of hypertrophic gastritis in 1922, by correlating with the gross features of fresh full-thickness mucosal biopsies procured during surgical procedures [25]. His description of hypertrophic gastritis, also known as Schindler's disease, is at the other extreme end of HG opposite to MD with morphological features fitting

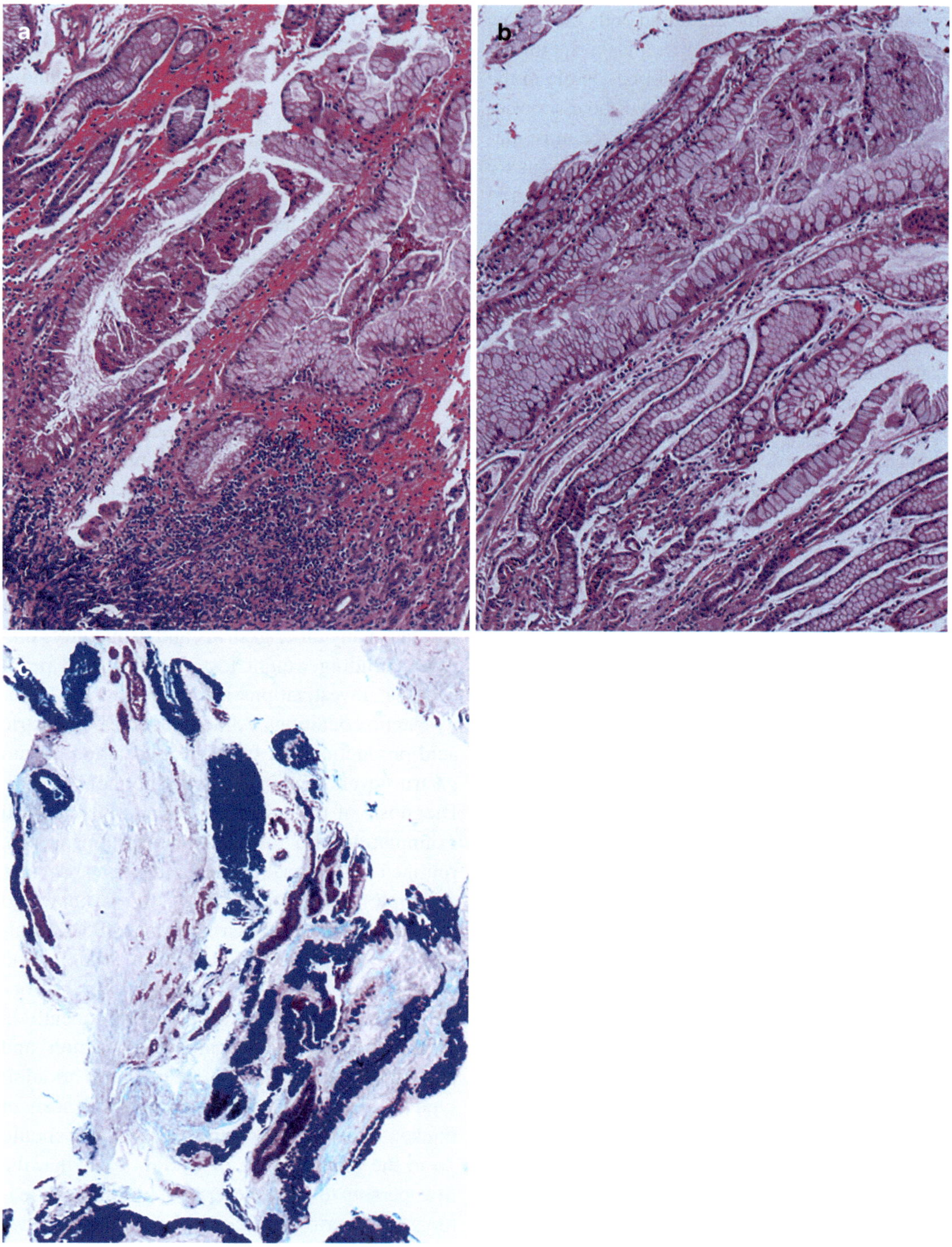

Fig. 20.3 (**a**) A low-power photomicrograph to show grossly disorganized hyperplastic glands with focal lymphoid aggregate in between. High proliferation of the epithelial cell is indicated by the presence of shredded cells within the hyperplastic glands (HE, x100). (**b**) Another area of the same polyp to show the varying sized foveolae, a few of which are lined by hyperplastic epithelium whereas others are lined by normal gastric foveolar epithelium. There is a total loss of the native gastric glands (HE, x200). (**c**) Another photomicrograph of the same polyp where special histochemistry staining had been done to highlight different characters of the mucin as indicated by the blue metaplastic mucin and purple colours normal gastric mucin (AB-PAS, x250)

into Ming's mixed mucous-glandular cell type [25]. Hypertrophic gastritis is characterized by enlarged and thick folds, a normal or increased gastric acid secretion with normal serum protein levels, along with parietal and chief cell hyperplasia, and a relative or absolute reduction in mucous cells. Hence, giant mucosal folds can be due to various conditions—it could be due to proliferation of primary intrinsic cells of gastric mucosa, or a long-standing inflammatory condition, or result of mucosal infiltrative disorders. All these conditions may produce a similar appearance in endoscopy irrespective of involvement of submucosa.

HG involves males more frequently and middle-aged individuals. It is occasionally seen in paediatric age group. The disease is believed to have an insidious onset and progressive. There are rare case reports with spontaneous regression. In paediatric age group, it has an acute onset and usually undergoes regression spontaneously. These patients can come with a variety of symptomatology which includes epigastric pain, weight loss, nausea, vomiting, gastrointestinal bleeding, diarrhoea and protein-losing gastroenteropathy. In hyperplastic gastropathy, the gastric epithelial cells that compose the foveolae glands become hyperplastic resulting in giant mucosal folds, which tend to be more than 5 mm in thickness. Hyperplastic gastropathies include Ménétrier's disease, hyperplastic hypersecretory gastropathy and Zollinger-Ellison syndrome. Infiltrative disorders resulting in increased mucosal fold thickness may be labelled as non-hyperplastic gastropathy, which will include various gastritidies, infiltrative disorders, infections and malignancy [18–20].

Ménétrier's disease (MD) is also known as hyperproliferative protein losing gastropathy associated with hypochlorhydria and hypoproteinaemia, was first described in 1888 by Pierre Ménétrier [26]. It has been reported more frequently in middle-aged males. Its pathogenesis and risk for gastric cancer are not completely understood. Increase in tight junction width has been described at ultrastructural examination, which seems to justify high mucosal permeability resulting in protein losing phenomena [27, 28]. It is a progressive disorder and common clinical symptoms are anorexia, pain in epigastrium, vomiting, weight loss, asthenia and GI bleeding. Upper gastrointestinal endoscopy is diagnostic and shows markedly thickened gastric mucosal folds sparing antrum relatively [27, 28]. Endoscopic differential diagnosis is broad and will include not only infective diseases but also infiltrative disorders like sarcoidosis and amyloidosis, malignancy like lymphoma and carcinomas, also occasionally gastric varices. Amongst the infective conditions, *Helicobacter pylori* gastritis will remain the commonest condition to be considered though in MD the gastric mucosal fold thickening will be more prominent. Another condition to be considered is Zollinger-Ellison syndrome and it often presents with gastric or duodenal ulcers. In portal hypertensive mucosopathy, the gastric mucosal fold bearing the varices have more serpentine form of fold thickening, tend to confine to cardia and fundus, though pylorus may also be involved. Thick folds in infiltrative conditions like sarcoidosis and amyloidosis are not diffuse and the infiltrative materials form aggregation resulting in grossly thicken folds with nodular appearance. Considerable differences in the natural history of the disease have been observed between adults and children [22, 27, 28]. In adults, it is insidious onset and a progressive disease. In the pathobiology of Menetrier's disease, a concept of transforming growth factor-α binding receptor upregulation due to overproduction of TGF-alpha has been proposed [29]. TGF-alpha is locally secreted by parietal cells and stimulates growth of epithelial cells and inhibits acid secretion [29–31]. But the molecular defect is not known. Basal and stimulated gastric acid secretion is low to normal in Ménétrier's disease and this variation is related to the time point of the disease course when the reading is taken. Mild to moderately elevated serum gastrin levels may be observed [28–30].

Normal gastric fundus and body mucosa are composed of two compartments, i.e. the superficial mucosa which includes the surface mucous cells and foveolar cells, and the deep compartment which is composed of specialized cells. Surface and foveolae are lined by mucous type of epithelial cells which also extends up to isthmus. The deeper half of the mucosa contains specialized glands lined by parietal, chief and few scattered D cells along with scattered enterochromaffin and enterochromaffin-like cells. Fold thickening is quite uniform and symmetrical, though there may be asymmetrical folds appearing as a polypoid lesion. Diagnosis is established on biopsy by the marked atypical changes observed in the oxyntic mucosa where the glands show marked hyperplasia in the form of mucous type of columnar lined elongated foveolae extending beyond the isthmus into the specialized glands replacing the specialized cells. Full-thickness thicken mucosal biopsy is required to demonstrate the classic changes. Any associated infection and other epithelial changes need to be looked for and commented upon.

Distinguishing Ménétrier's disease (MD) from disorders may be difficult. Polyposis syndromes are the most common mimics of MD. In a biopsy from the polypoidal mucosa in a case of syndromic presentation, there will be disorganization of the glands in their shapes and sizes, whereas in MD the glands are rather longer may be tortuous and mucous type of epithelial cells lining along the almost the whole length of the extended foveolae with minimal disorganization of the glandular architecture. Lamina propria component may not show much changes in contrast to the hyperplastic polyps where there will be increase in chronic inflammatory cell component. Erosions and ulcerations of variable degree with appropriate tissue response may be present in both types of lesions. May be study at the molecular level will be of help in difficult cases. In polyposis cases, there may be coexisting lesions in extra-gastric sites and family history may also be forthcoming [32–34].

Gastrectomy is the choice for treating those patients with intractable symptoms and who have not responded to medical therapy. MD though primarily is a disease that involves the oxyntic mucosa of the body and fundus, a total gastrectomy is the surgery of choice due to fewer surgical complications and better quality of life as compared with proximal gastrectomy. Natural history of MD is not well understood, though in adults, it is usually a progressive disease, although a few may respond to medical treatment. In children, it may resolve spontaneously or after treating the infecting agent if any. Risk of development of malignancy in the background of MD uncertain. In the past, all diagnosed cases of MD were subjected to total gastrectomy, thus cancer risk could not be accurately determined. More recently, an endoscopic surveillance program has been recommended, once every one or two years for early detection of dysplasia or carcinoma [28]. Hypertrophic and hypersecretory variant of MD is a very rare condition and is associated with high output gastric acid without significant hypergastrinemia. This group of patients may sometimes present with acid-peptic disease. On the whole clinical features are similar to MD. Proton pump inhibitor drugs control these variants of MD [28].

Zollinger-Ellison (ZE) syndrome is also known as gastric acid hypersecretion due to hypergastrinemia from a gastrinoma either sporadic or as a component of MEN type 1, or rarely it may also be associated with primary antral mucosal G cell hyperplasia. The patient usually presents with duodenal ulcer and diarrhoeal illnesses. It is a hyperplastic gastropathy involving gastric body and fundus. The cell which undergoes hyperplasia in ZE syndrome is parietal cell and it is the result of high level of gastrin observed in gastrinoma. Alternatively, this may also be seen in condition where the is increased expression of parathyroid hormone related peptide aberrently expressed by parietal cells. It may also be the result of increase histamine-secreting enterochromaffin-like cells as gastrin is trophic for these cells as well. Gastrinoma per se is a rare tumour and majority of the patients who present with ZE syndrome are between 20 and 50 years of age, higher incidence has been observed in males. Majority of gastrinomas are sporadic. More than 70% of cases of MEN1 have duodenal gastrinomas located in proximal duodenum [35, 36]. These gastrinomas are small in size ~ <1 cm, often multiple, unlikely to involve liver. Labelling of a tumour as a gastrinoma is based on clinical syndrome resulting from secretion of gastrin, not due presence of gastrin in the neurosecretory granules. To be noted is that not all patients with ectopic gastrin secretion have the symptoms associated with ZE syndrome. Excessive gastrin secreted results in high gastric acid output usually four to sixfolds and may be up to 10 folds. Apart from the duodenal ulcer, chronic diarrhoea in ZE syndrome is due to excess gastric acid exceeding the neutralizing capacity of pancreatic bicarbonates resulting in low pH of intestinal content further inactivating pancreatic digestive enzymes, failure to emulsify fat by bile acids. Further, high serum gastrin inhibits sodium and water reabsorption by damaged intestinal epithelial cells resulting in secretory components to the diarrhoeal disease [35, 37].

Secretin stimulation test is a good modality differentiating underlying aetiology for hypergastrinemia. Secretin stimulates the release of gastrin by gastrinoma cells in MEN1-associated ZE syndrome. Under normal situation, normal gastric G cells are inhibited by secretin. This test is not to be performed in patients who are on PPI. Both false negative and positive results can occur, especially in patients with achlorhydria induced by proton pump inhibitors. Antral G-cell hyperplasia unlike ZE syndrome is characterized by poor response to secretin stimulation test.

References

1. Dent TL, Kukora JS, Buinewicz BR. Endoscopic screening and surveillance for gastrointestinal malignancy. Surg Clin North Am. 1989;69:1205–25.
2. Viúdez LA, Córdova H, Uchima H, et al. Gastric polyps: retrospective analysis of 41,253 upper endoscopies. Gastroenterol Hepatol. 2017;40:507–14.
3. Turner JR, Odze RD. Polyps of the stomach. In: Odze RD, Goldblum JR, editors. Surgical pathology of the GI tract, Liver, biliary tract, and pancreas. 2nd ed. WB Saunders; 2009. p. 415–45.
4. Jain R, Chetty R. Gastric hyperplastic polyps: a review. Dig Dis Sci. 2009;54:1839–46.
5. Abraham SC, Singh VK, Yardley JH, et al. Hyperplastic polyps of the stomach: associations with histologic patterns of gastritis and gastric atrophy. Am J Surg Pathol. 2001;25:500–7.
6. Markowski AR, Markowska A, Guzinska-Ustymowicz K. Pathophysiological and clinical aspects of gastric hyperplastic polyps. World J Gastroenterol. 2016;22:8883–91.
7. Debongnie JC. Gastric polyps. Acta Gastroenterol Belg. 1999;62:187–9.
8. Islam RS, Patel NC, Lam-Himlin D. Gastric polyps: a review of clinical, endoscopic, and histopathologic features and management decisions. Gastroenterol Hepatol (NY). 2013;9:640–51.
9. Scott HW, Payne TP. Diffuse congenital cystic hyperplasia of stomach clinically simulating carcinoma; report of a case. Bull Johns Hopkins Hosp. 1947;81:448–55.
10. Littler ER, Gleibermann E. Gastritis cystica polyposa. (Gastric mucosal prolapse at gastroenterostomy site, with cystic and infiltrative epithelial hyperplasia). Cancer-Am Cancer. 1872;29:205–9.
11. Fonde EC, Rodning CB. Gastritis cystica profunda. Am J Gastroenterol. 1986;81:459–64.
12. Laratta JL, Buhtoiarova TN, Sparber LS, et al. Gastritis cystica profunda: a rare gastric tumor masquerading as a malignancy. Surg Sci. 2012;3:158–64.
13. Soares JB, Bastos P, Goncalves R. Menetrier disease with antrum polyposis and gastritis cystica profunda. Endoscopy. 2012;44(Suppl 2 UCTN):E56–7.
14. Lim JK, Jang YJ, Jung MK, et al. Menetrier disease manifested by polyposis in the gastric antrum and coexisting with gastritis cystica profunda. Gastrointest Endosc. 2010;72:1098–100.
15. Lee SJ, Park JK, Seo HI, et al. A case of gastric inverted hyperplastic polyp found with gastritis cystica profunda and early gastric cancer. Clin Endosc. 2013;46:568–71.
16. Franzin G, Novell P. Gastritis cystica profunda. Histopathology. 1981;5:535–47.
17. Odze RD, Greenson J, Lauwers G, et al. Gastritis cystica profunda versus invasive adenocarcinoma. Am J Surg Pathol. 2012;36:316.
18. Greywoode G, Szuts A, Wang LM, et al. Iatrogenic deep epithelial misplacement ("gastritis cystica profunda") in a gastric foveolar-type adenoma after endoscopic manipulation: a diagnostic pitfall. Am J Surg Pathol. 2011;35:1419–21.
19. Simson JN. Hyperplastic gastropathy. Br Med J (Clin Res Ed). 1985;91(6505):1298–9.
20. Park WD. Giant hypertrophic gastritis. Lancet. 1956;I:270–751.
21. Ming SC. Atlas of tumor pathology: tumors of esophagus and stomach. Washington, DC: Armed Forces Institute of Pathology; 1973. pp 115–119 and 153–154.
22. Kelly DG, Miller LJ, Malagelada JR, et al. Giant hypertrophic gastropathy (Ménétrier's disease): pharmacologic effects on protein leakage and mucosal ultrastructure. Gastroenterologia. 1982;83:581–9.
23. Weiber H, Borch K, Lindström C, et al. Hyperplasia of gastric antral beta-microseminoprotein endocrine-like cells and increased serum levels of beta-microseminoprotein in atrophic corpus gastritis. Scand J Gastroenterol. 1998;33:911–5.

24. Kraut JR, Powell R, Hruby MA, et al. Menetrier's disease in childhood: report of two cases and a review of the literature. J Pediatr Surg. 1981;16:707–11.
25. Almazar AE, Joshua D. Survival times of patients with Menetrier's disease and risk of gastric cancer. Clin Gastroenterol Hepatol. 2021;19:707–12.
26. Ménétrier P. Des polyadenomes gastriques et de leurs rapport avec le cancer de l'estomac. Arch Physiol Norm Pathol. 1888;1:236–62.
27. Coffey RJ Jr, Tanksley J. Pierre Ménétrier's and his disease. Trans Am Clin Climatol Assoc. 2012;123:126–34.
28. Huh WJ, Coffey RJ, Washington MK. Ménétrier's disease: its mimickers and pathogenesis. J Pathol Transl Med. 2016;50:10–6.
29. Dempsey PJ, Goldenring JR, Soroka CJ, et al. Possible role of transforming growth factor alpha in the pathogenesis of Ménétrier's disease: supportive evidence form humans and transgenic mice. Gastroenterologia. 1992;103:1950–63.
30. Bluth RF, Carpenter HA, Pittelkow MR, et al. Immunolocalization of transforming growth factor-alpha in normal and diseased human gastric mucosa. Hum Pathol. 1995;26:1333–40.
31. Nomura S, Settle SH, Leys CM, et al. Evidence for repatterning of the gastric fundic epithelium associated with Ménétrier's disease and TGF alpha overexpression. Gastroenterologia. 2005;128:1292–305.
32. Carmack SW, Genta RM, Schuler CM, et al. The current spectrum of gastric polyps: a 1–year national study of over 120,000 patients. Am J Gastroenterol. 2009;104:1524–32.
33. Lam-Himlin D, Park JY, Cornish TC, et al. Morphologic characterization of syndromic gastric polyps. Am J Surg Pathol. 2010;34:1656–62.
34. Worthley DL, Phillips KD, Wayte N, et al. Gastric adenocarcinoma and proximal polyposis of the stomach (GAPPS): a new autosomal dominant syndrome. Gut. 2012;61:774–9.
35. Mortellaro VE, Hochwald SN, McGuigan JE, et al. Long-term results of a selective surgical approach to management of Zollinger-Ellison syndrome in patients with MEN-1. Am Surg. 2009;75:730–3.
36. Gong S, Li Z, Liu XB, et al. Gastrinoma in multiple endocrine neoplasia type 1 after total pancreatectomy. Medicine. 2019;98:e18275.
37. Shao QQ, Zhao BB, Dong LB, et al. Surgical management of Zollinger-Ellison syndrome: classical considerations and current controversies. World J Gastroenterol. 2019;25:4673–81.

21 Peptic Ulcer, Gastric Ulcer and Gastropathy

Peptic ulcer disease (PUD) is a condition where there is a break in mucosa of stomach, duodenum or lower oesophagus [1, 2]. It is more of a chronic ulcer resulting from injury by acid peptic juices. Mucosal erosion refers to a breach in the superficial mucosa usually the surface lining of the mucosa. All ulcers possibly start as erosion and progress further to produce the deeper and full-thickness erosions along with inflammatory cell exudate covering the site of ulcer. But all erosions may not progress to ulcer. An ulcer depending on the duration may have active granulation tissue at the bed or sometimes it may be clean with no inflammatory response. Depending on the organ that is involved, it is called gastric or duodenal or oesophageal ulcer [1]. Peptic ulcer disease is a common disorder affecting about 4% of the general population [1]. This disease affects about 10% of individuals at one point of time [3]. Incidence has gown down in the last decade worldwide from 327,000 in 1990 to 267,000 in 2015 [4, 5]. The first peptic ulcer reported (in the year 1670) had perforation 1670 [1, 6]. *H. pylori* (HP) was identified as a causative organism for PUD by Barry Marshall and Robin Warren for which they were awarded Nobel Prize [7]. PUD is commonly seen involving antrum and lesser curvature at incisura; it may also be seen at GE junction, gastrojejunostomy site, adjoining ileal mucosa to Meckel diverticulum harbouring gastric mucosa. However, 98% of cases are located in stomach [8]. Common presenting symptoms are upper abdominal pain which is burning or dull aching, a few of the peptic ulcer patients may be asymptomatic. Common aetiological agents besides HP are intake of non-steroidal anti-inflammatory drugs, smoking, stress, Zollinger-Ellison syndrome usually with multiple ulcers related to excessive gastrin secretion; other factors that are related are reflux of duodenal content into pyloric antrum, excessive intake of alcohol, heavy tobacco use, steroid administration and ischemia/shock. Gastric ulcers do not have a strong association with hyperacidity [7]. Greater curvature ulcer is most likely related to intake of drugs like NSAID, which is related to accumulation of the chemicals due to gravity [8]. Gastric ulcers, not a peptic aetiology may also be seen in cancer, infections not related to HP, especially in immunocompromised patients [9].

What is an ulcer? Is it synonymous with erosions or mucosal infarction? All the three conditions have well-defined different definitions. Erosions, as have been discussed previously, is absence or denudation of the superficial mucosa or surface lining epithelium, which may be covered by a thin layer of acute inflammatory cell exudate with infiltration by neutrophils in the superficial lamina propria. Lamina propria in most of the situations will be showing oedema. Almost the whole thickness of the mucosa may be absent with no tissue response, which most likely is due to handling artefacts of the tissue during the process of endoscopic biopsy, tissue

K. Vaiphei, *Interpretation of Endoscopic Biopsy - Gastritis, Gastropathies and Beyond*,
https://doi.org/10.1007/978-981-16-6026-9_21

mounting or orientation on filter paper, or result of rough handling in the pathology lab. An ulcer is more extensive mucosal erosion extending up to muscularis mucosae or beyond covered by dense inflammatory cell exudate with granulation tissue along the ulcer bed (Fig. 21.1). Variable degree of inflammatory cell infiltration will be seen around the involved area with oedema and vascular congestion. Mucosal infarction is a situation where there is tissue necrosis involving full-thickness mucosa or beyond into submucosa or muscularis propria along with haemorrhages, vascular congestion and acute inflammatory cell infiltration. Mucosal infarctions are usually the result of vascular episodes, which may be prolonged shock or thromboembolization of fibrin in disseminated intravascular coagulation or septic thrombus [10–13]. Outside the boundary of the title of the book, a gross picture of a chronic peptic ulcer of the stomach has been added (Fig. 21.2).

Gastric ulcer may be considered under the following major paired headings—(1) benign or malignant, (2) peptic or non-peptic ulcer and (3) acute or chronic ulcer [14, 15]. Hence depending on the clinical situation where a gastric ulcer is observed, it is required to pay attention to the clinical history. Detailed documentation of the clinical history including history of any coexisting syndromic presentation will simplify many of the times. Approach to dyspeptic problems have revolutionized drastically in the last few decades parallelly with the advancement in upper GI endoscopic procedures and majority of the uncomplicated patients do not require to undergo any surgical resection of the involved segment, unlike before [14–16]. Endoscopic biopsies from the ulcer bed and ulcer margin and adjoining gastric mucosa help to clinch many of the diagnosis. This helps to exclude or confirm malignant ulcers, and also document the mucosal changes of inflammation, atrophy, metaplasia or dysplasia in the surrounding area with presence or absence of *H. pylori* infection. Biopsy from an acute ulcer will be dominantly showing acute inflammatory cell exudate neutrophil dominant inflammatory cell response. Active ulcers will show four typical zonation, i.e. neutrophil exudate, occasionally bacterial colonies, necrotic tissue debris and probably *Candida* colonies. The ulcer base and margins will show fibrinoid necrosis, granulation tissue formation with infiltration by mixed

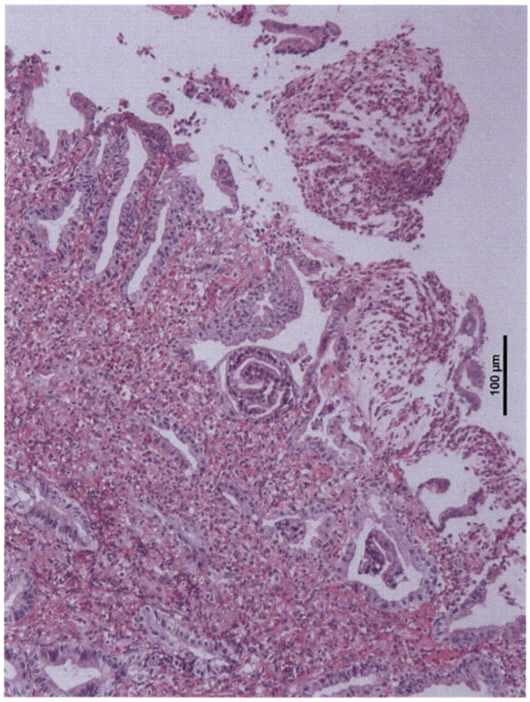

Fig. 21.1 Photomicrograph of an endoscopic biopsy taken from the margin of an antral ulcer showing heavily inflamed mucosa and oedema resulting in wide spacing of the gastric foveolae. The surface is superficially ulcerated and is covered by inflammatory cell exudate (HE, ×300)

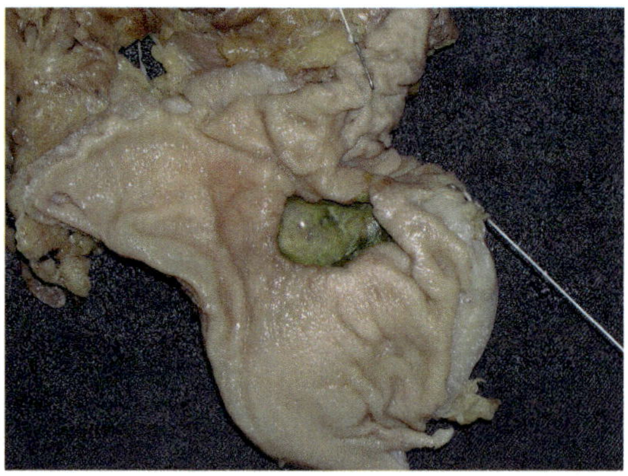

Fig. 21.2 A gross photograph of distal gastrectomy specimen showing a large ulcer of the size of 1.3 cms, deep seated, cleaned base with punched out margin. The surrounding gastric mucosa appears normal

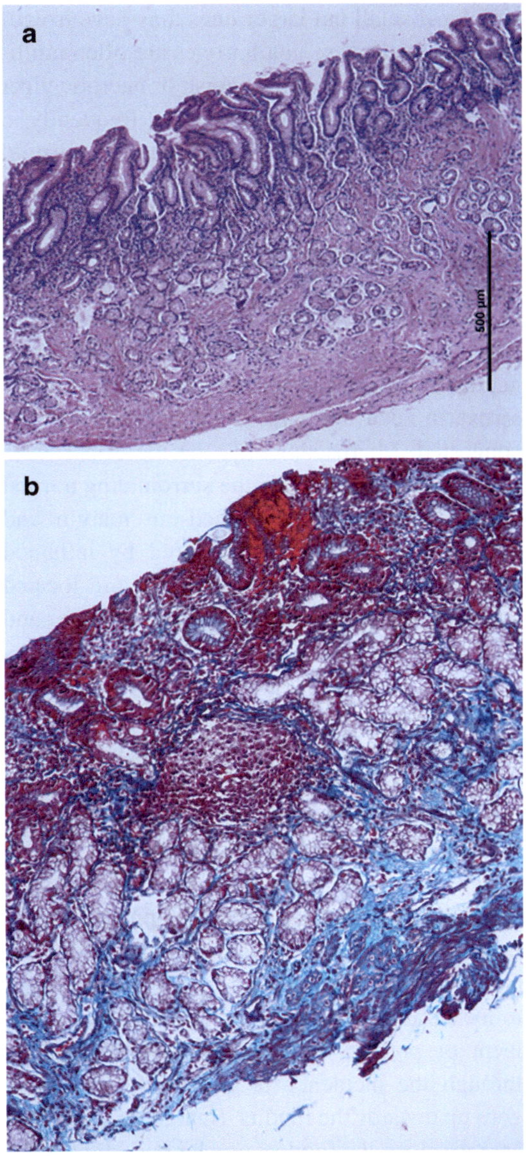

Fig. 21.3 (**a**) Photomicrograph taken from an old peptic ulcer from antral mucosa showing foveolar hyperplasia, lamina propria fibrosis extending deep in continuity with muscularis mucosae entrapping the pyloric glands, moderately heavy chronic inflammatory cell infiltration with lymphoid follicle formation (HE, ×300). (**b**) the same biopsy on which connective tissue histochemistry staining had been performed to highlight the collagenization (Masson's trichrome, ×300)

inflammatory cells including many lymphocytes, plasma cells, histiocytes and scattered eosinophils. As the ulcer tends to be deep seated, the fibrosis dominantly involving the submucosa extending to muscularis propria and replacing it with multiple thick blood vessels, some of with recanalized thrombus showing features of endarteritis obliterans. This chronic ulcer tends to have a clean base as bacteria rarely can grow in acidic medium and the surrounding mucosa will show evidence of regeneration, maybe with intestinal metaplasia [13]. In any setting, the histological finding of the surrounding non-ulcerated mucosa will be of much help in further management of the patient. In a given biopsy peptic and non-peptic ulcers will not reveal any difference and the biopsy only will not differ between the two conditions. According to the depth of the ulcer, the biopsy will reveal different layers of the gastric wall in the component, which is to be mention and document as important information to the treating physician. Inflammatory cell response in peptic ulcers tends to be sparse with minimal neutrophils whereas ulcers due to any other causes will have many heavy mixed inflammatory cell infiltrations. Biopsy taken from the ulcer margin may exhibit prominent fibrosis intermixed with lymphoid aggregates indicating chronicity of the ulcer. In such a case, the surrounding mucosa also will show chronicity (Fig. 21.3a and b), which may be accompanied by glandular atrophy and metaplastic epithelium. All forms of gastric ulcer may be complicated by either upper GI bleeding or perforation. Bleeding ulcers are due to erosion into submucosa blood vessels which sometimes may be identifiable in a biopsy exhibiting features of necrotizing vasculitis. These vasculitis per se may be a complication of the gastric ulcer or the gastric ulcer may be manifestation of a systemic vasculitis disorder. Acute ulcers are also referred to as stress ulcers as these ulcers may spontaneously undergo healing if the underlying stress or initiating condition resolves. Acute gastric ulcers are frequently observed at autopsy and have been associated with many conditions—drugs including NSAIDs, and steroids, sepsis, trauma, extensive burns (Curling's ulcer), increased intracranial pressure (Cushing's ulcer), radiation therapy and rarely can be the clinical manifestation for systemic amyloidosis. Grossly an acute gastric ulcers are usually <1 cm in size, sometimes maybe a few cms in size, tends to be circular if small but larger ones may have irregular shape and sizes; smaller ones are often multiple. These ulcers have brownish or necrotic ulcer bed and may present anywhere but frequently in pyloric antrum and fundus. There may be mild oedema in the surrounding mucosa otherwise there is no induration and the surrounding mucosa is normal in appearance. At autopsy, there may be many scattered pinpoint mucosal haemorrhages scattered diffusely in patients who died with septicaemia and shock. Ulcer may be of different depths, sometimes penetrating and the overlying serosa in such a situation will appear dull and congested. Microscopically, the ulcer margin is sharply demarcated from the surrounding normal gastric mucosa with punched-out margin and deeply located ulcer bed covered by inflamed necrotic debris. Acute peptic ulcers are located within 2 cms of the antro-duodenal sphincter and greater the distance from antro-duodenal sphincter, occurrence of peptic ulcers are lesser and they lie along the anterior and posterior walls, however, frequently, it may also be seen along the lesser curvature. Peptic ulcers are solitary lesions, occasionally an acute ulcer may be accompanied by a chronic ulcer with an indurated and thicken margin. Kissing ulcers locate in pre-pyloric antrum, occur when two ulcers are present face to face, i.e. one along the anterior and the other along the posterior wall. Acute gastric ulcers tend to locate along the lesser curvature and any segment or portion of stomach may be involved through the incidence is gradually lesser as it goes up towards the fundus. Benign gastric ulcers are rare along the fundus, greater curvature, anterior and posterior wall of the stomach. The susceptibility for chronic gastric ulcer along the lesser curvature has been hypothesized based upon the concept of Magenstrasse, which constitutes <5% of the total surface area of the stomach. Sometimes it is essential to differentiate benign from malignant ulcer irrespective of the site, size and clinical presentations. These ulcers are single, large and depressed. Benign peptic ulcers are long-standing chronically ongoing along with fibrosis along the ulcer bed and margins. Hence, these ulcers tend to be smaller, round or oval, clean base, elevated punched out margin with radiating gastric mucosal folds. Whereas a malignant ulcer tends to be large, irregular shape, shallow, necrotic base, irregular and indurated margins, nodular and heaped up, and flushing with surrounding mucosa. Ultimately the final diagnosis is to be established by histopathological examination of the representative blocks taken from the ulcers [10–14].

21.1 Gastritis Versus Gastropathy

A normal gastric mucosa, which we seldom get to see, contains rare scattered lymphocytes and rarely eosinophils in lamina propria. The contour of gastric pits or foveolae is a straight gland which is parallelly placed side by side. The proliferative zone is the zone of mucus neck cells corresponding to the basal region of gastric pits and these proliferative zone cells can divide and differentiate into different cell types. Cellular response to any form of injury is indicated by inflammation of the mucosa; corresponding morphological changes include degenerative change of the gastric epithelial cells, infiltration by acute inflammatory cells, epithelial cell regeneration along with oedema, haemorrhage, erosion or ulceration. Regeneration is indicated by proliferating mucus neck cells and elongated and tortuous gastric pits known as foveolar hyperplasia [15–17]. With time, in gastritis cases, the acute neutrophil infiltration will be replaced by mononuclear cells composed mainly of plasma cells, lymphocytes and scattered eosinophils, which eventually outnumbers neutrophils. In certain cases, gastric mucosal cell damage may not be associated with evidence of any epithelial cell regeneration or any significant inflammatory cell response. This condition has been defined as gastritis and may be seen in conditions associated with infection, autoimmune disorders, hypersensitivity reactions to chemicals including drugs or allergies of various conditions. On the other hand, gastropathy is usually seen in conditions like hypovolemia, stress, ischemia, alcohol, drugs, bile reflux and persistent congestion [15–17]. Histological morphology will help to differentiate between these two conditions. Active chronic gastritis most of the time gets referred to as non-specific chronic gastritis and is believed to represent more than one disorder.

Though maybe non-specific, histopathological features to suggest gastropathies are multiple and different segments of the stomach may show variable morphology, hence taking multiple biopsies from different areas is essential in establishing a definite condition [14–17]. Histological features in gastropathies are: (1) subnuclear vacuolization of mucous cells may favour bile reflux-related gastropathy, though the possibility NSAID cannot be excluded, though the history of intake is not coming forward; (2) lamina propria oedema, ectatic and congested capillaries and venules, occasionally with fresh or organizing fibrin thrombi may suggest the possibility of portal hypertensive mucosopathy or watermelon stomach; (3) epithelial atypia is a frequently seen feature as a part of reactive atypia may be due to regeneration, degeneration, effects of exposure to radiation or chemotherapeutic agent [14–17].

References

1. Najm WI. Peptic ulcer disease. Prim Care. 2011;38:383–94.
2. “Definition and Facts for Peptic Ulcer Disease” National Institute of Diabetes and Digestive and Kidney Diseases. Archived from the original on 2 April 2015. Retrieved 28 February 2015.
3. Snowden FM. Emerging and re-emerging diseases: a historical perspective. Immunol Rev. 2008;225:9–26.
4. Haidong W, Mohsen N, Christine A, et al. Global, regional, and national life expectancy, all-cause mortality, and cause-specific mortality for 249 causes of death, 1980-2015: a systematic analysis for the global burden of disease study 2015. Lancet. 2016;388(10053):1459–544.
5. GBD. Mortality causes of death collaborators (2015) global, regional, and national age-sex specific all-cause and cause-specific mortality for 240 causes of death, 1990-2013: a systematic analysis for the global burden of disease study 2013. Lancet. 2013;385(9963):117–71.
6. Milosavljevic T, Kostić-Milosavljević M, Jovanović I, et al. Complications of peptic ulcer disease. Dig Dis. 2011;29:491–3.
7. Wang AY, Peura DA. The prevalence and incidence of helicobacter pylori-associated peptic ulcer disease and upper gastrointestinal bleeding throughout the world. Gastrointest End Clin North Am. 2011;21:613–35.
8. Lin KJ, García Rodríguez LA, Hernández-Díaz S. Systematic review of peptic ulcer disease incidence rates: do studies without validation provide reliable estimates? Pharmacoepidemiol Drug Saf. 2011;20:718–28.
9. Morley J. The surgical pathology of peptic ulcer and gastric carcinoma. Edinb Med J. 1946;53:273–83.
10. Dore MP, Graham DY. Ulcers and gastritis. Endoscopy. 2004;36:42–7.
11. Brzozowski T. Experimental production of peptic ulcer, gastric damage and cancer models and their use in pathophysiological studies and pharmacological treatment--polish achievements. J Physiol Pharmacol. 2003;54(Suppl 3):99–126.
12. Yamagata S, Oshiba S, Hisamichi S, et al. Observations on benign gastric ulcer simulating gastric carcinoma. Gastroenterol Jpn. 1977;12:352–6.
13. The National Cooperative Group for Pathological Study on the Canceration of Gastric Ulcer. Clinicopathological study on 3441 cases of benign and malignant ulcers. Zhonghua Bing Li Xue Za Zhi. 1992;21:27–30.
14. McGregor DH, Haque AU. Gastric hyalinization associated with peptic ulceration. Arch Pathol Lab Med. 1982;106:472–5.
15. Carpenter HA, Talley NJ. Gastroscopy is incomplete without biopsy: clinical relevance of distinguishing gastropathy from gastritis. Gastroenterol. 1995;108:917–24.
16. Genta RM. Differential diagnosis of reactive gastropathy. Semin Diagn Pathol. 2005;22:273–83.
17. McQuaid KR. Gastritis & Gastropathy. In: Papadakis MA, SJ MP, Rabow MW, editors. Current medical diagnosis and treatment 2020. McGraw-Hill; 2020.

22 Gastric Mucosal Pathology in Kidney Disease

GI-related problems in patients with chronic kidney disease (CKD) is a frequent problem. About 80% of CKD patients will frequently complain of anorexia, nausea, dyspeptic symptoms and malnutrition [1–3]. Underlying aetiology is multifactorial such as—retention of endogenous and exogenous toxic substances in association with alteration in homeostasis of extracellular environment, influence by primary underlying condition for CKD, anxiety, depression, irritable bowel syndrome, the treatments given for the CKD per se and alteration in microbiota [2–6]. Gastroparesis is one condition that may be observed in uraemia which affects autonomic neuropathy, especially in CKD due to diabetes [2–5]. Improvement in the symptoms associated with gastroparesis is observed with a better control of the underlying disease [2, 5]. Gastric mucosal inflammation is frequently related to *H. pylori* infection having significant urease activity [6]. In addition, CKD patients tend to have increased serum gastrin, cholecystokinin and secretin levels correlating directly with renal failure [7–9]. Due to the associated biochemical changes in the blood of CKD patients, non-invasive test for *H. pylori* is less sensitive [7–9]. Peptic ulcer has a similar prevalence to the general population with an increasing prevalence of it has been associated with deterioration in renal function [10]. Risk of gastrointestinal bleeding in CKD patients may be various associated conditions; these patients have an inherent platelet dysfunction, intermittent administration of heparin, mucosal vascular ectasia giving the appearance of an angiodysplasia and frequent coexistence with peptic ulcers [11–14]. Angiodysplasia of small and large intestines is frequently encountered in elderly individuals, especially in autopsy setting.

Anaemia is a common complication of chronic kidney disease (CKD), severity increases with worsening of renal function. It has been associated with reduced production of erythropoietin, role of other factors like deficiency in iron, B12, folic acid and certain factors which may be responsible for less responsiveness to erythropoietin. Uraemia produces significant alterations in gastrointestinal system although pathogenesis is not well understood [15, 16]. Roughly about 40–90% of CKD patients have endoscopic abnormalities—acute lesions in gastric mucosa, angiodysplasias, diverticulosis, colonic polyposis and colorectal cancer, of which the most frequently described GI disease is angiodysplasia [15, 17, 18]. In the setting of CRF, like in chronic liver disease with portal hypertension, there are visible vascular markings in stomach and duodenum. Different percentages of angiodysplasia have been reported but the incidence of demonstrable angiodysplasia will definitely be higher in autopsy materials. Angio-ectasias are ectatic blood vessels usually lined by a single layer of endothelial cells which may be absent focally resulting in easy bleed. Persistent low-grade

K. Vaiphei, *Interpretation of Endoscopic Biopsy - Gastritis, Gastropathies and Beyond*,
https://doi.org/10.1007/978-981-16-6026-9_22

hypoxaemia is believed to induce neovascular growth factor propagating angiogenesis and formation of new vascular structures. These newly formed blood vessels may be either visible as tiny pinpoint punctate erythematous lesions which may be oozing or larger patchy erythematous areas. Angioectasias may be venous or arterial in origin. These newly formed vascular structures are found to be associated with high expression for VEGF compared to surrounding areas [14, 15, 19]. Apart from this, VEGF can be stimulated by various factors including hypoxia, cytokines, nitric oxide etc. Aetiopathogenesis of hindgut engiodysplasia is different from that of foregut angiodysplasia observed in a setting of CRF. In addition to vascular abnormalities, upper GI bleed in CRF patients may be related to intake of NSAIDS, stress and other medical complications the patient may have.

Due to high urea content in CRF patients, by default of the property of urea splitting by *H. pylori*, a high prevalence may be expected. CKD has been associated with systemic inflammatory response. There are various evidence supporting the presence of gastrointestinal barrier dysfunction responsible for systemic inflammatory response in uremic individuals and also in experimental animal models and increased permeability to large molecular weight polyethylene glycols in the intestinal mucosa due to loss of key proteins constituents in colonic epithelium in CKD rats [15, 20].

References

1. Usta M, Ersoy A, Ayar Y, et al. Comparison of endoscopic and pathological findings of the upper gastrointestinal tract in transplant candidate patients undergoing haemodialysis or peritoneal dialysis treatment: a review of literature. BMC Nephrol. 2020;21:444–53.
2. Cano AE, Neil AK, Kang JY, et al. Gastrointestinal symptoms in patients with end-stage renal disease undergoing treatment by haemodialysis or peritoneal dialysis. Am J Gastroenterol. 2007;102:1990–7.
3. Hammer J, Oesterreicher C, Hammer K, et al. Chronic gastrointestinal symptoms in hemodialysis patients. Wien Klin Wochenschr. 1998;110:287–91.
4. Grant CJ, Harrison LE, Hoad CL, et al. Patients with CKD have abnormal upper gastro-intestinal tract digestive function: a study of uremic enteropathy. J Gastroenterol Hepatol. 2016;32(2):372–7.
5. Hirako M, Kamiya T, Misu N, et al. Impaired gastric motility and its relationship to gastrointestinal symptoms in patients with chronic renal failure. J Gastroenterol. 2005;40:1116–22.
6. Osorio MS, Giraldo GC. Gastrointestinal manifestations of chronic kidney disease. Rev Colomb Nefrol. 2017;4:3–12.
7. Sheu BS, Huang JJ. Helicobacter pylori infection in hemodialysis patients. Int J Artif Organs. 2001;24:669–70.
8. Nakajima F, Sakaguchi M, Amemoto K, et al. Helicobacter pylori in patients receiving long-term dialysis. Am J Nephrol. 2002;22:468–72.
9. Fabrizi F, Martin P. Helicobacter pylori infection in patients with end-stage renal disease. Int J Artif Organs. 2000;23:157–64.
10. Huang JJ, Huang CJ, Ruaan MK, et al. Diagnostic efficacy of (13) C-urea breath test for Helicobacter pylori infection in hemodialysis patients. Am J Kidney Dis. 2000;36:124–9.
11. Liang CC, Muo CH, Wang IK, et al. Peptic ulcer disease risk in chronic kidney disease: ten-year incidence, ulcer location, and ulcerogenic effect of medications. PLoS One. 2014;9:e87952.
12. Yang JY, Lee TC, Montez-Rath ME, et al. Trends in acute nonvariceal upper gastrointestinal bleeding in dialysis patients. J Am Soc Nephrol. 2012;23:495–506.
13. Huang KW, Leu HB, Luo JC, et al. Different peptic ulcer bleeding risk in chronic kidney disease and end-stage renal disease patients receiving different dialysis. Dig Dis Sci. 2014;59:807–13.
14. Kalman RS, Pedrosa MC. Evidence-based review of gastrointestinal bleeding in the chronic kidney disease patient. Semin Dial. 2015;28:68–74.
15. Micic D, Sengupta N. Risk stratification of Angioectasia as a cause of gastrointestinal bleeding: untangling the spider's web? Dig Dis Sci. 2019;64:2693–5.
16. Babitt JL, Lin HY. Mechanisms of anemia in CKD. J Ame Society Nephrol. 2012;23:1631–4.
17. Mihai S, Codrici E, Popescu ID, et al. Inflammation-related mechanisms in chronic kidney disease prediction, progression, and outcome. J Immunol Res. 2018;2018:16.
18. Sabatino A, Regolisti G, Brusasco I, et al. Alterations of intestinal barrier and microbiota in chronic kidney disease. Nephrol Dial Transplant. 2015;30:924–33.
19. Chetcuti Zammit S, Koulaouzidis A, Sanders DS, et al. Overview of small bowel angioectasias: clinical presentation and treatment options. Expert Rev Gastroenterol Hepatol. 2018;12:125–39.
20. Verma PP, Pruthi HS, Thakur SK, et al. Upper gastrointestinal mucosa in chronic renal failure—an endoscopic and histological evaluation. Medical J Armed Forces India. 1999;55:307–9.

Gastric Microvasculature in Portal Hypertension

23

Blood flowing through blood vessels such as arterioles, capillaries and venules play a crucial role in the maintenance of physiological functional integrity and normal anatomical structure in all tissues in the body [1–6]. These microarchitectures maintain normal oxygen supply and other micronutrients, and help in the removal of toxic metabolites [1–6]. Gastric mucosa is normally composed of a dense capillary network. At the level of muscularis mucosa, submucosal arteries perforate through to give arterioles along the base of gastric glands. Arterioles divide further as capillary forming interconnected networks traverse towards the luminal aspect along the basement membrane of the gastric glands, ultimately converge to form the collecting venules just beneath the gastric mucosal lining epithelium. These interconnected collecting venules run downwards towards the muscularis mucosae carrying blood to submucosal veins [1–6]. Capillaries and venules (~ 0.5–1 μm thickness) are composed of a single layer of endothelial cells rest on fine basement membrane. Occasionally pericytes may be identified along the endothelial cells. Endothelial cells are interconnected by tight junctions and calcium-dependent molecules like adhesion molecule, integrin and cadherin forming a barrier [1–6]. These barriers prevent diffusion between adjacent endothelial cells allowing interchange of solutes, oxygen, CO_2 and nutrients. Endothelial cells generate various types of vasoactive substances including prostaglandins, nitric oxide and vascular endothelial growth factors responsible for the physiological contraction [1, 7, 8]. Unstimulated endothelium is impermeable to diffusion of substances from circulating blood acting as a selective barrier between luminal component and surrounding substances. Endothelial cells contain a specialized structure demonstrable at ultrastructural level called Weibel-Palade body which is the storehouse for many vasoactive chemicals including von Willebrand factor. Endothelial cells adapt rapidly to prevalent local environment under the effect certain vasoactive agents like histamine or serotonin, it loses its attachment to each other and retracts resulting in increased permeability and oedema [8]. This can be reversed within a few minutes time. Vascular endothelial cell growth factor regulates its permeability and nitric oxide along with prostacyclin having potent vasodilating properties protect gastric mucosa from ischemic injury by opposing mucosal damaging action of vasoconstrictors [9, 10]. Exposure to irritants or during acid back-diffusion, there is marked and rapid increase in mucosal blood flow facilitating removal of noxious agents and also dilution of back diffusing acid, thereby maintaining mucosal milieu and integrity [1]. Exposure to ethanol in rats has been found to result in microvascular injury as early as 1 min. Similarly, human gastric mucosa exposed to 40% ethanol shows exfoliation of surface lining epithelium

K. Vaiphei, *Interpretation of Endoscopic Biopsy - Gastritis, Gastropathies and Beyond*,
https://doi.org/10.1007/978-981-16-6026-9_23

and endothelial cell injury in 5 minutes time preceding glandular cell necrosis. Endothelial cell injury resulted in disruption of the physiological milieu of microvasculature resulting in disruption of integrity, dis-cohesion, breakdown of the vascular wall due to endothelial cell retraction, rupture and fibrin deposition resulting in ischaemia of the mucosal and mucosal erosion. This experiment indicates that endothelial cells are sensitive and vulnerable to toxic injury than epithelial cells. This differential response to ethanol probably is related to protective level of Survivin content by endothelial and epithelial cells. Toxic effect of alcohol could be reduced grossly by a pre-treatment of gastric mucosa with prostaglandin E2 [11, 12]. Virchow (1953) had proposed the hypothesis of ischaemia to be central factor in gastric mucosal diseases [13]. Though this hypothesis has remained unproven till date, there are multiple data characterizing the role of microcirculation in inducing mucosal injury [11–14]. Aspirin and NSAIDs are the important agents that have been proven to produce mucosal injury in the form of erosion, ulceration, haemorrhage and even perforation [14]. The underlying mechanisms include—(i) inhibition of COX-1 and COX-2 enzymes causing a reduction in prostaglandin E2 and I2 generations, (ii) increased gastric motility resulting compression on microcirculation and (iii) upregulation of selectins, integrins and ICAM releasing lysosomal enzymes and oxygen free radicals [14, 15]. NSAIDs are also known to produce mitochondrial damage inhibiting oxidative phosphorylation and increased apoptosis [15, 16].

23.1 Portal Hypertensive Gastropathy

Gastric varices and portal hypertensive gastropathy (PHG) are manifestations of portal hypertension. Both conditions may be seen together frequently. Varices refer to tortuous and distended collateral vessels that develop as the result of obstruction usually non-occlusive, to portal flow and the alternative blood vessels for the portal blood to drain to systemic circulation. These vessels may be located anywhere in the stomach but frequently are seen in gastric fundus and body. PHG involves the lining mucosa and develops as the result of increased resistance to portal flow. In this condition, gastric mucosa tends to be congested with prominent vascular markings. Endoscopically, gastric mucosa is oedematous and congested superimposed upon the mosaic pattern of mucosal vascular marking, which tends to be more prominent towards proximal stomach. Similar mucosal changes may be observed along the whole length of intestinal tract. In severe and longstanding cases, mucosa tends to be friable and bleeds easily. Frequently there may be multiple haemorrhagic spots. Palmer had proposed different mechanisms for the gastric mucosal pathology in cirrhotics as the result of mechanical venous back-pressure with the existing portal hypertension, rather than mucosal or intraluminal toxic factor [17]. Later on Sarfeh et al. documented the presence of distinct gastric mucosal haemorrhage in portal hypertension, termed it as portal hypertensive gastritis. They further recorded that mucosal changes in gastric mucosa could be reversed following portal decompression [18]. McCormack et al. differentiated gastric mucosal histology between portal hypertension and no portal hypertension, and used the terminology of congestive gastropathy in patients with portal hypertension [19], which was later on classified into mild or severe on endoscopic examination [20]. The underlying pathobiology of congested mucosopathy for the mucosal changes is not very clear whether it is the result of increased total blood flow to stomach or the congestion observed is the result of stasis due to increased resistance to the outflow. There are studies that reported decreased mucosal blood flow [21–24], similarly there are others who reported the reverse [25–29]. Severity of histological and gross morphological changes are related to degree and duration of portal hypertension [30–32].

Altered gastric haemodynamics possibly induce activation of various cytokines and growth factors. Gastric mucosa in PHG is reported to contain increased vascular endothelial growth factor [32, 33]. Tumour necrosis factor is implicated to play a major role in the pathogenesis of PHG for increase blood to gastric mucosa by stimulating nitric oxide (NO) production by inducing NO synthase. Administration of anti-tumour necrosis factor-alpha normalizes gastric blood flow [32]. Compromised gastric mucosa is more susceptible to any form of mucosal injury to any noxious substance including bile acids and NSAIDs [34, 35]. Factors to determine development and severity of PHG is per se related to presence of portal hypertension, however that may be related to its severity is still not very clear [36]. It has been suggested that the use of sclerotherapy or banding of varices associates with increased incidence of PHG, but again this does not relate to changes in hepatic venous pressure gradient [33, 36–39].

Diagnosis of PHG is established during upper GI endoscopy and grading is carried out at the same time. Documentation of severity grade is clinically important to predict as the risk of bleed is influenced by the severity [33, 38–42]. It is simply classified into mild having mosaic pattern without red spot and severe with red spots [41, 43, 44] and there are many endoscopic classifications exist with no consensus [41–44]. There are studies that had reported PHG to more frequently coexist with gastric and oesophageal varices as compared to solely oesophageal varices [41, 42]. Gastric biopsy in patients with PHG will reveal varied morphological features and the changes are more mark depending upon duration of portal hypertension and its complications of upper GI bleed. Usually, there will be diffuse mucosal oedema, prominence of the mucosal blood vessels in the form of dilatation of thin-wall vessels accompanied by a variable degree of lamina propria fibrosis, collagenization and splaying of smooth muscle randomly or as extension from muscularis mucosae. There may be surface erosions, ulcerations and thrombosed vessels of varying age [41–45]. Due to the basic underlying pathogenesis of PHG which is a hypo-oxygenated state, there may be basement membrane thickening along the surface ling epithelium, which shall not be misdiagnosed as a case of collagenous gastritis, until and unless there is clinically supporting features. Dilated vessels are prominently arranged along the surface lining epithelium in a chain-like fashion, vessels in between gastric glands will also be dilated and ectatic. Variable degree of extravasated RBCs, hemosiderin pigment deposition. Collagenization and smooth muscle splaying will be indicative of long-standing and complicated/treated varices. In addition, there may be a variable amount of both acute and lymphomononuclear cell aggregation including lymphoid follicle formation. These light microscopic changes are seen in different areas of the stomach, however, tends to be more prominent in fundus and body biopsies. When the biopsy includes deeper tissue like the submucosa or muscularis propria when there is associated deep mucosa ulcer, numerous larger vessels of both venous and arterial origin may be visible, and all these will exhibit variable degrees of dilatation, hypertensive changes and thrombosis [38, 39, 42, 46]. Sometimes eroding vessels, possible coming from the splurging bleeding vessel may also be included in a given biopsy, which may give the appearance of a Dieulafoy's artery. In a Dieulafoy's ulcer, besides the abnormal artery, there are many abnormally dilated vessels in and around the primarily abnormal blood vessel [47, 48]. Hence, background history, clinical profiles and endoscopic features will help to differentiate from a complicated mucosal ulcer in PHG. Besides, in PHG, there will be arterialization of the ectatic and tortuous submucosal veins, though these are softer point for differentiation. In PGH, there could be changes in hyperplastic or inflammatory polyps and atrophic gastritis with diffuse and prominent nodular gastric mucosal folds. Intestinal metaplasia may also be rarely identifiable. Superadded infection by any organism requires to be excluded in any given biopsy.

A condition that may simulate PHG closely is from GAVE (Gastric Antral Vascular Ectasia) and differentiating between the two conditions is important because they have distinct pathologic, clinical and endoscopic features, and different therapeutic measures [45, 49]. GAVE may be frequently seen in association with primary liver, cardiac or kidney diseases. It is selectively located in pyloric antrum with no known pathogenesis. Due to the coexistence of various other conditions that may cause upper GI bleed in chronic kidney and liver disease may be difficult to establish a diagnosis of GAVE syndrome and the frequent causes of GI bleed in both conditions can be vascular ectasia, peptic ulcer disease, oesophageal or gastric varices, and colonic and rectal ulcers [43, 47, 48]. Endoscopic appearance in PHG is a mosaic pattern around a polygonal area of erythema, briefly it may give appearance of a snake skin. GAVE erythema is linearly along antral mucosal folds and diffuse erythema is less common. Histology may of help to differentiate between PHG from GAVE. Characteristic histologic findings in endoscopic mucosal biopsy in PHG is dilation of the microvasculature in lamina propria, which may extend to the larger vessels in muscularis mucosae and submucosa. The dilated capillary network tends to form a chain-like interconnection along the sub-epithelium and the dilated draining venules positioned in between the gastric glands. Deeper arterioles present in between muscularis mucosae and submucosa will show dilatation and tortuosity with variable degrees of intimal proliferation and narrowing of lumen, which will be directly proportionate to the duration of the disease or post-treatment status of portal hypertension. Stromal fibrosis associated with disorganization of the glands and oedema of lamina propria are frequent phenomena. Inflammatory cells per se and fibrin thrombi are generally absent in an uncomplicated situation. There may be a variable amount of random smooth muscle proliferation within the lamina propria, which may also be seen in continuity with muscularis mucosae. The histology of GAVE shows splaying of smooth muscle fibres into lamina propria intermixed with many dilated thin-walled blood vessels. Many of them may contain fibrin thrombi in dilated capillaries. The proliferating fibromuscular tissue, like in cases of solitary rectal ulcer, extends from underlying muscularis mucosae suggesting a possibility of antral mucosal prolapsed to be the underlying initiating aetiological factor. And vascular ectasia to be the result of stasis and mechanical obstruction to blood flow in the affected site. In order to prove such hypothesis to be the cause for the development of GAVE, it will also be necessary to document mucosal fold size and status of the lumen of the pyloric channel and sphincter [47–50].

There are many endoscopic classifications for gastric varices, though some of them are preferably been in use. All patients who present with portal hypertension, irrespective of the underlying aetiology, undergo endoscopic examinations routinely to assess the status of gastric mucosa, to localize and classify the varices. Many of the times, gastric mucosal biopsy accompanies such routine endoscopic examinations. Only limited literatures are available in the English literature with respect to histopathological features in portal hypertension. Normal vasculature is complex and better understanding of the vascular supply of the mucosa and their drainage by the venules have been established largely by studying in experimental animals.

Morphological changes in gastric mucosa in portal hypertension have been described in the previous chapters. It will be of my intense interest to propose a grading system for the vascular changes observed in gastric mucosal biopsies. Routinely in a properly carried out endoscopic biopsies do have a component of submucosa many of the times, especially if the biopsy is from a patient with ongoing florid pathology. Hence, in a patient with thick gastric mucosal folds, the endoscopist possibly puts in extra effort to take a deep bite, hence submucosa becomes a frequent component of the mucosal biopsy. Presence of a few scattered dilated and congested capillaries in the lamina propria will be non-specific, which may be observed in many conditions including gastritis. The earliest or mild changes (grade I) observed in portal hypertension will be presence of prominent or dilated sub-epithelial capillaries arranged in interconnected chain-like patterns, which will

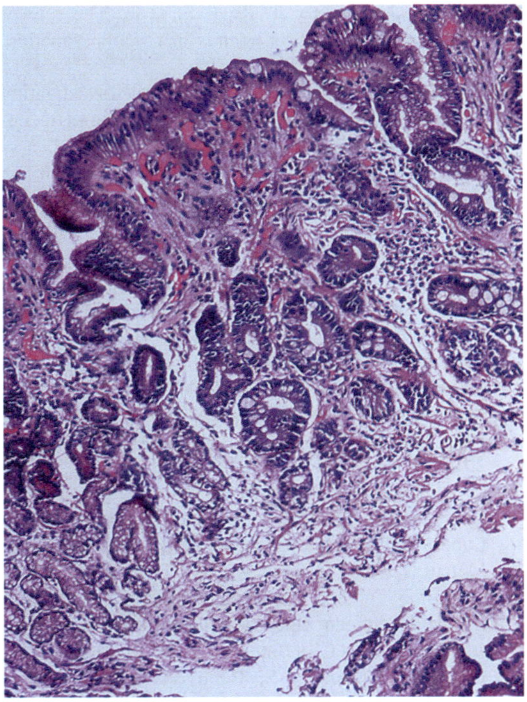

Fig. 23.1 Medium power photomicrograph showing multiple dilated and congested capillaries and venules along the basement membrane of surface lining epithelium as the result of portal hypertension. In addition, gastric mucosa shows loss of antral glands and intestinal metaplasia (HE< x250)

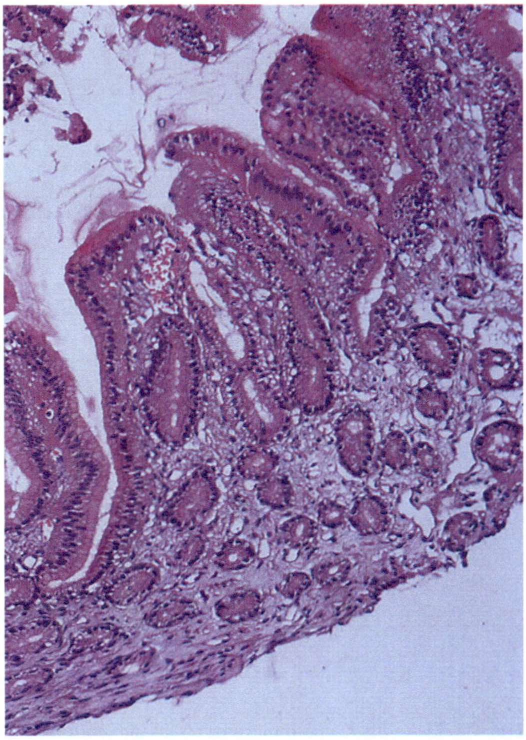

Fig. 23.2 A medium power photomicrograph of gastric biopsy showing changes of atrophy with lamina propria collagenization and many ectatic blood vessels (HE, x250)

be accompanied by dilated draining venules disperse in between the gastric glands (Fig. 23.1). Majority of the time, these dilated vasculatures in cases of portal hypertension do not show much congestion irrespective of the fact that the biopsies are from a congested gastropathy condition. In a slightly more advanced situation (grade II) there be the development of patchy lamina propria fibrosis, collagen deposition around the capillary network along the sub-epithelium associated with distortion, disorganization or loss of normal glandular pattern (Fig. 23.2). More advanced stage histological changes (grade III) will be all the above features and presence of proliferating myofibroblast randomly or in continuity with the muscularis mucosae (Fig. 23.3). In an uncomplicated situation, a component of inflammatory cells is minimal or there may be mild-to-moderate amount of chronic inflammatory cells in lamina propria. Though, the vessels are relatively non-congested, there may be extravasated red blood cells and hemosiderin pigment deposition in lamina propria at any stage of the mucosal changes. These biopsies may show features that may qualify for inflammatory gastric fundal pseudo-polyp due to the presence of distorted and hyperplastic fundic glands with pyloric gland metaplasia. The most extensive and severe most morphological grading will be grade IV where the biopsy shows an eroded and ulcerated mucosa exposing the submucosal vessels with eroded part of the vessel wall exhibiting splurging bleeding.

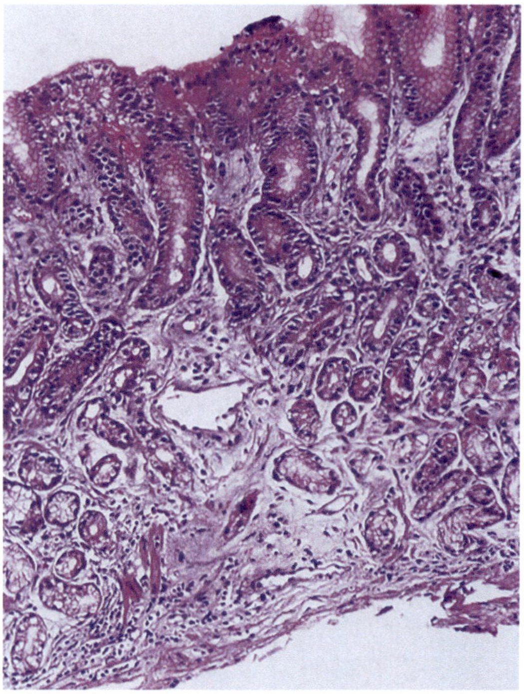

Fig. 23.3 Another photomicrograph of an endoscopic biopsy in a patient of portal hypertension to show fibrosis of lamina propria in continuity with muscularis mucosae entrapping ectatic vessels and sparse mononuclear cell infiltration and loss of gastric glands (HE, x250)

References

1. Tarnawski AS, Ahluwalia A, Jones MK. The mechanisms of gastric mucosal injury: focus on microvascular endothelium as a key target. Curr Med Chem. 2012;19:4–15.
2. Jacobson ED. The circulation of the stomach. Gastroenterol. 1965;48:85–109.
3. Delaney JP, Grim E. Canine gastric blood flow and its distribution. Am J Phys. 1964;207:1195–202.
4. Lundgren O. Gastric mucosal haemodynamic. Gastroenterol Clin Biol. 1985;9:26–9.
5. Gannon BJ, Browning J, O'Brien P. The microvascular architecture of the glandular mucosa of the rat stomach. J Anat. 1982;135:667–83.
6. Gannon B, Browning J, O'Brien P, et al. Mucosal microvascular architecture of the fundus and body of human stomach. Gastroenterol. 1984;86:866–75.
7. Kösem M, Tuncer I, Kotan C, et al. Significance of VEGF and microvascular density in gastric carcinoma. Hepatogastroenterol. 2009;56:1236–40.
8. Tarnawski AS, Ahluwalia A, Jones MK. Angiogenesis in gastric mucosa: an important component of gastric erosion and ulcer healing and its impairment in aging. J Gastroenterol Hepatol. 2014;29(Suppl 4):112–23.
9. Rochette L, Meloux A, Rigal E, et al. The role of Osteoprotegerin and its ligands in vascular function. Int J Mol Sci. 2019;20:705.
10. Vitovski S, Phillips JS, Sayers J, et al. Investigating the interaction between osteoprotegerin and receptor activator of NF-kappaB or tumor necrosis factor-related apoptosis-inducing ligand: evidence for a pivotal role for osteoprotegerin in regulating two distinct pathways. J Biol Chem. 2007;282:31601–9.
11. El-Abhar HS. Coenzyme Q10: a novel gastroprotective effect via modulation of vascular permeability, prostaglandin E2, nitric oxide and redox status in indomethacin-induced gastric ulcer model. Eur J Pharmacol. 2009;649:314–9.
12. Tarnawski AS, Ahluwalia A, Jones MK. The mechanisms of gastric mucosal injury: focus on microvascular endothelium as a key target. Curr Med Chem. 2012;19:4–15.
13. O'Brien PE. The nature of gastric mucosal defence against acid. In: Carter DC, editor. Peptic Ulcer. London: Churchill Livingstone; 1983. p. 28–43.
14. Matsui H, Shimokawa O, Kaneko T, et al. The pathophysiology of non-steroidal anti-inflammatory drug (NSAID)-induced mucosal injuries in stomach and small intestine. J Clin Biochem Nutr. 2011;48:107–11.
15. Bindu S, Mazumder S, Bandyopadhyay U. Non-steroidal anti-inflammatory drugs (NSAIDs) and organ damage: a current perspective. Biochem Pharmacol. 2020;180:114147.
16. Ivey KJ. Mechanisms of nonsteroidal anti-inflammatory drug-induced gastric damage. Am J Med. 1988;84(Suppl 1):41–8.
17. Palmer ED. Erosive gastritis in cirrhosis; influence of portal hypertension on the gastric mucosa. Am J Dig Dis. 1957;2:31–6.
18. Sarfeh IJ, Tarnawski A. Portal hypertensive gastritis. Gastroenterol. 1984;86:592.
19. McCormack TT, Sims J, Eyre-Brook I, et al. Gastric lesions in portal hypertension: inflammatory gastritis or congestive gastropathy? Gut. 1985;26:1226–32.
20. Taor RE, Fox B, Ware J, et al. Gastritis: gastroscopic and microscopic. Endoscopy. 1975;7:209–15.
21. Mezawa S, Homma H, Ohta H, et al. Effect of transjugular intrahepatic portosystemic shunt formation on portal hypertensive gastropathy and gastric circulation. Am J Gastroenterol. 2001;96:1155–9.
22. Gupta R, Sawant P, Parameshwar RV, et al. Gastric mucosal blood flow and hepatic perfusion index in patients with portal hypertensive gastropathy. J Gastroenterol Hepatol. 1998;13:921–6.
23. Iwao T, Toyonaga A, Ikegami M, et al. Reduced gastric mucosal blood flow in patients with portal-hypertensive gastropathy. Hepatology. 1993;18:36–40.
24. Kotzampassi K, Eleftheriadis E, Aletras H. Gastric mucosal blood flow in portal hypertension patients—a laser Doppler flowmetry study. Hepatogastroenterol. 1992;39:39–42.
25. Vyas K, Gala B, Sawant P. Assessment of portal hemodynamics by ultrasound color doppler and

laser doppler velocimetry in liver cirrhosis. Ind J Gastroenterol. 2002;21:176–8.
26. Shigemori H, Iwao T, Ikegami M, et al. Effects of propranolol on gastric mucosal perfusion and serum gastrin level in cirrhotic patients with portal hypertensive gastropathy. Dig Dis Sci. 1994;39:2433–8.
27. Ohta M, Hashizume M, Higashi H, et al. Portal and gastric mucosal hemodynamics in cirrhotic patients with portalhypertensive gastropathy. Hepatology. 1994;20:1432–6.
28. Chung RS, Bruch D, Dearlove J. Endoscopic measurement of gastric mucosal blood flow by laser Doppler velocimetry: effect of chronic esophageal variceal sclerosis. Am Surg. 1988;54:116–20.
29. Tomikawa M, Akiba Y, Kaunitz JD, et al. New insights into impairment of mucosal defense in portal hypertensive gastric mucosa. J Gastrointest Surg. 2000;4:458–63.
30. Gjeorgjievski M, Cappell MS. Portal hypertensive gastropathy: a systematic review of the pathophysiology, clinical presentation, natural history and therapy. World J Hepatol. 2016;8:231–62.
31. Tsugawa K, Hashizume M, Migou S, et al. Role of vascular endothelial growth factor in portal hypertensive gastropathy. Digestion. 2000;61:98–106.
32. Neri V, Tartaglia N, Fersini A et al. Gastroduodenal Lesions Associated with Portal Hypertension: An Extensive Review [Online First], IntechOpen, 2021. https://doi.org/10.5772/intechopen.96296. Available from: https://www.intechopen.com/online-first/gastroduodenal-lesions-associated-with-portal-hypertension-an-extensive-review
33. Cubillas R, Rockey DC. Portal hypertensive gastropathy: a review. Liver Int. 2010;30:1094–102.
34. Tsugawa K, Hashizume M, Tomikawa M, et al. Immunohistochemical localization of vascular endothelial growth factor in the rat portal hypertensive gastropathy. J Gastroenterol Hepatol. 2001;16:429–37.
35. El-Newihi HM, Kanji VK, Mihas AA. Activity of gastric mucosal nitric oxide synthase in portal hypertensive gastropathy. Am J Gastroenterol. 1996;91:535–8.
36. Lo GH. Mechanism of portal hypertensive gastropathy: an unresolved issue. J Gastroenterol Hepatol. 2009;24:1482–3.
37. Hartleb M, Michielsen PP, Dziurkowska-Marek A. The role of nitric oxide in portal hypertensive systemic and portal vascular pathology. Acta Gastroenterol Belg. 1997;60:222–32.
38. Iwao T, Toyonaga A, Oho K, et al. Portal-hypertensive gastropathy develops less in patients with cirrhosis and fundal varices. J Hepatol. 1997;26:1235–41.
39. Thuluvath PJ, Yoo HY. Portal hypertensive gastropathy. Am J Gastroenterol. 2002;97:2973–8.
40. Stewart CA, Sanyal AJ. Grading portal gastropathy: validation of a gastropathy scoring system. Am J Gastroenterol. 2003;98:1758–65.
41. Sarin SK, Sreenivas DV, Lahoti D, et al. Factors influencing development of portal hypertensive gastropathy in patients with portal hypertension. Gastroenterol. 1992;102:994–9.
42. Gupta R, Saraswat VA, Kumar M, et al. Frequency and factors influencing portal hypertensive gastropathy and duodenopathy in cirrhotic portal hypertension. J Gastroenterol Hepatol. 1996;11:728–33.
43. Kamath PS, Shah VH. Portal hypertension and bleeding oesophageal varices. In: Boyer TD, Manns MP, Sanyal AJ, editors. Zakim and Boyer's hepatology: a textbook of liver disease. 6th ed. Philadelphia: Elsevier Saunders; 2012. p. 296–326.
44. Burak KW, Beck P. Diagnosis of portal hypertensive gastropathy. Curr Opin Gastroenterol. 2003;19:477–82.
45. Payen JL, Calès P, Voigt JJ, et al. Severe portal hypertensive gastropathy and antral vascular ectasia are distinct entities in patients with cirrhosis. Gastroenterology. 1995;108:138–44.
46. Chandanwale SS, Gupta N, Sheth J, et al. Histopathological study of portal hypertensive gastropathy using gastric biopsy. Med J DY Patil Vidyapeeth. 2017;10:562–7.
47. Nojkov B, Cappell MS. Distinctive aspects of peptic ulcer disease, Dieulafoy's lesion, and Mallory-Weiss syndrome in patients with advanced alcoholic liver disease or cirrhosis. World J Gastroenterol. 2016;22:446–66.
48. Kalafateli M, Triantos CK, Nikolopoulou V, et al. Non-variceal gastrointestinal bleeding in patients with liver cirrhosis: a review. Dig Dis Sci. 2012;57:2743–54.
49. Ramai D, Linn S, Reddy M. Gastric Antral Vascular Ectasia and Portal Hypertensive Gastropathy, Stomach Disorders, Jianyuan Chai, IntechOpen, 2017. https://doi.org/10.5772/intechopen.70610. Available from: https://www.intechopen.com/books/stomach-disorders/gastric-antral-vascular-ectasia-and-portal-hypertensive-gastropathy
50. Rockey DC. An update: portal hypertensive Gastropathy and Colopathy. Clin Liver Dis. 2019;23:643–58.

24 Paediatric Gastritis and Peptic Ulcer Disease: *H. pylori* and Non-*H. pylori*-Related Conditions

Here I repeat again that understanding of normal anatomy, histology and embryology is an essential step in understanding diseases. Descriptive embryology of human gastrointestinal tract published more than a century ago has remained the same, however, in other aspects dealing with ultrastructure, histochemistry, immunohistochemistry and molecular biology have advanced grossly in the last one or more decades [1]. Endoscopic biopsies are of big help in determining the illness type, stage and response to treatment. It is a very aspect of collaborating with a clinician while evaluating endoscopic biopsies [2]. In addition to clinical and laboratory information of the patient, knowing the endoscopic appearance of the lesion is equally important. Clinician and pathologist should learn to use the same language and same terminology. It is equally important for the clinician to understand what the pathologist implies to; at the same time pathologists should know the approach of the clinician (repetition of the biopsy, endoscopic resection, surgery) [2].

Helicobacter pylori (HP) is a Gram-negative inverted S-shaped organism, has the tendency to reside and grow gastric mucosa specially aggregated in pyloric antrum. Due to inbuilt biochemical and physiological properties, it is capable of producing tissue injury and inflammation resulting in the development of chronic gastritis [3, 4]. HP is almost always acquired in childhood and if untreated, it is a lifelong infection [5]. Almost half of the human beings in the world harbours HP in their stomach and the prevalent rate in developing countries is almost 80% amongst the paediatric population [1, 3]. Risk of developing peptic ulcer disease in this infected group of population is 10–15% and the risk for gastric cancer is less than 1% [5]. WHO classifies HP as a group 1 carcinogenic agent [6]. HP gastritis in terms of GI symptoms is indistinguishable from other conditions of acid peptic diseases. Routes of transmission are through gastro-oral and direct human-to-human contact through faeco-oral routes [7]. Most frequent reservoir possibly is contaminated water. Major risk factors for the transmission of the infection are low socioeconomic status, poverty, crowding and poor hygiene [8]. Pathobiology and pathology of gastric mucosa in HP infection in paediatric age group are similar to that observed in adults. Children tend to have a less severe form of gastritis compared to adults with a similar bacterial load. This is probably related to increased activity of regulatory T cells (Tregs) that downregulate the inflammatory response in children [9].

Anatomic zonation in adult stomach is also applicable to a child with subtle differences. Mucosal glands help in defining different regions of the stomach. In the cardiac region, the glands are simple tubular type containing neutral mucin, occasionally there may be scattered parietal cells without the chief cells. Acid mucin is frequently identified in paediatric cardia mucosa as opposed

K. Vaiphei, *Interpretation of Endoscopic Biopsy - Gastritis, Gastropathies and Beyond*,
https://doi.org/10.1007/978-981-16-6026-9_24

to adult mucosa comprising mainly of neutral mucin of the glandular and surface columnar epithelial cells. This acid mucin may persist into childhood and should not be misinterpreted as evidence of intestinal metaplasia unless the acid containing cells are true goblet cells, as surface alcian blue (PH 2.5) positivity is well known in gastric columnar lining epithelium. Any pancreatic acinar tissue at cardia or antrum in children with no significant changes of chronic gastritis should be taken as developmental rest [10]. Gastric body mucosa has thick mucosal folds or rugae and areae gastricae. Fundus and body mucosa have similar morphology with more flatter surface than more villiform cardia and antrum. Distal one-third of the stomach is referred to as the antrum ending at pyloric junction. Gastric pits or foveolae comprise one-quarter or more of mucosal thickness overlie the glandular zone containing parietal, chief and mucus glands. Gastric biopsies in paediatric age group are handled similarly to adult cases.

In spite of the fact that a child may be presented with clinical symptoms, the clinician and the endoscopist tend to underestimate the disease condition that may be affecting the stomach. Gastritis in paediatric age group is under-recognized, the histological parameters are poorly defined as majority of the patients are assessed on endoscopic appearance associated with apparent reluctance on the part of the endoscopist to subject the child to biopsies [11, 12]. Certain conditions like stress-induced erosion can be adequately evaluated only by endoscopy. Discrepancy between gross and microscopic findings in gastric biopsy is well known. Hence, in a symptomatic child, it is advisable to accompany the endoscopic examination by mucosal biopsy [13, 14]. Histological spectra of gastritis are similar to adults, especially infective associated gastritis as it is environmental dependent. Amongst the non-infective causes, celiac disease (CD) is one condition that affects frequently preschool and school going children. In this condition, there is an increased number of T-cell infiltration of the duodenum along with or without villous atrophy. Extra-duodenal mucosal inflammation is a frequent finding in CD patients including the gastric mucosa, though the child may not have any specific symptom that can be related to stomach. The usual histological form of gastric mucosal changes in CD is lymphocytic gastritis which may be associated with or without basement membrane thickening. Unlike duodenal biopsy, any number of lymphocytic infiltration along the surface lining and also in the lamina propria in gastric biopsy, especially in a child may be interpreted as significant. As CD is an autoimmune or cell-mediated allergic disorder in response to gluten, there may be scattered eosinophils intermixed with the dominant lymphocytic population. In a situation where eosinophil becomes dominant, it is required to be considered a separate distinct entity, not related to CD, re-evaluating the clinical history in such situation may be of immense help. Hence, being a pathologist does not exclude you from listening or knowing the clinical profiles of a patient in detail. In addition to lymphocytes, there may be neutrophil infiltration, which will be a warning sign to exclude any superadded infection in the background of lymphocytic gastritis. A close differential diagnosis for lymphocytic gastritis with or without basement membrane thickening will be autoimmune gastritis where the patients require more attention to differentiate between the two by further examination of the clinical profiles and serology evaluations. In a patient with autoimmune disorder, intestinal biopsies including biopsy from duodenum may reveal lymphocytosis. In addition, though it is a rare situation, gastric involvement by Crohn's disease in paediatric age group is considered to be of higher proportion compared to adult Crohn's disease [9, 12].

24.1 Pathogenesis of HP Associated Peptic Ulcer Disease

HP adheres to the surface of epithelial cells making the cells to be leaky, which results in enhancement and facilitation of passing of nutrients and other effector molecules essential in the development of peptic ulcer disease (PUD) [15]. HP virulence is determined by pathogenicity island present in HP called cytotoxin-associated gene or cag. Cag-positive strains are closely associated with PUD and gastric cancer and the effector protein is the cagA which gets translocated into the epithelial cell cytoplasm. It then disrupts the signalling pathways resulting in abnormal epithelial cell proliferation and motility, and changes the cellular cytoskeletal system [16]. VacA is also a protein present in HP and is believed to be a responsible factor for HP colonization in gastric mucosa [16]. VacA is present in all different strains of HP and only 50% can express the mature protein and it helps to increase intracellular permeability. HP by adhering to gastric epithelial cells produces cytotoxicity and stimulates the release of cytokines via its cell wall lipopolysaccharides (LPS) resulting in further cell injury. HP also produces urease and helps the bacteria to survive in the stomach by creating a less acidic environment. The associated morbidity with HP infection will only be manifested in adulthood in these countries [3]. It is also important to realize the distinct differences between HP infection per se and associated disorders like gastric and duodenal ulcer diseases, gastric malignancies and development of these conditions in adulthood is not predictable by the time of acquisition of infection and have been seen to be influenced by factors like the bacteria, the host and the potential environmental exposures [3]. Majority of the infected individuals will not develop any significant disease and it is not practical to treat all who acquire HP infection in their childhood. Hence, it is important to realize important indicators of disease outcome [3]. Despite the various epidemiological evidence explaining the relationship between peptic ulcer diseases and HP infection, HP infection during childhood has seldom been associated with peptic ulceration and gastric atrophy [17, 18]. These observations indicate different underlying mechanisms for the histopathological changes and clinical expression of HP infection between children and adults, and are still poorly understood.

24.2 Pathogenesis of Non-HP Peptic Ulcer Disease

Any agent that produces disruption in the balance between gastric acid, pepsin and gastric mucosal protective layer formed by the mucus, bicarbonate secretion and gastric blood flow, can result in gastric ulcer or gastritis. Frequently causative known agents are NSAIDs, alcohol, caustic agents, bile reflux, pancreatic enzymes and haemodynamic shock. Many other varieties of ingested food particles may also disrupt the balance. Chemical gastropathy, also known as chemical or reactive gastritis, is characterized by foveolar lining epithelial cell hyperplasia, vascular congestion, oedema of the lamina propria and splaying of smooth muscles of muscularis mucosae origin in the absence of any significant mucosal inflammation [19]. Duodeno-gastric bile reflux and NSAIDs are well-established common causes for chemical gastropathy, gastritis and peptic ulcer diseases, but the incidence of such pathology is much less frequently observed in paediatric age group compared to adults. NSAIDs used in children for short term as a pain reliever and fever are well tolerated. However, chronic NSAID therapy is usually associated with significant gastric injury and more than 75% of children having pain abdomen while taking NSAIDs have associated gastritis, antral erosions or ulcers [20, 21].

References

1. Blecker U, Mehta DI, Gold BD. Paediatric gastritis and peptic ulcer disease. Indian J Pediatr. 1999;66:725–33.
2. Kayaçetin S, Güreşçi S. What is gastritis? What is gastropathy? How is it classified? Turk J Gastroenterol. 2014;25:233–47.
3. Drumm B, Day AS, Gold B, et al. Helicobacter pylori and peptic ulcer: Working Group report of the second World Congress of Pediatric Gastroenterology, Hepatology, and Nutrition. J Pediatr Gastroenterol Nutr. 2004;39(suppl 2):S626–31.
4. Suerbaum S, Michetti P. Helicobacter pylori infection. N Engl J Med. 2002;347:1175–86.
5. Czinn SJ. Helicobacter pylori infection: detection, investigation, and management. J Pediatr. 2005;146:S21–6.

6. IARC Working Group on the Evaluation of Carcinogenic Risks to Humans. Schistosomes, liver flukes and Helicobacter pylori. Lyons, 7–14 June. IARC Monogr Eval Carcinog Risks Hum. 1994;61:1–241.
7. Gold BD, Colletti RB, Abbott M, et al. Helicobacter pylori infection in children: recommendations for diagnosis and treatment. J Pediatr Gastroenterol Nutr. 2000;31:490–7.
8. Fujimoto Y, Furusyo N, Toyoda K, et al. Intrafamilial transmission of Helicobacter pylori among the population of endemic areas in Japan. Helicobacter. 2007;12:170–6.
9. Harris PR, Wright SW, Serrano C, et al. Helicobacter pylori gastritis in children is associated with a regulatory T-cell response. Gastroenterology. 2008;134:491–9.
10. Krishnamurthy S, Integlia MJ, Grand RJ, et al. Pancreatic acinar cell clusters in pediatric gastric mucosa. Am J Surg Pathol. 1998;22:100–5.
11. Dahshan A, Rabah R. Correlation of endoscopy and histology in the gastroesophageal mucosa in children: are routine biopsies justified? J Clin Gastroenterol. 2000;31:213–6.
12. Carpenter HA, Talley NJ. Gastroscopy is incomplete without biopsy: clinical relevance of distinguishing gastropathy from gastritis. Gastroenterology. 1995;108:917–24.
13. Bertges LC, Dibai FN, Bezerra G, et al. Comparison between endoscopic findings and histological diagnosis of antral gastritis. Arq Gastroenterol. 2018;55:212–5.
14. Sheiko MA, Feinstein JA, Capocelli KE, et al. The concordance of endoscopic and histologic findings of 1000 pediatric EGDs. Gastrointest Endosc. 2015;81:1385–91.
15. Maeda S, Mentis AF. Pathogenesis of Helicobacter pylori infection. Helicobacter. 2007;12(suppl 1):10–4.
16. Basso D, Zambon CF, Letley DP, et al. Clinical relevance of Helicobacter pylori cagA and vacA gene polymorphisms. Gastroenterology. 2008;135:91–9.
17. Cover TL, Blanke SR. Helicobacter pylori VacA, a paradigm for toxin multifunctionality. Nat Rev Microbiol. 2005;3:320–32.
18. Whitney AE, Guarner J, Hutwagner L, et al. Helicobacter pylori gastritis in children and adults: comparative histopathologic study. Ann Diagn Pathol. 2000;4:279–85.
19. Pashankar DS, Bishop WP, Mitros FA. Chemical gastropathy: a distinct histopathologic entity in children. J Pediatr Gastroenterol Nutr. 2002;35:653–7.
20. Mulberg AE, Linz C, Bern E, et al. Identification of nonsteroidal antiinflammatory drug-induced gastroduodenal injury in children with juvenile rheumatoid arthritis. J Pediatr. 1993;122:647–9.
21. Ashorn M, Verronen P, Ruuska T, et al. Upper endoscopic findings in children with active juvenile chronic arthritis. Acta Paediatr. 2003;92:558–61.

25 Congenital Anomalies—Gastric Outlet Obstruction, Microgastria, Duplications and Gastroschisis

Individuals who are born with congenital anomalies of GIT usually have a clinical manifestation in early post-natal life, some may manifest late in their life, maybe in adulthood [1]. The role of endoscopic biopsy is limited and does have practically any role in the definitive diagnosis of such condition. Malformations of GIT represent some of the most common anomalies where clinicians come across during their lifetime of clinical practices [1]. Primitive gut in its earliest form is a simple tubular structure composed of endoderm, muscle and connective tissue developing from splanchnopleuric mesoderm [2–5]. Primitive foregut gives rise to respiratory system, oesophagus, stomach, proximal duodenum to the level of ampulla, liver and pancreas. The tubular structure of the foregut distal primitive oesophagus forms the stomach slinging from dorsal or posterior wall of the body with the help of dorsal mesentery and anteriorly by the ventral mesentery from septum transversum. The dilated portion forming the primitive stomach undergoes a rapid differential growth resulting in a 90° rotation along its long axis. Dorsal mesentery develops into greater omentum and the ventral mesentery develops into falciform and coronary ligaments of the liver attached to diaphragm and lesser omentum [2]. Congenital abnormality affecting stomach is rare and it can be structural, functional or both. Structural anomalies may be due to embryological defects or associated with in utero complications like ischaemia. Structural anomalies can be atresia, malrotation and duplication [6–8]. Functional conditions will be due to associated conditions like meconium plug syndrome or intestinal hypoperistalsis. Conditions where both structural and functional anomalies may contribute in the development of the clinical problem will be—midgut volvulus, aganglionosis and hypertrophic pyloric stenosis [6–9].

Gastric outlet obstruction. This can be due to one of the following conditions, i.e. atresia or microgastria, pyloric stenosis or atresia, obstruction of the lumen by pyloric/pre-pyloric membrane or by an antral web [6–9]. Gastric atresia can be of three types—(1) complete atresia where there is no communication between stomach and the duodenum, (2) complete atresia, however, the blind end of the two atretic segments (proximal stomach and distal duodenum blind end) are interconnected by a fibrous band and (3) presence of a thin membrane or diaphragm that can be composed of a fold of the mucosa occluding the lumen completely [6–10]. Completely occluded outlet is seldom observed condition and is the result of atresia, seen in <1% of all congenital GI obstruction. Atresia if occurs, involves antrum and pylorus [11]. Outlet obstruction may be associated with extrinsic compression by a peritoneal band or by annular pancreas. Outflow tract stenosis may be the result of localized ischaemia in foetal life, rather than a failed canalization of the primitive endoderm [12]. Atresia may be in a familial form or acquired in association

K. Vaiphei, *Interpretation of Endoscopic Biopsy - Gastritis, Gastropathies and Beyond*,
https://doi.org/10.1007/978-981-16-6026-9_25

with epidermolysis bullosa. Affected children and neonates present with regurgitation with no bile in the vomitus and this may happen within the first few hours after birth. A plain abdominal X-ray will show the distended stomach with a single bubble present within the stomach proximal to the site of obstruction, along with no visible gas shadow in small bowel and colon [7, 10]. Almost all affected and diagnosed patients require surgical intervention. In addition to the characteristic radiology appearances, endoscopy may sometimes help to type the obstruction, i.e. either a blind end or presence of a membrane or a web. This may present as an isolated non-syndromic sporadic case or with a family history with autosomal recessive inheritance pattern in the association of multiple stenoses of GIT. There can be segmental stenosis in the body region giving hourglass appearance. Gastric atresia is usually associated with history of polyhydramnios. Clinically, the neonate will present with vomiting which is non-bilius and persistent usually after the first feeding of the neonate. Sometimes it may be accompanied by excessive salivation and a lesser amount of stool volume which subsequently will disappear [10–12]. However, a neonate with less severe degree of stenosis will be associated with milder symptoms and delayed clinical symptoms even up to several years. This type of presentation is difficult to differentiate from the acquired type of gastric outlet stenosis. Hypertrophic pyloric stenosis is an infantile disease with distinct clinicopathological features in the immediate postnatal period with normal intrauterine and neonatal imaging studies [13, 14]. A barium meal study will reveal string and shoulder signs. Histological examination of the hypertrophic segment will show concentric layers of smooth muscles, increased amount of fibrocollagenous tissue and elastic fibres, the overlying mucosa may be eroded or ulcerated. The child will present with vomiting which is projectile in nature, at 3–5 weeks of postnatal life. Abdominal examination will reveal gastric peristaltic waves and a palpable epigastric mass usually as large as an olive. Ultrasound examination shows distinctive features [15]—(1) thicken echo poor pyloric muscle and elongated pyloric channel, (2) "doughnut appearance" reflective the central lumen surrounded by the mucosa, submucosa and echo poor muscular layer, (3) the pyloric antrum length tends to be longer 15 mm, the thicken muscle layer measuring more than 3 mm, if less than 2 mm in thickness, is considered to be unequivocally normal, between 2 and 3 mm is considered abnormal, not diagnostic and (4) thickness across the pylorus from serosa to serosa greater than 15 mm is diagnostic.

Microgastria. In this condition, small and tubular stomach lies along the midline. It is believed to be result of failure in gastric rotation during development [14]. The affected child suffers from failure to thrive and has other anomalies presenting as a syndrome. Other associated anomalies are malrotation, asplenia and anomalies of renal, cardiac, limb and vertebral (VACTERL syndrome) [8, 9, 14]. Intrauterine ultrasound examination may be non-specific, frequently results in misinterpretation as a case of oesophageal atresia as the stomach is not well visualized. During upper GI endoscopy, there will be dilatation of the oesophagus accompanied by a midline tubular stomach with an ill-defined or incompetent gastro-oesophageal junction. It may be associated with oesophageal dysmotility due to its massive dilatation [8–14].

Gastrointestinal duplication. It is also known by many other terminologies [16]. Condition is also known by many other terms depending on the site where it occurs. Simply they are usually referred to as duplications and neuro-enteric (dorsal enteric) cysts or remnants. Gastric duplication cysts constitute about 4–9% of GI duplication cysts [17]. Duplication cysts as the name suggests are located along the mesenteric border of the involved segment sharing the mesentery and blood supply. It may be closed or open, round or tubular [18]. Gastric duplications are seen along the greater curvature. It may be a closed cyst or may have a mouth or opening that is communicating with adjoining normal gut segment and section from the wall of the cyst will have all the layers of the gut wall including the nerve plexuses, and the mucosa tends to be similar to the adjoining segment with heterotopic tissue of any other type of mucosa may be present

[19]. The cyst may contain proteinaceous debris, crystal formations or engulfed histiocytes. Gastric mucosa is frequently observed in oesophageal and small intestinal duplications. A large mesenteric lymphangioma located in upper abdomen was misdiagnosed for gastric duplication cyst [20].

Gastroschisis is a birth defect present as a linear dehiscence present along the paramedian of anterior abdominal wall adjacent and right to umbilical cord insertion, separated by a narrow band of skin with underlying tissue [21]. Through the dehiscence, loops of intestine extrude into amniotic cavity resulting in a kind of irritation to the part of the exposed intestine. It is usually observed in foetus whose mother is <25 years of age. Gastroschisis develops during the first or early second trimester as the result of improper development of abdominal muscle. There is a formation of a gap through which the intestine along with other abdominal organs extrude out. As the protective layer of the intestine is not present, it gets exposed to unnatural environment of amniotic fluid resulting in intestinal irritation [22–25]. This constant irritation causes shortening, twisting or swelling. Hypothetical pathogenesis of gastroschisis—possible exposure to vasoactive drugs, mother suffering from thrombophilic disorder, result of early disintegration of right umbilical vein, or intrauterine disruption of right omphalomesenteric artery.

References

1. Santulli TV, Amoury RA. Congenital anomalies of the gastrointestinal tract. Paed Clin North Am. 1967;14:21–45.
2. Kim TH, Shivdasani RA. Stomach development, stem cells and disease. Development. 2016;143:554–65.
3. Fukamachi H, Mizuno T, Takayama S. Epithelial-mesenchymal interactions in differentiation of stomach epithelium in fetal mice. Anat Embryol (Berl). 1979;157:151–60.
4. McCracken KW, Catá EM, Crawford CM, et al. Modelling human development and disease in pluripotent stem-cell-derived gastric organoids. Nature. 2014;516:400–4.
5. San Roman AK, Shivdasani RA. Boundaries, junctions and transitions in the gastrointestinal tract. Exp Cell Res. 2011;317:2711–8.
6. Wright V, Walker-Smith J, Sanderson I. Congenital abnormalities of the gastrointestinal tract. In: Oxford textbook of medicine. Oxford: Oxford University Press; 2020.
7. Ramachandra SP, Bydder M, Gurjar N et al. Congenital anomalies of the gastrointestinal tract: a radiological review. Presented in the Congress of European Congress of Radiology, poster no C-1669. Burton on Trent, UK. 2010.
8. Teresa Berrocal T, Torres I, Gutiérrez J, et al. Congenital anomalies of the upper gastrointestinal tract. Radiographics. 1999;19:855–72.
9. Davoud B, Aslanabadi S, Faramarzi M. Vacterl association with hypertrophic pyloric stenosis. 2018;4. https://doi.org/10.22037/irjps.v3i3.13917.
10. Gupta AK, Guglani B. Imaging of congenital anomalies of the gastrointestinal tract. Indian J Pediatr. 2005;72:403–14.
11. Singleton EB, Wagner ML, Dutton RV. Radiology of the alimentary tract in infants and children. 2nd ed. Philadelphia, Pa: Saunders; 1977.
12. Brown RP, Hertzler JH. Congenital prepyloric gastric atresia: a report of two cases. Am J Dis Child. 1959;97:857–62.
13. Russo P, Ruchelli E, Piccoli D. Pathology of Pediatric gastrointestinal and liver disease. In: Odze RD, Goldblum JR, editors. Surgical pathology of the GI tract, liver, biliary tract and pancreas. New York: Springer; 2004. p. 29.
14. Jeziorczak PM, King A, Warner BW. Chapter 67—surgical disease of the stomach and duodenum in infants and children. In: Yeo CJ, editor. Shackelford's surgery of the alimentary tract, 2 volume set (eighth edition). Elsevier; 2019. p. 770–85.
15. Maheshwari P, Abograra A, Shamam O. Sonographic evaluation of gastrointestinal obstruction in infants: a pictorial essay. J Pediatr Surg. 2009;44:2037–42.
16. Doepker MP, Ahmad SA. Gastric duplication cyst: a rare entity. J Surg Case Rep. 2016;2016:rjw073.
17. Wang B, Hunter WJ, Bin-Sagheer S, et al. Rare potential pitfall in endoscopic ultrasound-guided fine needle aspiration biopsy in gastric duplication cyst: a case report. Acta Cytol. 2009;53:219–22.
18. Liu R, Adler DG. Duplication cysts: diagnosis, management, and the role of endoscopic ultrasound. Endosc Ultrasound. 2014;3:152–60.
19. Napolitano V, Pezzullo AM, Zeppa P. Foregut duplication of the stomach diagnosed by endoscopic ultrasound guided fine-needle aspiration cytology: case report and literature review. World J Surg Oncol. 2013;11:33.
20. Xv FY, Sun A, Gan Y, Hu HJ. Gastric duplication cyst mimicking large cystic lymphangioma in an adult: a rare case report and review of the literature. World J Clin Cases. 2019;7:2087–93.
21. Rentea RM, Gupta V. Gastroschisis. [Updated 2020 Nov 12]. In: StatPearls [Internet]. Treasure Island (FL): StatPearls Publishing; 2020 Jan. Available from: https://www.ncbi.nlm.nih.gov/books/NBK557894/.

22. Kirby RS, Marshall J, Tanner JP, et al. For the National Birth Defects Prevention Network. Prevalence and correlates of gastroschisis in 15 states, 1995 to 2005. Obstet Gynecol. 2013;122:275–81.
23. Jones AM, Isenburg J, Salemi JL, et al. For the National Birth Defects Prevention Network. Increasing prevalence of gastroschisis—14 states, 1995-2012. MMWR Morb Mortal Wkly Rep. 2016;65:23–6.
24. Bird TM, Robbins JM, Druschel C, et al. And the National Birth Defects Prevention Study. Demographic and environmental risk factors for gastroschisis and omphalocele in the National Birth Defects Prevention Study. J Pediatr Surg. 2009;44:1546–51.
25. Feldkamp ML, Reefhuis J, Kucik J, et al. And the National Birth Defects Prevention Study. Case-control study of self reported genitourinary infections and risk of gastroschisis: findings from the National Birth Defects Prevention Study, 1997-2003. BMJ. 2008;336:1420–3.

GPSR Compliance

The European Union's (EU) General Product Safety Regulation (GPSR) is a set of rules that requires consumer products to be safe and our obligations to ensure this.

If you have any concerns about our products, you can contact us on ProductSafety@springernature.com

In case Publisher is established outside the EU, the EU authorized representative is:

Springer Nature Customer Service Center GmbH
Europaplatz 3
69115 Heidelberg, Germany

Batch number: 10296506

Printed by Printforce, the Netherlands